Making Things Happen

Catastrophes in Context

General Editors:
Robert E. Barrios, University of New Orleans
Crystal Felima, University of Kentucky
Mark Schuller, Northern Illinois University

Catastrophes in Context aims to bring critical attention to the social, political, economic, and cultural structures that create disasters out of natural hazards or political events and that shape the responses. Combining long-term ethnographic fieldwork typical of anthropology and increasingly adopted in similar social science disciplines such as geography and sociology with a comparative frame that enlightens global structures and policy frameworks, *Catastrophes in Context* includes monographs and edited volumes that bring critical scrutiny to the multiple dimensions of specific disasters and important policy/practice questions for the field of disaster research and management. Theoretically innovative, our goal is to publish readable, lucid texts to be accessible to a wide range of audiences across academic disciplines and specifically practitioners and policymakers.

Volume 5
Making Things Happen: Community Participation and Disaster Reconstruction in Pakistan
Jane Murphy Thomas

Volume 4
Constructing Risk: Disaster, Development, and the Built Environment
Stephen O. Bender

Volume 3
Going Forward by Looking Back: Archaeological Perspectives on Socio-ecological Crisis, Response, and Collapse
Edited by Felix Riede and Payson Sheets

Volume 2
Disaster Upon Disaster: Exploring the Gap Between Knowledge, Policy and Practice
Edited by Susanna M. Hoffman and Roberto E. Barrios

Volume 1
Contextualizing Disaster
Edited by Gregory V. Button and Mark Schuller

Making Things Happen
Community Participation and Disaster Reconstruction in Pakistan

Jane Murphy Thomas

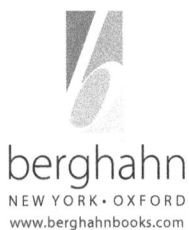

berghahn
NEW YORK • OXFORD
www.berghahnbooks.com

First published in 2022 by
Berghahn Books
www.berghahnbooks.com

© 2022, 2024 Jane Murphy Thomas
First paperback edition published in 2024

All rights reserved. Except for the quotation of short passages for the purposes of criticism and review, no part of this book may be reproduced in any form or by any means, electronic or mechanical, including photocopying, recording, or any information storage and retrieval system now known or to be invented, without written permission of the publisher.

Library of Congress Cataloging-in-Publication Data

A C.I.P. cataloging record is available from the Library of Congress
Library of Congress Cataloging in Publication Control Number: 2022016051

British Library Cataloguing in Publication Data

A catalogue record for this book is available from the British Library

ISBN 978-1-80073-561-3 hardback
ISBN 978-1-80539-340-5 paperback
ISBN 978-1-80073-281-0 web pdf
ISBN 978-1-80073-562-0 epub

https://doi.org/10.3167/9781800735613

The electronic open access publication of *Making Things Happen* has been made available under a CC BY-NC-ND 4.0 license as a part of the Berghahn Open Migration and Development Studies initiative.

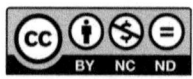

This work is published subject to a Creative Commons Attribution Noncommercial No Derivatives 4.0 License. The terms of the license can be found at http://creativecommons.org/licenses/by-nc-nd/4.0/. For uses beyond those covered in the license contact Berghahn Books.

Dedicated with love to Sarah
and with love in memory of my parents and grandparents
for their hints of social justice

Contents

List of Illustrations	viii
List of Anecdotes and Ethnographies	ix
Preface. Stakeholder Remarks	xii
Acknowledgments	xv
List of Abbreviations	xvii
Introduction. Disaster Strikes	1
Chapter 1. The Moment the Quake Struck	15
Chapter 2. Contexts of a Reconstruction Site	38
Chapter 3. Community Participation: What Has Happened to It?	82
Chapter 4. The Social Component	115
Chapter 5. Social and Technical Integration	175
Chapter 6. PERRP Design and Construction	211
Chapter 7. The Library Challenge	252
Chapter 8. The Social Anthropology of Reconstruction	265
Conclusion	280
Appendix. Schools and Health Facilities Constructed in the Pakistan Earthquake Reconstruction and Recovery Project (2006–2013)	290
References	292
Index	308

Illustrations

Figures

1.1. A Collapsed School	17
1.2. Mohandri School	19
1.3. Reconstruction in Mountainous Areas	32
2.1. Contexts of a Reconstruction Site in PERRP	39
2.2. The School above the Clouds	52
4.1. Committee-Organized School Activities	164
5.1. Voting on a Willingness Resolution	179
5.2. School Inauguration	190
5.3. Communication Protocol with Grievance Procedures	192
7.1. The Book Fairs	259

Tables

4.1. Power Structure—The Blocs of Power in PERRP Communities	126
4.2. PTC/SMC Guideline Changes to Shift and Share Power	132
4.3. Stakeholder Analysis	143
4.4. Capacities/Vulnerabilities and Conflict Sensitivity Analysis: The Findings	147
4.5. "What Could Go Wrong?" Analysis: The Findings	153
4.6. Monitoring—Social Steps Tracking Chart: Monthly Progress	156
5.1. PERRP's Step-by-Step Process	177
5.2. Working Together—Stay in Your Lanes	201
8.1. Negative or Positive Effects for Construction and the Local People	269

Anecdotes and Ethnographies

Throughout these pages there are about seventy short stories, anecdotes, and more detailed ethnographies recounting some things that happened in the project. These are included to show a wide range of realities and challenges, as well as successes and surprises.
Note: * indicates pseudonym

Introduction
"Making Things Happen" 13

Chapter 1
"As We Watched the Construction, It Was a Symbol" 33
Ethnography: Government Girls' High School at River View* 33

Chapter 2
Serious Cultural Breach 68
"All It Takes Is One Person" 69
Who Are the Powerful People? Depends on Whom You Ask and When 69
Power and the School above the Clouds 70
Low-Caste Families Pooling Subsidy Funds 71
Low-Caste Son Becomes a Leader 71
Landowner Suddenly Claims Encroachment; Shunning Threatened 71
"What? Now I Have to Learn the Folk Songs and Wear Traditional Clothes?" 72
"Why Didn't You Just Tell Them They Had to Change the Culture?" 73
Who Should Attend the Meeting? 74
Land Issues? Perspective Matters 75
Ethnography: Government Girls' School Sabaz Zameen* 76

Chapter 3

An Embankment Alignment in Bangladesh	104
Syria—"We're Not Too Happy You're Here"	107
Ontario, Canada—The Potato Patch	109
No to Community Participation!	110
Myanmar—"What Is This?!"	111
Afghanistan—Afghan NGOs Start Up in Refugee Camps in Pakistan	112

Chapter 4

"Participate? Nobody Had Ever Asked Us to Do That Before"	166
See the Difference? Participation versus No Participation	166
An Elite's Demands—Attempting to Capture Benefits	167
Blocked Access to Construction Site	167
"My Parents Never Set Foot in My School"	168
Parents Locked the School and Led a Protest against the Head Teacher	168
Community Helping Construction Drew Attention to Girls' Education	169
Brother Who Refused to Lend Land after His Family Agreed to It	170
Meeting a Main Stakeholder on the Snow-Blocked Road	170
Why We Want This School	171
Bherkund Snake Infestation	171
Ethnography—Government Girls' High School Long Valley*	172

Chapter 5

Sample Willingness Resolution	204
Introducing Grievance Procedures	205
"How Do You Do It? Be a Catalyst in Dispute Settlement"	205
Camel in a Tent School	206
A Deliberately Broken Water Pipe	206
Construction Steel Stolen and Hidden in a Corn Field	207
Fight Over the Road Being Blocked	207
"We Never Hear Complaints about this Project"	208
Two Views—Listening to the People	208
Rough First Year	209
"Look Who Is in the Graveyard! Ha, Ha, Ha!"	209

Engineers Say, "Having a Social Team Saves a Lot of Time and Trouble" — 210

Chapter 6
Architect—"There's Nothing about Culture in a Modern Building" — 239
Official—"Village People Don't Know Anything about Design" — 240
Toilet Orientation — 240
Boundary Walls — 240
Unwanted Visibility — 241
Glass Blocks in Windows — 242
Don't Waste the Land — 242
Respect for Graves — 243
"My School Is My Life" — 243
Flash Floods and Local Knowledge — 244
Honor the Committee-Contractor Agreement — 244
"Construction Here Is an Uphill Battle" — 244
Mohandri School, Mountainside Boulders — 245
Hostel for Students from Farthest Valleys — 246
Trouble over the Word "Local" — 246
Pouring Concrete Roof, Community Members Stood By Overnight — 247
Locals Threaten to Be Given Jobs — 247
Two Contractors in a Road Dispute — 248
Ethnography: Boys' Primary and High School Glacier Way* — 248

Chapter 7
First Student Donation to the Library Challenge — 262
"Look! I Can Read This!" — 262
First Books Ever Owned — 263
Roadside Chat about Books — 263
"But My Sons Won't Even Read Their Syllabus Books!" — 264

Chapter 8
Ethnography—Government Boys' High School in Flat Land* — 274

Preface
Stakeholder Remarks

During informal visits to or at community meetings in PERRP project locations, stakeholders frequently made remarks about the project to me. I have included many such comments and opinions in this book's chapters, but here are a few other samples quite representative of what people said.

Vice Principal and Committee General Secretary at Government Girls' High School Kheral Abbasian: With the first jolt, I ran out of the office and the school building collapsed just behind me. I turned back and was terrified to see fallen rubble with so many students buried beneath. It was a horrific scene when we found eighty-six students of this school dead and many others were seriously injured. Now with the new school we have learned a little about earthquake resistance in buildings. If we'd had it before the quake many of the departed souls would have not met this fate. Students' parents have seen that the new building is being constructed according to the earthquake code and this helps them shed their fears. (PERRP 2011/12: 10)

Teacher at Government Boys' Higher Secondary School Jared: Since 2005 when the earthquake happened, many NGOs have been visiting us and saying that they would rebuild our school, but then nothing would happen. So we are very happy that the PERRP project did make this happen for us. The children here are very eager to have a roof over their heads to study again. (PERRP 2011/12: 19)

Student at Government Girls' High School Behali: We hardly remembered anything teachers told us when we were studying in the open air because there were so many distractions but now with this new building we can focus on what teachers tell us. (PERRP 2011/12: 19)

Committee Chairman at Government Girls' High School Jaglari: What we like about this project is that it is open and transparent, we know the construction details, schedule and quality of material being used. This kind of standard of construction we are seeing for the first time. (PERRP 2011/12: 15)

Principal at Government Girls' High School Chatter #2: Community participation has led our people to be aware of standards and transparency. (Murphy Thomas 2013b: 12)

Student at Government Boys' Chaknari, AJ&K: After our old school collapsed and before this school was constructed we were attending class by sitting on stones on the ground, and in the rainy season it was a big problem. Now we have a beautiful new building and a library with interesting story books. We love our school very much! (PERRP 2013: 13)

Coordinator of the KP Provincial Earthquake Reconstruction and Rehabilitation Authority (PERRA): This USAID project has worked very well in post-earthquake reconstruction in this district. The project started construction by involving the stakeholders and partners and completed its work in the stipulated time. It will be remembered due to the quality buildings and excellent social coordination among stakeholders. This model should be replicated by every donor-funded construction project because due to community involvement, people have a sense of ownership and this helps ensure their durability and proper maintenance. (PERRP 2013: 15)

Lady Health Visitor at Basic Health Unit Harighel: This new Basic Health Unit (BHU) building is much better than the previous one. It is facilitating patients from far-off areas. (PERRP 2013: 14)

Student at Government Boys' High School Pinyali: When the earthquake struck, everybody rushed outside and I fell down in the stampede and then my school building collapsed. To my luck, I survived but got wounded badly. Since then we have been studying under the sky, but now I am graduating. I am very happy to see the new school constructed thousands of times better than the previous building. (PERRP 2013: 17)

Community Member at Dhal Qazian: In this project we have set up School Management Committees that we now think are necessary because they act as coordinating bodies between the people and school management. They discuss how the education system can be improved, what kinds of difficulties are faced by the teachers and what types of problems contractors face during construction. These bodies help resolve all problems. (PERRP 2013: 20)

Manager at Manshera District Reconstruction Unit: This project was unique due to its coordination with all departments, including ERRA, the District Reconstruction Unit, KP's Provincial Earthquake Reconstruction and Rehabilitation Authority and especially communities. This enabled the construction to go smoothly and on time as there were efforts for conflict resolution at every stage. PERRP succeeded in completing construction well in time. (PERRP 2013: 15)

Mr. Saradar Qamar-Uz-Zaman Khan, Minister of Health and Bagh District Member of Legislative Assembly: I made a presentation about this project in a session of the AJ&K Legislative Assembly which led to the up-grading of some of these newly constructed schools, because they are spacious buildings constructed in accordance with international standards. For example, the Government Girls' Inter-College at Rerra has been up-graded to a degree college which means that girls can continue the education into a degree granting institution without leaving home, a major advantage for them and their families. Another is the government girls' High School at Thub, located in such a far-flung area. It has been upgraded to an Inter-College and several other upgrades are underway. (PERRP 2013: 16)

Teacher at Government Girls' School Juglari: This was the first time that the community was involved in construction and we found that the engineers gave weight to our opinion, and sometimes adjusted the design according to our wishes. Reciprocating their initiative of giving us importance, we extended all possible help including provision of extra land and water to help facilitate this construction. (PERRP 2013: 18)

Student at Government Girls' High School Chatter #2: The number of students in our school was sharply dropping as we were being taught in the open air after the earthquake destroyed our school. Even our desks [had] been ruined, so we sat on the ground or on stones, and it was miserable for all of us attending class like this in the rains. Many of my school fellows left the school and some families migrated out to the city for the sake of education. But with construction of this school, now the number of students has risen more than even before the earthquake. That's because it has been constructed so well, with all facilities that are now attracting students not only from this village but from the nearby places too. (PERRP 2011/12: 9)

Acknowledgments

This is one of those books that took quite a while to make happen.

Thanks to Dr. Anthony Oliver-Smith for recognizing this project was a story that should be told and for your patience with my figuring out how to tell it.

Thanks to Robert MacLeod, director (2006–2010) of the USAID/Pakistan Earthquake Reconstruction Program, Islamabad, and to his colleagues, for originally building "community" into this project concept.

Very special thanks to Tarek Selim, the PERRP chief of party, or head of project and main engineer, because every day for six years on this project he managed to juggle the technical and social elements so successfully and set an example of leadership and respect. In my long career of project work, PERRP was the most effectively managed project, due largely to his abilities and style. He regularly asked staff, "How can I support you?" It is rare for a project to have such low staff turnover, such a high level of pride in the project, and such teamwork. Thanks also to the other project engineers, construction managers, designers, drivers, and other support staff, as well as to PERRP and CDM Smith administrators (in Pakistan and the USA) and contractors who built such wonderful buildings.

PERRP's social mobilizers: It is hard to imagine this project without these social team members, all from the same districts as those affected by the 2005 earthquake and survivors themselves. Thanks to them for their deep knowledge, strong desire to help in the disaster recovery, ability to work even in tense times, and immeasurable enthusiasm and dedication. For Bagh district, Azad Jammu and Kashmir: Ghayour Abbas (coordinator), Asya Tabassum, Sadaf Batool, Zia Ahmed, Zaheer Khan, and senior consultant Afzal Mir. For Mansehra district, Kyber Pakhtunkhwa province: Kaleem Rehman (coordinator), Nasir Mehmood, Niaz Ahmed, M. Farooq, and Fakher Zaman.

To the over six hundred committee members in the communities who took up PERRP's challenge to participate, and did it with such enthusiasm, goes my extra special admiration and thanks. To the thousands of people in the communities, the men, women, girls, and boys who participated and said they would always remember those of us in PERRP and the help received from the other side of the world: here is remembering you too.

And with love to my daughter Sarah and all my family from Murphys' Corners, where so much of my experience started. This is in gratitude for all your support and encouragement, and it might help explain what I was doing all those years away.

In Gratitude

I am honored for the professional recognition by:

- The Rockefeller Foundation, for the 2018 award of a fellowship and writing residency at the Rockefeller Bellagio Center, Italy, to write part of this book.
- The Washington Association of Professional Anthropologists, for the 2021 Praxis Award for excellence in translating anthropological knowledge into action in the Pakistan Earthquake Reconstruction and Recovery Program.
- Knowledge Unlatched, for selecting this book in 2022 to place it in Open Access so that it can be read, shared, and used freely by anyone, anywhere, to help alleviate some of the problems in future disasters.

Abbreviations

AJ&K: Azad Jammu and Kashmir province, or, for short, Azad Kashmir
BHU: Basic Health Unit
CDM Smith: Camp, Dresser & McKee Smith
DRR: disaster risk reduction
ERRA: Earthquake Reconstruction and Rehabilitation Authority
IAK: Indian Administered Kashmir
ISAF: International Security Assistance Force
KP: Khyber Pakhtunkhwa province
LOC: Line of Control
NATO: North Atlantic Treaty Organization
NESPAK: National Engineering Services Pakistan
NGO: nongovernment organization
PAK: Pakistan Administered Kashmir
PERRA: Provincial Earthquake Reconstruction and Rehabilitation Authority (for province of KP)
PERRP: Pakistan Earthquake Reconstruction and Recovery Project
PTC: Parent Teacher Council
SERRA: State Earthquake Reconstruction and Rehabilitation Authority (for the state of AJ&K)
SMC: School Management Committee
UN: United Nations
UNOCHA: United Nations Office for the Coordination of Humanitarian Affairs
USAID: United States Agency for International Development

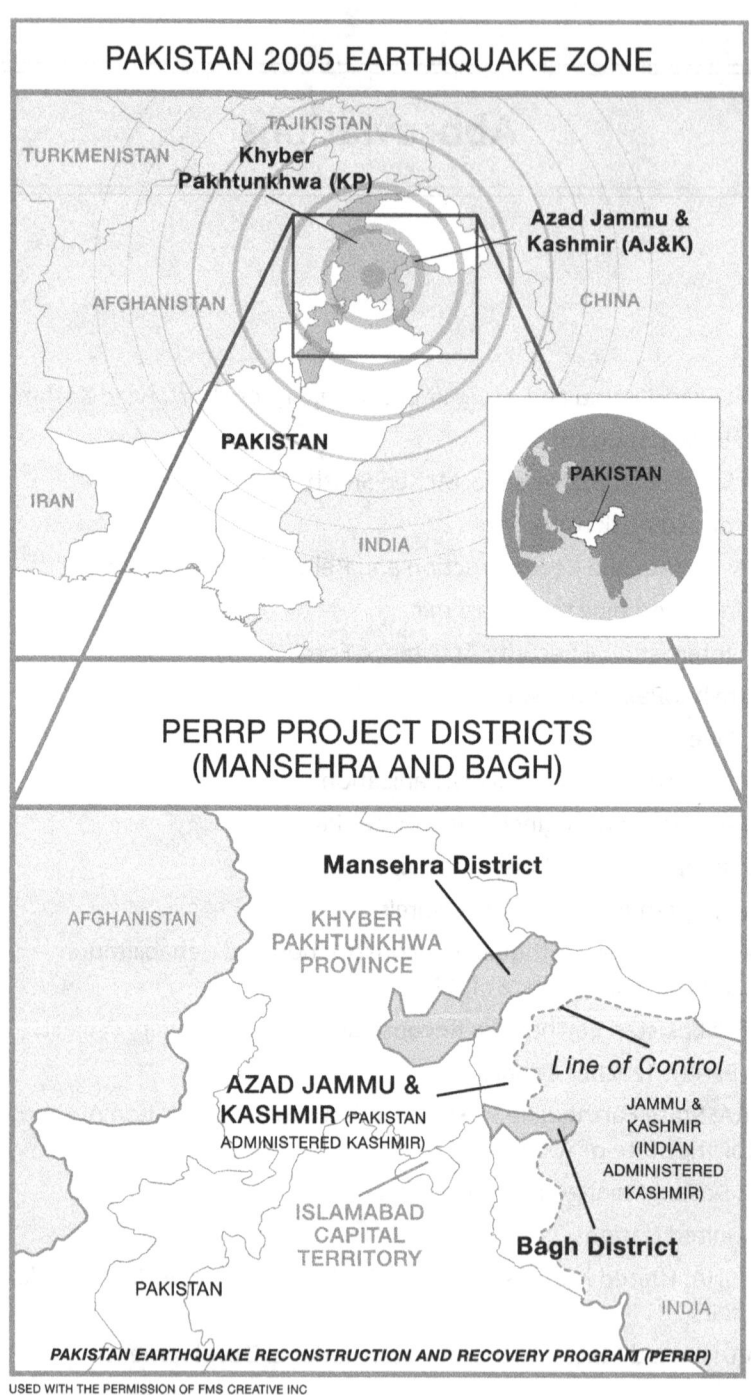

Maps: Pakistan 2005 Earthquake Zone; PERRP Project Districts (Mansehra and Bagh).

INTRODUCTION

Disaster Strikes

When disaster—an earthquake, flood, hurricane, wildfire, or tsunami—strikes, help rushes in from around the country and the world. For decades, this kind of assistance has been provided in both developing and developed countries; a great deal of study has been conducted to learn lessons and apply them when considering the next crisis. The main concern is that disasters are increasing around the world.

Disaster Studies, Future Disasters

Accordingly, disaster studies has grown into a worldwide field with specialized university departments for graduate and postgraduate programs around the globe. There are scholarly publications and conferences; nongovernmental organizations (NGOs), donors, United Nations programs, and national and local agencies specializing in disasters; and international, national, and local agreements, policies, strategies, plans, budgets, programs, and projects to analyze and implement in anticipation of, or in response to, disasters. And there are many specializations in the fields of disaster emergency preparedness, relief, recovery, reconstruction, and long-term development that cover a wide range of concerns and sectors: policy, planning, funding, health, education, housing, water and sanitation, livelihoods, environment, food security, infrastructure, administration, agriculture, human rights, human trafficking, climate change, and so on.

However, despite a great deal of study, it is widely recognized that the lessons learned are often not applied, resulting in assistance that too often is weak or failed. Many of these same organizations and analysts often observe and express disappointment with the gaps between theory and practice. This is discussed in detail in another book in this Berghahn Books "Catastrophes in Context" series entitled *Disaster Upon Disaster: Exploring the Gap Between Knowledge, Policy and Practice* (Hoffman and Barrios 2020).

The reality remains: "Disasters, both natural and technological, are becoming more frequent and more serious as communities become more vulnerable. They are impacting ever-larger numbers of people around the world" (Oliver-Smith and Hoffman 2002: 5). While disasters—and the losses and destruction they bring—will grow, so too will the need for physical reconstruction. With disasters also having major impacts on lives, livelihoods, and communities, there will be an intensified need to address social concerns as well. A main question is: can that increasing need for physical rebuilding, and the process to achieve it, also be a vehicle for social restoration and development? Better yet, how can the reconstruction and social development benefit each other while also reducing risks and vulnerabilities?

Making Things Happen offers some answers to the above questions, drawing on the experience in PERRP (Pakistan Earthquake Reconstruction and Recovery Project). It shows how a structured, representative, guided community participation program can help improve project efficiency and effectiveness while also significantly building on local capacities that can be used in further recovery and development. For this kind of participation program to occur in infrastructure reconstruction projects, a social component needs to be included, and that is the main subject of this book.

Other Literature

Given that postdisaster reconstruction of public infrastructure is such a widespread and common need, one might reasonably expect there would be a commensurate amount of research and literature about it—but this is not so. While there is mushrooming literature on the constituent parts of postdisaster reconstruction—hazards, construction, and the people whom construction is meant to benefit—these subjects are siloed, and there is a shortage of published work about many other aspects of disaster reconstruction. In the vast literature on construction in nondisaster times and contexts worldwide, there is a dearth of content about end users, while in the literature on disasters, there is scarce coverage of reconstruction, particularly of infrastructure, in this project location—especially in the Azad Jammu and Kashmir (AJ&K) region.

While there is a fair amount of literature about shelter and how it may be rebuilt by local people, there is little discussion of how local people can play highly important roles in large-scale public infrastructure reconstruction. Here, public infrastructure refers to facilities from which the public benefits, which are usually government owned and operated: schools, health facilities, roads, energy grids, and water systems.

The sources used in this text come from academic research in disaster studies, development studies, and community participation and development; scholarship in engineering and construction project management; the worldwide construction industry; organizations involved in hazard- or disaster-related agreements, policy, and planning; and institutions and groups such as governments, NGOs, donor agencies, the United Nations (UN), and international financial institutions (e.g., the World Bank). At times when disasters occur, the media also play a role as sources of information, as reconstruction is often highly politicized. While there might very well be a general assumption or even direction that the local people should be involved in reconstruction, how this could occur almost always remains vague.

Of particular note is the construction industry and its sources of funding or financing. Due to scale and demand for specialized know-how, public facilities are usually rebuilt by commercial construction firms or NGOs with advanced construction skills. This is not likely to change. As disasters increase, it is a safe bet that demands for their technical expertise will grow. The trouble is, while the construction industry is also generating a large amount of information and literature, it includes relatively little about disaster reconstruction. Furthermore, as discussed in more detail in chapter 6, stakeholders in the construction industry are often considered to be only the companies and financing sources involved—excluding local people, even when they will be the main users of the new facilities.

The kinds of consequences that come from this lack of awareness were frequently demonstrated in the Pakistani context discussed in this book. As observed by the social team of PERRP, other reconstruction projects, agencies, and contractors frequently were ineffective in dealing with the problems involving local people. This ineffectiveness was largely due to not anticipating the issues and how they could be prevented or mitigated, including contractor-community conflict, cultural insensitivity, land issues, access to the construction site, and contractor use or overuse of water, electricity, or other resources. Missing also was an understanding of the communities—the realities of their existing frictions, tensions, and conflicts—and of how outside assistance projects, including reconstruction, could exacerbate these kinds of situations, as well as what a project needed to prevent or handle them. In general, there was a lack of awareness that some construction problems have underlying social causes; such problems were one main reason for Pakistan's delayed reconstruction.

The fact is that the construction industry and those with humanitarian concerns are seen as having competing or contradictory interests, when in fact they can have parallel goals. Collaboration would benefit both construction firms and humanitarian groups and, most importantly, the end users. Chapter 5 discusses more bringing these two sets of expertise together to build understanding and cooperation in what would be a new field of study and practice: the social anthropology of construction.

Overview of PERRP, Including Anecdotes and Ethnographies

As introduced in detail in chapter 1, *Making Things Happen* is a case study of a disaster reconstruction project called the Pakistan Earthquake Reconstruction and Recovery Program. Running from 2006 to 2013, PERRP responded to the October 2005 earthquake that struck northern Pakistan. In PERRP, lessons and theories were put into practice, resulting in a project considered unusually successful by stakeholders—from the donor agency to the local governments, affected communities and people, and the design and construction companies involved.

While much of the other infrastructure reconstruction in this postdisaster scenario was slow, stalled, or even abandoned, in PERRP seventy-seven large, earthquake-resistant schools and health facilities were reconstructed in only six years, with almost all the construction completed on or ahead of schedule—a rare if not unprecedented feat in Pakistan. The project achieved these outcomes despite being in a highly complex security and sociocultural setting: a disaster site, in a part of the world with a long history of tension and conflict, in conservative rural communities on mountainous Himalayan terrain. The project accomplishments were attributed mainly to an unusual combination of strong construction management, structured community participation, and respect for local culture.

This book—like the steel and concrete construction project it investigates—is multidisciplinary, written in detail from several perspectives about intersecting subjects. It is about a construction project considered through the lens of disaster reconstruction, community participation and development, culture, social structure, peace and conflict, and relief and development. It also includes the rarely discussed challenges involved in sociocultural experts, engineers, and other technical people working together effectively, and it presents the processes developed to achieve this cross-disciplinary collaboration. Together with unprecedented community participation in the reconstruction of government-owned facilities, PERRP's social and technical coordination worked to "make things happen"—an expression used daily throughout the project.

Included at the end of each chapter are over seventy anecdotes and ethnographies which recount some of the project's complexities on a day-to-day basis. These and other stakeholder remarks capture the voices of some of the people involved and show a range of activities and incidents. The reader might like to read all of these anecdotes and ethnographies first, to get a sense of the range of issues and activities, as well as an understanding of how these illustrate points made in the other content.

What This Book Offers

While the rebuilding of destroyed houses, roads, bridges, schools, hospitals, and all aspects of the physical infrastructure is essential, desired, and welcomed, this book focuses on one aspect of reconstruction: the all-too-frequent negative reputation of construction. In many parts of the world, specifically in relation to the people in the vicinity of the reconstruction sites—who are most often the main end users of the completed facilities—the process of construction is often associated with missed opportunities, frustration, disappointment, damage, loss, conflict, legal proceedings, injustice, and more.

Disaster reconstruction, and even construction without a disaster, is infamous for being planned but never started. When it does start, it is slow, stalled, or even abandoned; even years later, much of what was destroyed has not been rebuilt, which was especially the case in the Pakistan disaster. Such failed construction may add to existing losses of trust, hope, and opportunities for the future. In contrast, as we will demonstrate in PERRP, the reconstruction process can be positive and productive, and it can even have dual achievement: not only speeding along construction, but also mobilizing communities, restoring hope, strengthening local recovery and increasing local capacities for further development. This book lays out this process in detail.

While problems for construction are numerous and the reasons for such delays and incompleteness vary widely, the central discussion of this book is about one of the main causes: the interactions between the reconstruction project and the local people. They can have very strong negative or positive effects on each other, and some of the problems for construction have underlying social causes. Conflict and long, costly court cases are a common result.

In other words, this book is about the sociocultural side of disaster reconstruction. It presents the many possible challenges to reconstruction and gives an example of how a structured community participation process was set up in a reconstruction project. In PERRP, a small social team was included for this purpose; we worked to develop an understanding of each community. Some of our strategies included identifying the social structure, social challenges, and possible underlying causes of conflict;

the community's strengths or capacities in dealing with conflict; and the community's capacities for participation and responsibility in the reconstruction project.

As any project needs to do, this social team also led the project to foresee potential problems and plan ahead. As shown in chapter 4, the PERRP social team started out by consulting with the various stakeholder groups, from community members to construction contractors and government officials, and then, from these different perspectives, identified the most common problems between communities and contractors. With this list, as shown in "What Could Go Wrong" (see table 4.5), the social team—in cooperation with project construction managers—worked backward through preventative measures and solutions. From these analyses, we developed several tools, including protocols, agreements with and between committees and contractors, lines of communication, and an integrated step-by-step technical and social process. Our later project assessments identified these approaches and tools as main ways that much conflict was prevented—they were, along with the way construction was managed, the reasons for the project going smoothly.

Importantly, this book sets out how community participation can be planned and implemented. Here, community participation is incorporated in a way that is specific, highly visible, structured, systematic, step-by-step, sometimes measurable, and integrated with the technical factors to help meet a project's overall goals more effectively.

More detail is laid out on these subjects as we move from chapter to chapter. Chapter 1 discusses the Pakistan disaster and PERRP's start there. Chapter 2 advises on what any project needs to do: understand the many contexts in which it will exist. Those contexts are factors that may affect the project, and which the project may have an effect upon in turn. These include other disasters; international relations and policy; conflict and collaboration; social structure, power, and culture; and resources, especially land. Chapter 3 explores the ideas of community and participation, their histories, and critical perspectives on them in construction development and disaster areas. Chapter 4, which discusses PERRP's social component, is set out in three parts: what was found upon arrival; the social team and its process; and how the communities worked and contributed. To encourage these components to work together, chapter 5 frankly addresses the infrequently discussed challenges of sociocultural specialists, engineers, and other technical specialists working together, and how these were managed in PERRP. Chapter 6 is about design and construction, and how community involvement benefitted both. Chapter 7 is about the Library Challenge, an activity not included in the original project plan, but one taken up by the schools, parents, communities, committees, local officials, the media, police, book publishers and sellers, construction contractors, engineers, and the general public. The Library Challenge was a culmination of all the local cooperation and became a symbol of collaboration, fun, and hope. Chapter 8 is about the social anthropology of construction.

The conclusion to this book gives a final analysis of the project, with much of the content coming from focus group discussions by the project's social mobilizers and most experienced construction engineers and managers, who had, collectively, over five hundred years of experience in social mobilization and construction in Pakistan and other countries. In those sessions, the social mobilizers were asked, drawing on all their experience (including that in PERRP), to suggest improvements for reconstruction projects in future disasters.

That being said, I still feel compelled to provide a few words of caution. PERRP could have lessons for other disaster reconstruction projects, but it was only one project in one area of one country, and it was developed in response to one particular disaster. As situations and projects can vary greatly from country to country, in different times and circumstances, it must be stated that PERRP is not being presented as a universal recipe or blueprint for disaster reconstruction or community participation. It also must be said that, while there were some innovations, no claim is being made that PERRP invented new ideas. Those of us in the project drew on the cumulative centuries of experience among PERRP staff, and from many others from earlier times and from different disciplines. Project ideas went back to the basics—adopting, adapting, or combining innumerable other sources of expertise—and those ideas were simply put into practice.

Who Is This Book For?

Given the predicted growth of disasters and need for reconstruction, there is a tremendous need to examine what can be done to improve the reconstruction processes, which can also reduce the risks and vulnerabilities not only of the new buildings, but of the people. This book emphasizes the need to bring sociocultural, technical, and other expertise together in addressing this need.

For this purpose, this book is offered especially to practitioners, researchers, academics, and students in both the sociocultural participatory and technical realms such as architecture, engineering, and construction management, as well as to planners, aid and policy makers, and funding agencies preparing for future reconstruction. This book provides detailed exposure to one cross-disciplinary project in a particularly challenging situation, written from a practitioner's point of view.

This book aims to raise awareness about disaster reconstruction, social complexities around reconstruction sites, and the need to include a social component with sociocultural specialists in reconstruction work, which frees technical staff to concentrate on their own specializations. For social specialists, this book also suggests raising awareness about the complexities of construction in postdisaster situations and how the sociocultural skills in community participation can be applied to benefit both the people and construction. Importantly, the book urges readers working from either perspective—the sociocultural or the technical, including engineering and construction—to look ahead and plan for frank discussion on how to cooperate and complement each other's work.

Due to the multidisciplinary nature of its content, *Making Things Happen* may also be relevant to a broad range of linked interests and specializations of individuals and organizations related to disaster reconstruction: governments, NGOs, consultants, social activists, community leaders, design and construction planners, and managers in both the nonprofit and business sectors, as well as other scholars, researchers, and practitioners in fields of study such as disasters, peace, conflict and security, international development, community participation and development, land issues, culture, sociology, and social or applied anthropology.

This Book's Geographical Focus

In Pakistan, PERRP was carried out in two adjoining locations, Khyber Pakhtunkhwa (KP) province and Azad Jammu and Kashmir (AJ&K), which is a disputed territory. Although some detail of PERRP's work in KP is included, this book is mainly about PERRP's work in AJ&K for a number of reasons. Destruction from the earthquake was concentrated in AJ&K; consequently, the government of Pakistan requested the United States Agency for International Development (USAID) to undertake reconstruction mainly there. Accordingly, PERRP's main field office and staff were placed in Bagh district of AJ&K so as to work in the most locations and communities, with a second field office and staff in the Mansehra district of KP province. From the beginning, it was planned that most of the construction and activity would be in AJ&K.

This book's content, therefore, is mainly about AJ&K—not only because the project's main operations and the communities involved were located there, but also because KP and AJ&K are quite distinct from each other. I have chosen to focus mainly on the location with most activity to avoid developing a cumbersome comparative analysis of PERRP's social processes in relation to KP's and AJ&K's particular cultures, histories, political and power structures, and cultural norms and practices.

Special Recognition

I have already mentioned this in my acknowledgements, but it cannot be emphasized enough that thousands of people contributed to this project. Despite the many challenges of the project area—the aftereffects of the disaster, the ongoing risks of conflict, and the hierarchical social structure with divisions, differences, and competing blocs of power—PERRP's results demonstrated how communities and people's willingness to collaborate can be very powerful, contrary to some arguments that claim that community is a myth (see chapter 3). Dedicated people, led by about six hundred committee members, helped make it all happen: teachers, students, parents, health facility staff, project staff, contractors, construction workers, and local officials, among many others.

Although they were from some of the poorest communities in the country, community members called on what strengths and resources they had to support the PERRP reconstruction and made it the right and popular thing to do. This was also a reflection of what any project can choose to do: treat the people with respect and confidence.

Project Key Terms

"Program" and "Project"

USAID's main assistance in response to this earthquake was in the form of the Pakistan Earthquake Reconstruction and Recovery "Program," to address needs in four sectors: reconstruction, health, education, and livelihood. Reconstruction was the flagship activity carried out using the umbrella name of the Pakistan Earthquake Reconstruction and Recovery Program, but this reconstruction work on the ground, as in this writing, was known interchangeably as a "program" or a "project."

Construction and Reconstruction

In the context of disasters, the word "reconstruction" is used as a catchall term to describe the act of putting back together the physical and sometimes intangible things that had been damaged or destroyed. In PERRP, we usually avoided using the word "reconstruction." The buildings would be new, not repaired or retrofitted, and the word implied redoing or repeating construction in the dangerous ways that had led to so much destruction in the first place. As design and construction in PERRP were based on the international building standards and codes for earthquake resistance, it was not repeating mistakes from the past. Other than all the extra challenges created by the disaster, this reconstruction was still "just" construction. For these reasons, the reader will see throughout the word *construction* used frequently, and for variety, *reconstruction*.

Implementing Agency and Contractors

Construction projects can be carried out numerous ways. When construction is needed, owners may do the construction themselves, or they might contract others to do it. In large scale commercial construction, especially involving governments and international donor agencies, it is common for projects to be tendered for competitive bidding by interested companies. The winning bidder is then contracted to do the job, and they may do it all themselves, or subcontract parts of the work to other companies. In any construction project, any number of contractors or subcontractors may be involved. As part of the United States government's response to Pakistan's request for postearthquake assistance, a request was issued for proposals and bids from qualified companies to carry out PERRP. The winning bid was from CDM Constructors Inc. (CCI), a subsidiary of CDM Smith, an American engineering and consulting firm. The company's role was overall project management, direction, and supervision of the Pakistani firms contracted to carry out the design and construction.

Although CCI was the main contractor, for the sake of clarity in this book it is referred to as PERRP's "implementing agency," while all the companies it hired are referred to as "contractors," who in some cases subcontracted. Also, while the contract was with CCI, on the ground in Pakistan the implementing agency was known as CDM.

Committees

In PERRP, groups were activated with different names according to location. In AJ&K, the groups were School Management Committees (SMCs) or Health Management Committees (HMCs), where health facilities were being built. In KP province, the groups were Parent Teacher Councils (PTCs) or Advisory Groups to the PTC. To simplify language, the reader will see the acronyms SMC, PTC or HMC used, or more often just the word "committee," referring to any of these groups.

Social and Technical Components

The project had two main components. The social component consisted of a team of social mobilizers—also called the sociocultural team—who were responsible for all the community participation and related activity. The technical component referred to engineers, architects, construction contractors, and design and construction managers.

Author's Reflections

For thirty years, I lived and worked full-time in conflict- and disaster-prone areas in Afghanistan, Pakistan, Bangladesh, and Azad Jammu and Kashmir, specializing in community participation in various forms and sectors of reconstruction and recovery.

My earliest learning experience about communities began in my early teen years in my family's remote sawmill community at Murphys' Corners in Ontario, Canada. This rural community consisted of my parents, grandparents, siblings, aunts, uncles, cousins, as well as sawmill workers, their families, and a few other community members. There, I frequently played the role of leader to all the kids in the community—organizing fun activities such as games or swimming at the lake because, in such a rural area, if we didn't organize activities ourselves, they would not happen.

I was aware of how among families, including my own, there were tensions over old differences. I saw how some were better-off and others were poor, and I wondered what might have been the causes of all these differences. Our great-grandfather had immigrated to Canada from Ireland at the time of the Irish famine in the mid-1800s, and so did the forebears of most of our neighbors, bringing with them the old political and religious differences between the Protestants and Catholics. Although by then a century had passed for our families in Canada, the differences had subsided, and we had practically no knowledge of them, there still was a clear separation, and some animosity and discrimination. My extended family members were the only Catholics in all the surrounding townships of Protestants. As such, my family was in the dichotomous position of being in the minority, even though my grandfather's sawmill was a main employer in the area. This was my introduction to community organizing in divided communities, and in retrospect, to arrangements of power at the community level.

Over time, I figured out what made people want (or not want) to participate in activities. I continued to be a community organizer as the founder and manager of clubs, associations, events, and projects through high school and art college, and in my first career in the visual arts. But after a few years, my interests in making art and organizing activities around it were overtaken by my interests in the world. In 1984, I made a planned career change to international development and was assigned by an international development education NGO to work in Pakistan in an Afghan refugee urban enclave, which led to working in the Afghan refugee camps along the border of Afghanistan and Pakistan. There I worked with the refugees to mentor and train them to become their own community organizers, which played a lead role in the start-up of the first ever Afghan NGOs.

As the reader will see, this book frequently addresses the highly important subject of power and arrangements of power, especially at the community level. For a total of fifteen years before the 2005 earthquake in Pakistan, I lived and worked full-time with Afghans in the refugee camps; then, after the USSR withdrew their troops in 1989, I worked in communities in east, north, and west Afghanistan, and lastly in Kabul. This experience immersed me not only in the realities and complexities of conflict but also in the related arrangements of power within hierarchical, heterogenous, conservative communities with many divisions. These divisions had become more pronounced in the refugee camps—and perhaps even more so upon return to home villages. In the war period, parts of the social structure were in a state of quick change, from hereditary power (by ethnicity, sect, etc.) to the power gained by political alliances and weapons. In the villages, the elders had always held sway, but now it was younger men with weapons and outside connections. In such work, one learns that knowledge of and sensitivity to the culture is not only essential; it is a crucial part of conflict sensitivity—how to help without contributing to more conflict. Such work also benefits from not only knowing such challenges but also from seeking out the existing skills and strengths among the local people in any location.

In 1995, I took a break from this project work to study at the School of Oriental and African Studies in the University of London, receiving my MA in the Social Anthropology of Development—the work I had been doing all along. In 1997, I returned to Asia, this time to Bangladesh to head up a flood control embankment construction project, and later returned to Afghanistan. Over the years I worked as an independent practitioner, consultant, project manager, and social anthropologist in projects for UN agencies, NGOs, governments, donor agencies, and consulting firms, specializing in community participation applied to many sectors—agriculture, forestry, water management, education, health, land mines, construction, land issues, rangeland management, livelihoods, microfinance, forestry, refugee camp management, and conflict prevention and resolution—as stated, all in conflict- and disaster-prone areas.

Back in Afghanistan in 2002, following the invasion of that country by US and other foreign forces and the fall of the Taliban government, I worked as a consultant, researcher, and adviser to NGOs and the new government of Afghanistan. In 2006 in Kabul, I was recruited by CDM Smith to design and manage the PERRP community participation program and be part of senior project management.

In this kind of work, one project and its lessons lead into another. That experience has not made writing this book easy, as so many perspectives are possible. Even so, from this one project alone, I have written from my various roles—not as a visiting researcher, but as a full-time member of the senior management team, social anthropologist, participant observer, and social program designer and manager.

From all this experience, if there was only one lesson I have learned to pass on, it would be this: participatory and anthropological approaches help solve real-world problems, but that require knowing, from multiple perspectives, not only what exactly the problems are in the first place, but also what the "best" solutions are. It is such approaches—mainly observing and listening to the people—that can lead to participation and the people themselves identifying what is "best." In aid projects, this means being able to work within the overall power structure, but especially for those with the greatest stake: those for whom the benefit is intended.

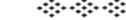

"Making Things Happen"

The title of this book, *Making Things Happen*, comes from that expression used daily among PERRP project staff and community members as an affectionate, joking, catchall phrase to encourage and explain to one another the work being done. When going to a community meeting, mobilizers might say to each other, "Time to make things happen." Or, to explain being late back from the field, one might say, "Things were happening." A community-based committee member would point out something new, saying, "See, we made it happen like we said we would." An architect signed off a note, adding, "Made things happen."

As head of the social program, I frequently visited the communities, sitting down with committees, head teachers, teachers, and school children. One of my favorite discussions was to ask students what they saw happening in their community now that construction of their new school was underway. What could they see happening? Did they notice who is making it happen? And did they themselves, as students, ever make things happen? In such school settings, where learning is by rote and discussion is not yet part of the teaching style, such questions opened a floodgate of observations and more questions. "When will construction be finished?" "What's the big hole in the ground?" "Will we have a computer room?" "We hear about shear walls and earthquake resistance, but can we get someone to explain that to us?" About the Library Challenge (see chapter 7), many wanted to know how they could help to get books.

These being far-flung rural areas, any construction site stood out, let alone one as big as a school or health facility—becoming the center of attention. Almost all the children had stories about walking by the construction site every day to their temporary tent school, how they would see the engineer and others working on the site and how they waved hello at each other. Many talked about going with friends, family members, and visitors after school to watch the workers digging in the ground, pouring concrete or carrying the steel rods up on the roof, the big trucks coming and going. As students and community members were briefed to stay out of the construction site for safety reasons, they and other visitors often sat on nearby hillsides, watching construction just for the fun of it. In one place, teachers talked about how their contractor sometimes worked at night even when it was snowing, using big lights run from generators. Some talked about project engineers coming into their classroom with the social mobilizer and teacher, to tell them about the construction. Students, and even many adults, watched how people were making things happen that they had never seen before.

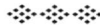

CHAPTER 1

The Moment the Quake Struck

Introduction

I will always carry the guilt for this, the way I was talking to the girl and what happened. Class was already underway, and I was going desk to desk, checking my students' homework. As usual this one girl had not done her homework and I was getting angry with her, demanding to know why. According to custom here, she was standing for me to speak with her, when all of a sudden there was a violent jolt and blast of sound when the earthquake hit and, already standing and likely stressed from my speech, she bolted for the door. She was the first to reach the door and as the building started to break apart, the instant she went through the door, something heavy fell off the building from above, killing her on the spot. Many others in our school were injured but she was the only one to die.

—A teacher

When the quake hit, I was at my relative's place farther up the mountain. As all the cell phone connections were broken, we had no way to know what happened at my home in the valley or anywhere. After a couple of days of not knowing, but hearing terrible stories, my cousins and I started walking down the mountain road, and it was like going down into a nightmare. All along the road, bodies were placed, wrapped in blankets for shrouds, waiting to be taken to cemeteries.

—A shopkeeper

When the Pakistan earthquake struck, I was in Kabul, Afghanistan, in my office on the ground floor. I had my door open to get some sun. I was at my computer, finishing some materials for the Government of Afghanistan's Ministry of Rural Rehabilitation and Development—which had engaged me to draft the plan for the country's first rural development training center—when I heard a roar off in the distance. At first I discounted it as another noise from the nearby military airport, but I soon felt the floor move. My colleagues and I ran outside, realizing the roar was the sound of an earthquake arriving. People already outside were crouched down on the ground, feeling it move with their hands in disbelief. About three hundred miles away from the epicenter in Pakistan, the Kabul buildings we were in suffered no damage, and there was relatively little damage in the rest of Afghanistan. A few days later, looking out from my same office door, I watched an unusual formation of army helicopters flying eastward over Kabul. These were later reported to be the first International Security Assistance Force (ISAF) helicopters on their way to Pakistan for emergency relief. Little did I know that I would also be in Pakistan a year later, working on the reconstruction project for the earthquake I had felt that autumn morning.

It was 8 October 2005 at 8:52 a.m. when the earthquake struck northern Pakistan, India, and Afghanistan. Although concentrated in north-central Pakistan, the shaking reached out over an area of about eighteen thousand square miles. The Asian Development Bank (ADB) and World Bank (WB) described this earthquake "as arguably the most debilitating natural disaster in Pakistan's history" (ADB and WB 2005: 4). Not only was the scale unprecedented in the country, the United Nations Emergency Relief Coordinator, Jan Egeland, stated that the organization had "never seen such a logistical nightmare," referring to the scale and urgency of assistance needed, with tens of thousands of people affected over a large area at high elevation with few roads and winter setting in ("Quake" 2005).

The Geological Impact

According to the US Geological Survey, the quake measured a magnitude of 7.6 on the Richter scale. The epicenter was near the town of Balakot, about one hundred twenty-five miles north of Islamabad, Pakistan's capital city, from which destruction was concentrated in a hundred-mile-wide circle reaching across two administrative units of the country. The damage occurred across the north-central part of Khyber Pakhtunkhwa (KP) province to the west of the epicenter, while the highest destruction rate occurred in the east, in the internationally disputed territory of Pakistan-administered Kashmir, known as Azad Jammu and Kashmir (AJ&K) or Azad Kashmir.

The quake zone was located in the Indian plate and Asian plate's subduction region, where tectonic movement—compression and bending—was responsible for the creation of the Himalayan mountain ranges (Durrani et al. 2005: 12). The quake was attributed specifically to a "rupture of the northwest-southeast oriented Muzaffarabad thrust fault . . . [with its] hypocenter located at a depth of 20 kilometers" (Bulmer et al. 2007: 53). Due to its scope, this quake has different names in the literature—it has been called, variously, the Pakistan Earthquake, the Kashmir Earthquake, the Balakot Earthquake, and the Balakot-Kashmir Earthquake.

Over the following weeks, more than a thousand aftershocks reaching up to 6.0 on the Richter scale caused innumerable landslides and severe rock falls, resulting in even more destruction. Roads were blocked by the landslides and, in a few places, rivers also were blocked, creating new lakes. Visible in many locations even years later were mountain slopes with fresh, lightly colored scars that were created when rock faces broke away, taking forest cover with them. In many locations with steep slopes, rocks and boulders were dislodged, which then rolled or bounced downward, destroying roads, villages, markets, and anything in their way. One of the schools rebuilt in this USAID-funded reconstruction had been destroyed when an enormous boulder crashed down the steep mountainside and through the roof of the school, killing four students and seriously injuring several more.

Much of the quake area is of similar typography, covered with mountains on the southern edge of the Himalayas. Few roads exist, and those that do are narrow, barely wide enough for two vehicles to pass when they meet. These roads were treacherous even before the quake. The only way for most inhabitants to get to markets or seek services of any kind has always been through long walks on footpaths, up and over the mountains, through riverbeds and across narrow wood-and-rope suspension bridges. In this part of Pakistan, it is not uncommon for children to have to walk

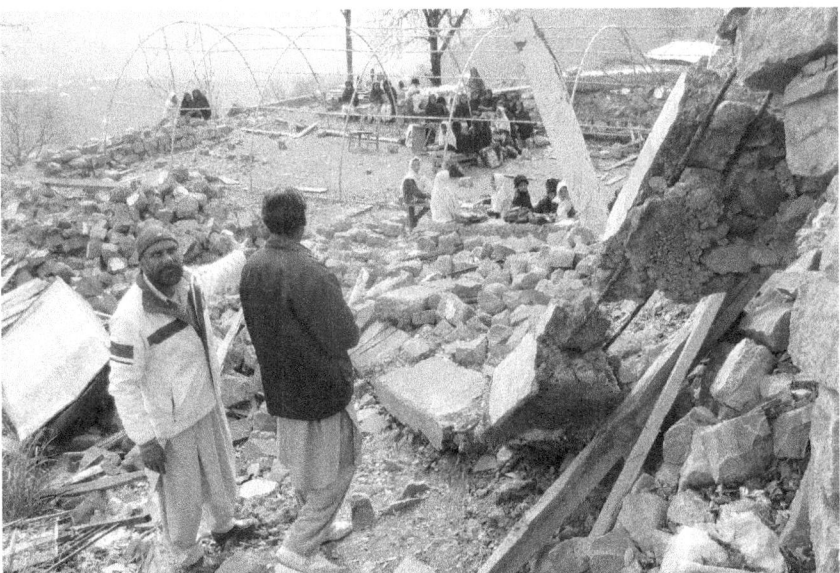

Figure 1.1. A Collapsed School. A community member indicates how, in the earthquake, the Government Girls' High School Kheral Abbasian collapsed. Students continued attending class in the rubble. 2010. © Jane Murphy Thomas.

at least one to two hours one way to attend school. Heavily damaged bridges and roads made accessing help and getting help to local inhabitants challenging.

While Balakot was almost completely destroyed, so also was the AJ&K capital city of Muzaffarabad, which is only twelve miles away. From both those densely populated urban areas, the destruction spread out across eight neighboring districts—mainly the districts of Mansehra in KP and Bagh in AJ&K. In this disaster, with many victims trapped far away from damaged roads, accessing help posed extra challenges. The USAID-funded PERRP was carried out in both KP and AJ&K.

The Human Impact

While estimates varied, damage from the quake claimed more than 74,000 lives, and injured an additional 70,000 people. Figures on the rate of destruction varied widely, but early assessments reported about 272,000 buildings had been levelled, including 574 healthcare facilities and at least 7,669 schools. About 84 percent of the houses were destroyed, leaving 2.8 million people without shelter, scattered over 15,000 villages (ADB and WB 2005).

Greatly complicating the government's response, especially in Muzaffarabad, was that the destruction of government buildings rendered the civil administration unable to function effectively. There was also large loss of life among civil servants and their families. An early assessment reported:

> [The area] suffered extensive damage to economic assets and infrastructure, with social service delivery, commerce, and communications either debilitated or destroyed. Vulnerable groups, mainly women and children living in inaccessible mountain areas with low levels of income and service provision, have borne the brunt of the earthquake's impact. (ADB and WB 2005: 2)

Even places relatively close by the city were on their own, as expressed by a school teacher one hour north of Muzaffarabad. Her school had collapsed, trapping teachers and 110 students. As she and others scrambled to try to rescue the trapped, they shouted for others to come help. Later, she wrote:

> About five hours [after the quake], a man arrived from Muzaffarabad and we asked him, "Where is the government? Where is the army? They should come and help us." And he said, "What are you talking about? Muzaffarabad is destroyed too. There is nothing left—hospitals, schools, government buildings are all destroyed. No-one can help us." (Kokab 2015)

At Muzaffarabad, AJ&K's Prime Minister Sikander Hayat Khan (2005) explained the tragic scene to gathered international media representatives: "For the first two days we have been either digging in the ground to recover bodies or digging to bury them. I have become premier of a graveyard."

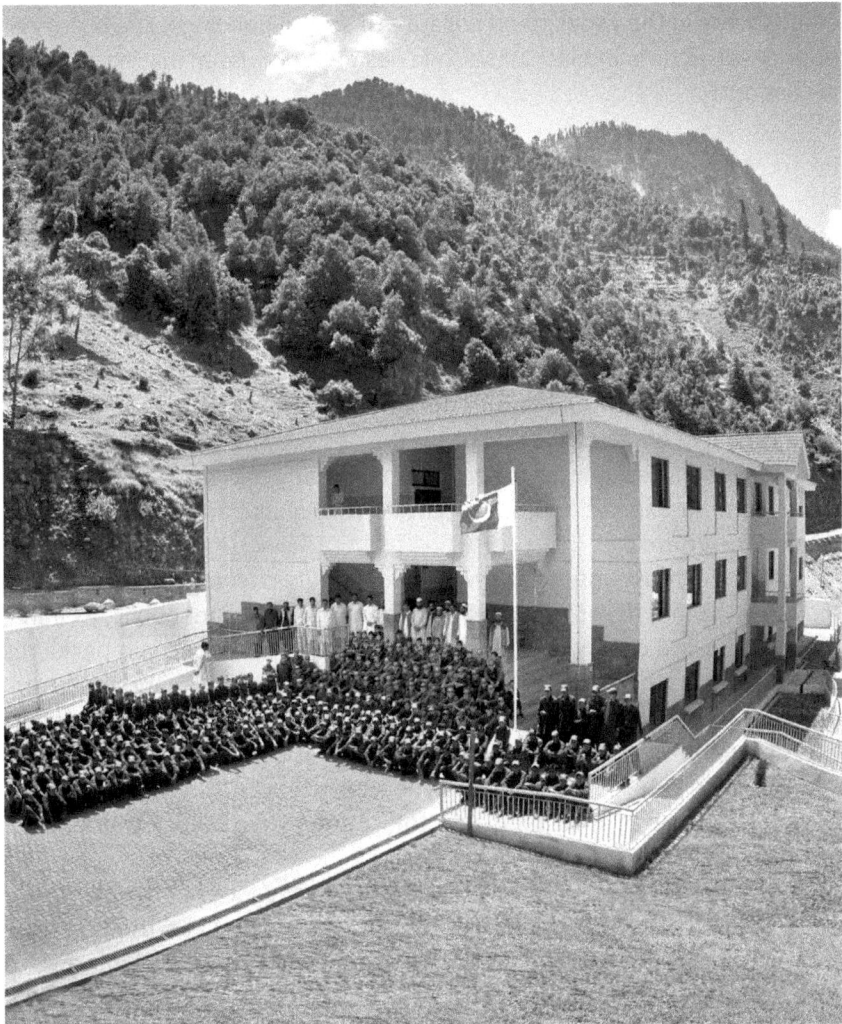

Figure 1.2. Mohandri School. At this location, the earthquake dislodged boulders, which rolled down the nearby steep mountain slope, smashing into the school, taking several lives. Here, students and teachers pose in front of their new school constructed by the PERRP project. Government Boys' Primary and Secondary Schools, Mohandri village, Khaghan Valley, KP. See anecdote in Chapter 6: "Mohandri School, Mountainside Boulders." 2011. © Umar Farooq.

The high death rate was attributed to two main factors: timing and the poor-quality construction of buildings. It was Ramadan, and that morning—after their predawn meal—many people were busy in their homes. The quake struck so suddenly that there was no time for them to escape their collapsing houses. It was also a school day, and classes had just started. The Government of Pakistan estimated that seventeen thousand children and eight hundred teachers died in the quake, and that most of these deaths were in the widespread collapse of school buildings. The history of poor construction and lack of seismic design is discussed in greater detail in chapter 6.

Local, National, and International Assistance

Within hours, news of the earthquake was known around the world. Word of the disaster and destruction was made known first by the local private TV and the region's only FM radio station, the Voice of Kashmir, which had operated out of a family's house amidst heavily destroyed buildings. Then "it took a couple of hours before the state-owned electronic media broke the news" (Rehmat 2006: 1). But by the very next day, the mainstream Pakistani and international media outlets already had their journalists on the ground in Balakot and other parts of the quake zone, reporting live around the world.

With the almost immediate worldwide media coverage, levels of help did come from different sources, first from the Pakistani public, as initiatives across the country were taken to collect and deliver aid packages directly to the stricken areas. Groups of friends, neighbors, and faith communities formed, collecting food, clothing, medicines, and other goods, and delivering them personally to the quake-hit areas on damaged roads jammed with other vehicles doing the same. It was "the largest philanthropic response by Pakistanis that the country [had] ever experienced" (Wilder 2008: 4).

One such group, composed of friends and colleagues in the city of Lahore, called themselves the Pakistan Azad Kashmir 2005 Earthquake Devastation and Relief Camp. This group managed to deliver an impressive forty tons of relief goods. However, as spokesman Aizad Sayid (2012) said, "organizing [the] purchase of tents, essential goods, medicines and then transport[ing] them turned out to be much harder than expected." Besides trying to acquire quantities of relief goods when so many others were doing the same, getting the goods to the quake site was another major challenge. As the NGOs and donor agencies found out early on, the quantity of relief goods—especially winterized tents, needed immediately in the hundreds of thousands—exceeded the world supply.

The Pakistani private sector also played an important role with cash donations and in restoring and rapidly expanding telecommunications. Before the quake, cell phone usage in these remote areas was limited; after 8 October 2005, providers joined the rush to help, and in only months, new cell phone towers appeared throughout the area. Within the next couple of years, even the poorest extended families or villages owned at least one cell phone.

The Pakistan earthquake was then on the world stage through the media. It was the headline story, featured by major TV personalities from the BBC, CNN, and other media outlets from the USA, Canada, Europe, Australia, Japan, China, the Gulf States, and Latin America. Such reporting played the essential role of bringing news of this disaster into homes and workplaces, sparking interest to help from around the world. But, as happens frequently in such disasters, other world events arose and the international media focus changed. Within about three weeks of the quake, "the global broadcasters [had] packed up their satellite dishes and moved on" ("Kashmir's Earthquake" 2005).

Two days after the quake, the UN secretary-general, Kofi Annan, spoke at a press conference, saying, "Every hour counts, and I urge the world to respond and respond generously and willingly" (2005). Two weeks later, on 26 October 2005, the UN issued a world-wide urgent appeal for $550 million[1] for immediate assistance for the tens of thousands of survivors stranded in remote areas. Annan reminded reporters of the urgent need "to prevent a second shock wave of deaths and prevent further suffering." As severe winter conditions were setting in, which would cut off access to the remote mountain areas even by helicopter, he added, "[i]n the next few days, weeks, we literally remain in a life-saving phase" (Sengupta 2005).

On 19 November 2005, at the UN-convened donor conference in Islamabad, eighty countries and agencies pledged a total of $5.8 billion to reconstruction and rehabilitation programs (Naqvi, 2005). In the first few days, UN agencies already present in Pakistan initiated large-scale relief operations. These agencies included the World Food Program, World Health Organization, United Nations Development Program, UN-Habitat, the United Nations Children's Fund (UNICEF), United Nations High Commission for Refugees (UNHCR), United Nations Office for the Coordination of Humanitarian Affairs (UNOCHA), and United Nations Educational, Scientific and Cultural Organization (UNESCO).

Hundreds of local, national, and international NGOs arrived to provide relief aid for the short-term emergency phase only, while others arrived for this early phase as well as for the long-term reconstruction, recovery, and development. They provided a wide range of assistance, including large-scale food shipments, support to staff of destroyed health facilities, treatment of the injured, and water purification and sanitation, and they helped to set up temporary shelters. They also provided priority items such as winterized tents, blankets, generators, diesel, tarpaulins, ground sheets, stoves, fuel, and kitchen sets. Organizations there for the longer term implemented projects in such fields as seismic construction, agriculture, water management, sanitation, livelihood restoration incentives, environment, health, nutrition, child protection, critical psychosocial support for the trauma, and capacity building in education and health, with teacher and medical staff training.

Many parts of the world responded to the crisis: the European Union and European countries individually, including Denmark, France, Italy, Germany, Poland, Sweden, Turkey, and the United Kingdom; Australia, Canada, Russia, and the USA; and many Asian and Middle Eastern countries including Afghanistan, Cambodia, China, India, Indonesia, Iran, Japan, Jordan, Kuwait, Malaysia, and Nepal. Only hours after the quake, specialized canine search and rescue teams arrived from England, France, Russia, Poland, Canada, and other countries. One of the largest foreign contingents of medical workers to rush to Pakistan's aid was Cuba: "Within two weeks of the quake, two hundred Cuban doctors, nurses and paramedics were at work on the ground" ("Cuba" 2005).

Perhaps the most unusual source of help came from the nearby large-scale international military presence across the border in Afghanistan. As part of the so-called War on Terror, troops from fifty-one countries—members of the North Atlantic Treaty Organization (NATO)—were stationed close to the west side of the quake zone in Kabul and the eastern provinces of Afghanistan. This NATO-led security mission, the International Security Assistance Force (ISAF), sent two hundred medical personnel and another thousand engineers and support staff on a three-month emergency mission to assist (NATO 2010). It was these ISAF helicopters that I had watched fly east from Kabul a few days after the earthquake. This mission also set up an air bridge, lifting thousands of tons of emergency supplies of tents, stoves, and blankets from Europe to Pakistan. Their helicopters delivered goods to remote villages and evacuated the injured. Many NATO countries provided services on the ground, including a field hospital, water purification teams, and a fuel farm to refuel the many helicopters being used. They also helped to clear rubble and set up temporary shelters, and provided other specialized workers such as a British unit of engineers specialized in high-altitude relief work.

Response from the US Government and Government of Pakistan

The US government pledged $510 million for relief and reconstruction efforts to assist the government of Pakistan's relief operations. This total included $300 million in humanitarian relief and reconstruction assistance, and $110 million in military support of relief operations, especially to supply goods needed immediately for the onset of winter: shelter, relief supplies, health, water, sanitation, and logistics. The US also responded to Pakistan's request for helicopter support, ferrying over five thousand tons of food, shelter materials, and rescue equipment to the disaster area. A US Army mobile surgical hospital at Muzaffarabad provided urgent care. In the first few months, American private charitable donations for earthquake assistance topped $73 million (US Department of State 2005).

For assistance in long-term recovery, the US funded four projects handled by the United States Agency for International Development (USAID). The flagship project was PERRP, with a budget of $120 million to rebuild a number of schools and health facilities. This budget was increased to $137 million in 2011 to reconstruct more schools in both of the quake-hit districts (Hagan and Shuaib 2014). The three other projects were the RISE (Revitalizing, Innovating, Strengthening Education) project to improve educational capacities and quality; PRIDE (Primary Healthcare Revitalization, Integration and Decentralization in Earthquake-Affected Areas) project to enhance capacities in health; and I-LEAD (Improving Livelihoods and Enterprise Development) to assist in reestablishing income sources.

To carry out PERRP, USAID tendered the project and selected CDM Constructors Inc. (CCI), a subsidiary of CDM Smith, an American engineering and construction firm. With operations in several countries around the world, the company provides environmental, transportation, water, and energy-related engineering and construction services in a range of sectors to public and private clients.

The government of Pakistan, led by President General Musharraf, the former army general who had gained power in a coup d'état in 1999, took on the role of leading the emergency and long-term reconstruction, with such efforts alternatively lauded or condemned. The government, which had been without a national body responsible for disasters, almost immediately established the Federal Relief Commission to take charge of coordinating and monitoring relief efforts. Two army divisions—approximately twenty-thousand troops—were dispatched to the affected areas to set up staging posts and facilitate the delivery of relief goods.

Later that same month, the government of Pakistan established its Earthquake Reconstruction and Rehabilitation Authority (ERRA), which was an extension of the military led by former and active military officers. ERRA was given the mandate to plan, lead, coordinate, monitor, and oversee reconstruction, incorporating "building back better" approaches to ensure that "all reconstruction would be seismically resilient so that future earthquakes would have a less damaging effect" (World Bank Group 2014: 4). Over the next years, the army's own Frontier Works Organization also rebuilt the roads and bridges.

Studies conducted by foreign organizations in the early months following the quake tended to praise the efforts of the government of Pakistan and ERRA. One early study by the Mid-America Earthquake (MAE) Center at the University of Illinois reported, "The impact on healthcare and education has been severe. Nonetheless, recovery has been more rapid than observed by members of the MAE Center–Rice University Team who have studied several previous earthquakes worldwide. The response of government organizations, the Pakistan Army and private companies was impressive" (Durrani et al. 2005: 7). Similarly, the World Bank Group stated that "strong leadership within ERRA was a key reason for the success of post-earthquake reconstruction. While Pakistan has incurred many high intensity natural disasters before and after the 2005 earthquake, none of the recovery responses by the public sector have come close to matching the uniquely successful 2005 reconstruction program" (World Bank Group 2014: 27).

However, within Pakistan and in the quake zone, opinions generally were—and still, years later, are—highly critical, blaming ERRA for mismanagement and a wide range of failures in reconstruction. For example, when PERRP arrived to start rebuilding destroyed schools and health facilities a year after the quake, we at first had major problems with distrust. People in the communities were angry with both ERRA and the NGOs because so little reconstruction had happened. In PERRP's social mobilizer meetings in communities that first year, remarks were consistent in almost every village, with people saying, "Many of these agencies have come and asked us a lot of questions and made promises of help to us, but then never came back. Why should we believe you [PERRP] people?" A main role of the social team throughout the project was to build trust and protect it.

At the village level, some sources at first also expressed extreme worry about foreign money and foreign organizations, and the unwanted influence this could bring. This concern was partly due to foreign NGOs not being present in AJ&K before the earthquake, and largely due to the prevailing security situation. As discussed in chapter 2, the project area was not far from the border of Afghanistan and Taliban strongholds. In introductory meetings in a few villages, the occasional speaker said, "American money, we don't want it." Or they expressed suspicion such as, "Why are you planning to build such strong buildings here? You are just going to build these as forward bases, preparing for Americans to invade here, just like they did in Afghanistan [after 9/11]." The few times such sentiments were expressed, others in the same meetings responded with embarrassment, putting down such ideas. PERRP social staff used such remarks to reinforce the project's request for the people to organize and participate, so they would know what was happening and share responsibility for it.

In that early period, many survivors were especially angry with the Pakistani government and army, from whom they had expected help. They too had heard that international assistance was being provided, and they blamed the government when they did not see it arrive. Unfortunately, even years later, many never received assistance, and not all promised reconstruction was completed.

Reconstruction Status: "Concrete Skeletons of Unfinished Schools"

By the tenth anniversary of the quake in 2015, tens of thousands of students still sat in the open air to learn, winter and summer. One such student was Abid Bashir, an eighth-grade student in a state-run school in Hattian Bala, south of Muzaffarabad. He had never had a school roof over his head: "Since he can remember, he has been studying under the open sky. He is not alone; some 450 other students learn with him" (Naqash 2015). Even a dozen years after the quake, international humanitarian crisis analysts reported that thousands of schools were still not rebuilt. The public was left to wonder what had happened to the twelve years and $6 billion of donor pledges (Naviwala 2017).

From the start, the overall political power structure and ruling style was reflected in government involvement in earthquake reconstruction. As a full-fledged province, KP has enjoyed the security, rights, and national and international identity of being part of Pakistan, while AJ&K's status as a disputed territory perpetuates uncertainty. While KP inherited and sustains the many-layered hierarchy of the British bureaucracy, with its fixed procedures and chains of command, AJ&K's bureaucracy is relatively ad hoc. Although reconstruction was a federal jurisdiction, the province and disputed territory often had different policies and practices; many actors gave different directions—a situation made all the more complex by the lack of coordination of NGOs and other implementing agencies.

By 2015, donor assistance had plunged, and the rate of construction was still stymied. Tenth anniversary commemorations condemned the government and ERRA for the lack of progress. Mohammad Zaffar Khan, secretary for the AJ&K branch of ERRA, expressed his dissatisfaction with having at least 150,000 students still studying year-round in the open air due to the lack of completed buildings (Naqash 2015). Although data on the proportion of destroyed schools that had been rebuilt remained widely inconsistent, the reality on the ground, which could be seen on a daily basis, was best described by one analyst as "the concrete skeletons of unfinished schools [that] litter northern Pakistan" (Naviwala 2017).

Reliable, consistent data on construction starts and completions was never available, beginning with the original estimates of the number of schools destroyed being wildly inconsistent, from six thousand to fifteen thousand. As discussed further in chapter 4, the reason for the divergent information was largely due to a breakdown of data sharing by governments, donor agencies, ERRA, NGOs, and others. At one point about five years after the quake, ERRA officials reported informally that in KP province, 65 percent of the started schools were stalled, and in one AJ&K district, 100 percent were stalled. Even without official reliable studies, the destruction was so visible and widespread that a relatively reliable survey could be conducted by simply driving down the roads and watching for reconstruction activity, a daily activity of PERRP staff moving between the project's own job sites.

Why were so few schools being completed? When asked this question, Secretary Khan explained the reason for this was poor cash flow, saying "a severe financial crunch had virtually paralyzed the reconstruction programme since April 2010" (Naqash 2015). In my own interviews with ERRA staff members, funding from government and problems with contractors were major issues, but other problems included "intercommunal disputes, community issues over land and access to construction sites, and court cases." One of the officials reported, "There are so many court cases that ERRA has had to hire a full-fledged legal team to represent ERRA in court over all the issues" (Murphy Thomas 2012b: 7).

With all the challenges there are in construction at any time, as discussed in chapter 6, those listed by ERRA representatives could be valid, but at least part of the challenges go beyond funding problems. As I will discuss in more detail in the chapters to come, some of the problems for construction come from how construction is managed in relation to local people. As shown in PERRP, it is possible to manage construction so that it can prevent or mitigate issues such as intercommunal disputes, land issues, and long, costly court cases by involving the local people. Results can benefit both construction and the people.

Introduction to PERRP

Any such development or reconstruction projects have official and unofficial metrics by which to assess their success—and these metrics usually bring up the challenges or weaknesses the projects had, and if and how they were addressed. Below is a summary of PERRP's construction and work with communities, with details to be found in each chapter.

In contrast to this earthquake's wider reconstruction scenario—in which much of the work had never been started, was slow, stalled, or even abandoned—PERRP completed almost all its assigned construction sites either on or ahead of schedule, despite a major but temporary aid policy shift discussed below. The PERRP work saw the construction of seventy-seven large health and education facilities. For construction in Pakistan—even in normal times, without a disaster—such a completion rate is rare if not unprecedented. This achievement was attributed to the project's strong construction management, a respect for local culture, and a level of community participation not undertaken by the other projects.

With much of this earthquake's other reconstruction incomplete, PERRP was well known in the local earthquake reconstruction field: it stood out from the others because, once started, construction proceeded steadily with virtually no stoppages. The highly visible slow pace of much of the other reconstruction had innumerable causes such as social issues and financial, technical, management, or logistical factors.

To meet its reconstruction goals, PERRP introduced some innovations. Of all the other donor and ERRA reconstruction projects, PERRP was the only project with a dedicated social team to mobilize community participation in a structured, step-by-step program to facilitate construction. A few years later, one other reconstruction project modeled on PERRP was carried out in the area by the same implementing agency for another donor. From such experience, this book shows how a well-organized community participation program can help reduce many of the problems that hold up reconstruction.

Gaps in understanding between construction contractors and people living in affected communities can lead to lack of cooperation and even conflict. Underlying social, cultural, and political differences need to be understood in order for such gaps be bridged. To help avoid long costly delays in construction, the local people must be involved in shaping the work; to ensure effective community involvement, it was necessary to understand the people and the challenges involved.

Having a social team in PERRP enabled us to bring together key stakeholders, community committees, construction contractors, PERRP engineers, and others—and, using participatory methods, to conduct joint analyses to assess needs, foresee problems, and consider prevention and solution options. Several approaches and management tools used in the project were developed jointly by these stakeholders.

While ERRA and and the respective government departments responsible for education had to deal with halted work at innumerable construction sites due to conflict, and had a backlog of court cases over land and reconstruction issues, in PERRP, only eight of our fifty thousand construction days were lost due to conflict, and not a single court stay order was issued. Such problems were prevented in PERRP by a participatory, step-by-step process in which all parties had agreed-upon roles.

As detailed in chapters 4 and 5, PERRP's social approach was to propose to communities that they activate a committee to work in partnership with the project, with both the community and the contractors contributing to shared responsibilities. The experienced social team members were already well versed in the challenges, risks, and problems exacerbated by the disaster. Most social team members were from nearby villages and were earthquake survivors themselves, so they knew firsthand about the complexity of this work: the poverty, heterogeneity, long-standing differences, and history of conflict, which were now added to by the losses and trauma of the disaster. Yet social mobilizers were also encouraged to recognize the local knowledge and the powerful, productive attitudes, skills, and resources that had existed in the same locations before the disaster, and that could now be called on again in design and reconstruction work.

Taking this capacities approach—rather than the much more common vulnerabilities or hand-out approach—was also new to the communities. Until the arrival of PERRP a year after the quake, people in these communities had been treated in the ways common in all disaster situations: as poor aid recipients with many problems that needed to be taken care of. This conventional, vulnerability-focused approach emphasizes loss and weakness. However, from lessons learned in countless other disasters, PERRP's social team knew that, although top-down assistance is essential to save lives in the early postdisaster emergency phase, such handouts become counterproductive, even damaging. A vulnerability-focused approach, if continued too long or in the wrong places—whether in the form of decision-making or the distribution of physical goods—can build dependence and other serious disincentives. As a result, in some of the first communities we approached, we were met with demand for individualized handouts. However, this expectation changed almost immediately when we announced an alternative strategy: instead of bringing gifts, we were asking communities to become partners with PERRP, and for them to contribute to having a new school or clinic built.

Showing confidence in the local people and challenging them with a capacities approach not only got their strong buy-in but also resulted in problem-solving, accessing and providing resources, and other contributions far in excess of what had been anticipated, as documented in chapter 4. In addition to helping prevent many of the community-related problems experienced in other reconstruction efforts, the committees, as part of their duties to also help improve education, worked with teachers to introduce activities at the schools. In some schools, these often were the first activities ever involving students, teachers, parents, and the public. They raised their own funds to start each school's library and the wildly popular Kashmir bookfairs. Although it was new for all involved to share responsibility with such an outside project, the general effect was an unusual level of collaboration and enthusiasm. This helped to avoid problems, and it kept the project's step-by-step process in action by meeting the construction schedule and deadline.

In these rural areas, each construction site became a landmark—a center of attention and community activity. Each new PERRP site garnered attention in the surrounding communities, among both the public and officials, who noted that the projects were progressing without the interruptions common in other reconstruction efforts. PERRP's "reconstruction activities were unique [in that they included] significant community involvement—probably the first time that an infrastructure development project in Pakistan took the community onboard," said Sahad Hamid, program manager for ERRA's District Reconstruction Unit for Mansehra district of KP. "This helped the project and revived the spirit of the communities. They took ownership of this reconstruction project" (Hagan and Shuaib 2014: 2).

A Department of Education official frequently made remarks about how PERRP differed from other reconstruction projects underway: "In our office, we are constantly contacted by community members about problems with construction in their villages, but we have never had a single complaint about the PERRP project" (Murphy Thomas 2012a: 38). He wanted to know how the project took care of people's complaints so they did not have to take them to the government. He especially wanted to know about the project's grievance procedures, and so accompanied social mobilizers to several meetings to observe how they worked. He expressed surprise at how social mobilizers successfully tackled even some of the toughest problems around land issues, while the government itself was inundated with court cases and work stoppages over the same things (Murphy Thomas 2012b).

Challenges

Outlined in individual chapters are the many challenges PERRP faced. For construction, they included the technical factors of topography and weather. Roads most often were single-lane dirt roads with mountain switchbacks, and in some places, they were blocked by landslides, making transport of equipment and materials difficult. High-altitude variations in weather, from deep snow in some areas to monsoons in others, complicated construction scheduling. Construction challenges are discussed in detail in chapter 6.

The security situation was a considerable challenge. The earthquake and PERRP occurred at a time of especially high insecurity in Pakistan, as detailed in chapter 2. There were also the realities of heterogenous communities where disputes and conflict are common and how these might be manifested, even exacerbated, at the community level when a construction project arrives on scene.

PERRP was an unusual mix of technical and social specialists, engineers, and social mobilizers who were figuring out how to work together for the first time, and it did not always go smoothly. As detailed in chapter 5, it took about a year to understand each other's roles and be able to coordinate using the protocols established.

One of the main challenges, although temporary, was about a major change in aid policy, a possible hazard in projects anywhere. The reality is that aid programs are subject to international, political, and security conditions, and they can bring changes that have their own devasting effects, causing projects to falter or fail. Such a policy change occurred during PERRP, but fortunately it was reversed about a year later. In the interim, especially from the perspective of the beneficiaries, failure appeared to have happened.

In 2009, three years into PERRP, a major change in aid strategy to Pakistan was implemented by the US government in the form of the Kerry-Lugar bill. In recognition of the newly elected civilian government, the US government allocated $7.5 billion directly to the government of Pakistan for "development assistance," bypassing the usual route through USAID. Now the Pakistani government would make the decisions on how and where to spend the funds, having an immediate negative impact on USAID-funded projects in Pakistan, including PERRP, as it changed the decision-making. Until the new government's decisions would be known, USAID directed a number of its projects to close down, and others were put on hold at least temporarily. With roughly half the construction completed or underway, and the second half ready to start, USAID directed PERRP to complete any construction underway, but not to start any new construction. In the communities readied for construction to start anxiety was high. Would the government ask PERRP to complete the work? Or would those places be contracted to others? Or, like at so many other stalled reconstruction sites, would reconstruction happen at all? With all the communities and contactors already prepared, it was the social mobilizers' role to break the news to the communities and stay in touch with them. Fortunately, about one year later, the US government announced a reversal, and USAID directed PERRP to go ahead with all the remaining planned construction, even adding to the budget to build five more schools. Trust by the communities had been seriously shaken, but participation continued to be high, and the construction was still completed within the time allowance for each contract.

Being put on hold added about one year to the project's duration, but preparations held in abeyance were rapidly put into action. In all but two places, the construction at each site was still completed in the planned amount of time. People were thrilled to get their school, but the experience may have reinforced their reasons to doubt even when promises are made.

PERRP in Numbers

PERRP constructed seventy-seven schools and health facilities. At an average size of 17,000 square feet, the sixty-one schools ranged in size from 4,987 to 84,000 square feet, while health facilities included a 69,367 square-foot hospital and fifteen Basic Health Units each around 6,000 square feet. These steel-reinforced concrete buildings were designed and constructed to international codes for earthquake resistance. While a few were in dense urban areas, most were in remote mountainous locations with an average elevation of 5,500 feet.

Beneficiaries of the work numbered over 1,000,000 local people. Out of the total facilities constructed, sixteen were health facilities, including Basic Health Units and a hospital that served a total population of 300,000. The sixty-one schools constructed were for students from primary to high-school levels, with a total enrollment of 17,000 students from 556 villages with a combined population of about 800,000. Beneficiaries of these government-owned health and education facilities were from some of the poorest families in the quake-struck region.

At its peak, the project had 207 staff, including ninety-three engineers with various specializations and a twelve-person social team—myself included. The balance of staff—all but five of whom were Pakistanis—carried out duties in administration, finance, procurement, communications, logistics, security, transport, information technology, and all other responsibilities. The central office was in Islamabad, but the large majority of staff were located at the field offices or on the construction sites in Bagh, AJ&K, and Mansehra, KP province. All design and construction were carried out by Pakistani firms engaged by the project.

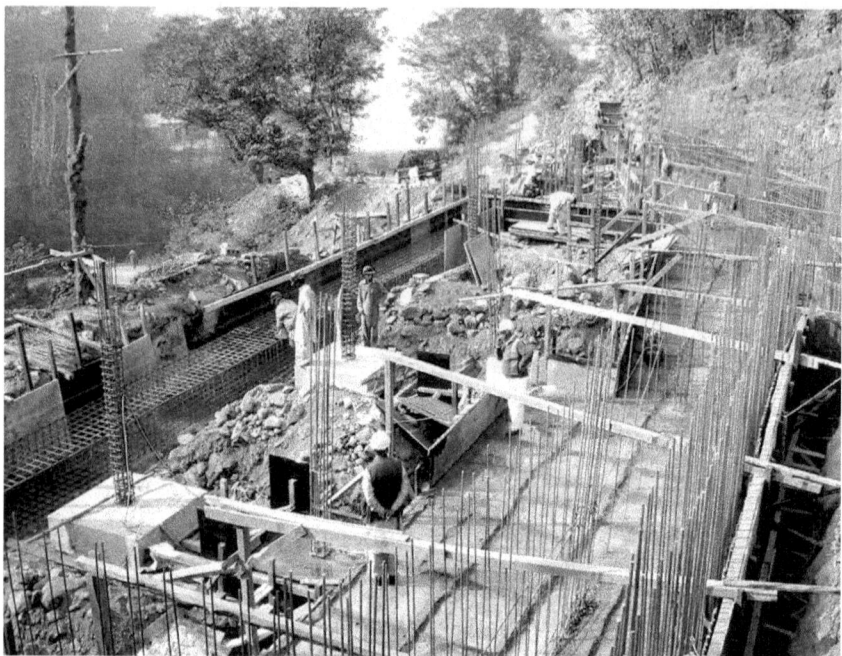

Figure 1.3. Reconstruction in Mountainous Areas. Most of the reconstruction in this project was in mountainous areas on small plots of land, such as this AJ&K location. Here, construction work underway was being inspected. Government Girls' Middle School Kahna Mohri. 2007. © Zahid Ur Rahman.

PERRP Emphasis on the Construction Schedule

The project objective was to complete construction on a number of assigned facilities as soon as reasonably possible, while also building local capacities that could lead to further community development. All this work needed to be completed within a preset time limit, according to good management practice, as well as for the following reasons.

First, the earthquake had destroyed the health and education physical infrastructure, making it much more difficult for millions of people to access these basic services. Students, even the youngest children, were attending classes in the outdoors, in rough tents or hastily constructed sheds, even in high rainfall, snow, and freezing temperatures. The sooner the schools could be rebuilt, the sooner many more students and teachers would be encouraged to return to school and be served in a safe and comfortable environment.

Second, the construction schedule meant contracted firms were given a specified number of days to complete each construction job. Moreover, the contractors worked on a firm fixed-price contract—meaning budgets would not be increased if they went past their deadlines—and so the sooner they completed the work, the fewer their expenses, and the greater their profit.

Third, the social team also emphasized the strict construction schedule in public and with committee members, informing them of the number of days their contractor was allotted to complete construction. This helped emphasize to the committees the need to focus on the urgency and the responsibility they had to prevent community-related problems that might interfere with construction. The construction schedule was commonly known and days were counted down as progress was made.

"As We Watched the Construction, It Was a Symbol"

"When PERRP construction started here, we were surprised, as we thought we'd never get our school rebuilt. But then, when construction went ahead so steadily, we were even more surprised. All around here, so many other schools were destroyed but they are not being rebuilt, or they have problems so construction is stopped. We would watch all the activity on the PERRP construction site, and it helped us think more positively. Since the disaster we had lost all hope, but seeing the new building going up, it was like a symbol of hope for us, that things were going to get better after all."

—Community elder

Ethnography: Government Girls' High School at River View*

River View is a pseudonym. To maintain confidentiality, the names of schools and villages have been changed.

This account is about PERRP's initial visit to the first community and its earthquake-destroyed school to conduct technical and social assessments and have discussion with local key people. It describes what was discussed, what was found there, and the community's main challenge of land issues. It also reviews why and how the process to settle the land issues was rationalized and integrated into the project.

Within two weeks from the day that PERRP started, we had hired two highly experienced Pakistani social mobilizers. Between them, they already had decades of experience being community organizers farther north in the country, and their familiarity with similar communities, cultures, social structures, and issues meant the three of us could move quickly in our project area. By the end of the first month of the project, we had made our first visits to three communities to consider rebuilding schools there.

At the first meeting at the first school, the government girls' high school at the village of River View, we, along with three project engineers, met with the head teacher and some of the community elders. Seated facing each other in a circle around a low table, we explained why we were there and asked the head teacher and elders about what had happened there in the quake and how the school was still running, although the school building had been destroyed. By this first visit, all the rubble of the destroyed building had been removed from the site and the place we were sitting in the open air was on the footprint of the old school. Behind us, students were seated in lines on plastic chairs facing away from us, writing their exams in the chilly November weather. Further beyond the students was an open wood-frame shed covered with corrugated steel sheets, built by community members from materials donated by an aid agency in the previous months. It was being used for storage of the chairs and books and for safekeeping of records and other materials saved from the collapsed building.

We explained that USAID and ERRA had sent us to this school as part of an assessment to see if it was socially and technically feasible to build a school here or not. Although the head teacher and elders were instantly eager for this to happen, the engineers were already pointing out it might not be feasible, as the site had no road to it, and it was located on cliff a few hundred feet above the main road that passed below the cliff. The only way to get to the site was by a steep rocky footpath up the cliff, which students and teachers used coming and going. While the land on which the school had stood was government-owned land, it was blocked in, with the several small plots of land surrounding school land being privately owned, from high up on the mountainside down to the main road.

Since this school was on the list provided by ERRA to USAID for this project to consider building, and since each place required an official, justified response to explain feasibility or not, over the next couple of weeks, the engineers carried out a detailed technical and environmental assessment, having a geotechnical survey and soil testing conducted. All those aspects indicated it was technically feasible to build again on the site itself, even though new building standards would require a much larger building. But there were two major issues: besides there being no road access so that a contractor could transport materials to and from the construction site, it had also emerged that the exact location of the boundary line of the school was in question. It was not marked and there were different opinions among local people about it, as people remembered the line only by natural indicators: e.g., from that rock to that house wall, or to that big stone.

While the technical feasibility was being explored, the social assessment in this site was carried out, easily passing the criteria we had set. This high school had been in full operation, with attendance of about two hundred girls long before the quake; the head teacher was well known and respected in the community for her management abilities and caring for the students; and community members showed strong interest in having this girls' school rebuilt. They were enthusiastic about forming a committee to help and committed to whatever volunteer work would be needed.

But we were stuck. Here was the start of the land issues that had many of the other reconstruction projects already stalled or stopped. How could PERRP avoid getting into the same situation?

How would we handle land issues in PERRP?

As the senior social mobilizers and I made first social assessment visits to potential sites for PERRP to build, such as River View, we were also conceptualizing the whole social component, what would need to be done, what would priorities be, and how to proceed. Land issues were clearly the priority, since these were problems that existed long before the earthquake, but with so many of the other reconstruction projects delayed or stalled indefinitely we were determined to not let that happen in PERRP. With the three of us collectively having decades of community mobilizing experience in northern Pakistan, including for the demanding partnerships formed with communities in the Aga Khan Rural Support Program (AKRSP) in northern Pakistan, we could see that part of the problem with land issues in the other projects was because the aid agencies put no expectations at all on the affected communities to settle the issues. Indeed, among the other agencies the idea may never have been considered, or assumptions were made that this would not be possible. But the experience of the senior social mobilizers and myself had shown that even the poorest villages can successfully take on what at first might seem impossible; if the agency listens, facilitates, and encourages people respectfully, people become motivated. In the AKRSP, the challenge for communities was building their own link roads or irrigation channels in almost unsurmountable locations across mountain faces, rather than in the PERRP project area. From another construction project in Bangladesh, I also brought experience and a process for settling similar land issues, which, until that project, was also treated as undoable. It all depended on how the agency treated people and how the undertaking matched the people's own priorities.

The postearthquake situation was a time when community abilities were seriously underestimated by other projects. From our experience, we had come to know that if people are treated as if they cannot do something, they are more likely to act as if that is so. At the same time, knowing from our experience that even the poorest communities have strong capacities such as skills, ideas, wishes, goals, and resources, even if there are differences among the people, we knew that if people are treated as if they can achieve something and are encouraged to do so, they are more likely to achieve it. The three of us concluded that taking the positive approach was the way to go:

given the characteristics and capacities of these earthquake-affected communities, it would be entirely feasible for the people at potential PERRP sites to settle the land issues, and it would be a fair and reasonable expectation of communities to do it as a condition for design and construction to then go ahead. The project would offer to form a partnership and proceed with these communities on that and other conditions. Rather than hope there would be no land issues, we chose the preventative approach.

To do so, we would have the project treat this issue head-on, first having all the issues put on the table in a public process where we invited anyone with land issues to make them known. We would ask the elders, landowners, and anyone in the community: Is there any encroachment? Who owns adjoining land? Who are the owners and co-owners? Is there agreement or disagreement among owners? Where exactly are the boundary lines? Has there ever been a cadastral survey? Are there up-to-date land ownership records that are registered in the responsible government offices? Do you have copies of those records? Are there any claims on the land, its use, or its boundaries by anybody for any reason? We would say: If there are any issues, let us hear all of them now.

But first, to put this strategy into action, there had to be buy-in from project management and the technical side to have land issues settled first. Until now, PERRP had not discussed what we would do if there were land issues. None of the other projects had any such conditions or requirements of the communities, and none of the engineers had any experience with setting such conditions. The social team would facilitate the making and formalization of agreements with villagers, owners, and respective government departments.

We set about to convince project engineers this had to be done—long before construction would start—otherwise we would be in the same situation as the other projects. Some were concerned that raising land ownership issues and settling boundary lines this early in a project would be opening a can of worms that would delay the start of construction. With further discussion about the realities of land issues in these locations, and how it was an even bigger risk to wait until construction started, common understanding developed. If construction was already underway and land issues cropped up, that could almost certainly bring construction to a halt, leading to costly delays. Project management and engineers then agreed to go along with this approach and to have the social team address this subject head-on. Dealing with land issues then became part of the social team's scope of work throughout the project, coordinating with communities to prevent such issues or to deal with them if they still happened, which frequently happened.

Community members at River View, as elsewhere, were well aware of the other slow or stalled reconstruction and that land issues were a common cause of it. In retrospect, this was the ideal community in which to start this approach. As there was no conflict about the land, only differences in opinion about boundaries, this allowed the social team to set up and test the decision-making process. This community was composed of one large extended family from one of the higher castes and was known for being relatively collaborative, not known for conflict. While innumerable land issues and disputes about land still cropped up during the project, this approach established the processes for handling all those conflicts that did occur.

When we announced there that it would be PERRP's policy at all sites to have land issues settled first and expeditiously, before construction would proceed, there was wide agreement. The same was true at all the schools and health facilities constructed by PERRP, not even one community opposed the general idea or expressed concern that it might be too difficult to achieve. This clearly was an example of how other projects had underestimated the importance of attempting to do this, as well as the community's willingness to participate in this matter and get solutions.

The next step was to get local government involvement. Social team members visited the district's head official—the Deputy Commissioner or District Coordination Officer—to get his support for PERRP having the land issues settled and for him to help by requesting the responsible land authorities—that is, the Board of Revenue, commonly known as the Revenue Department—to send its land records representative, a *patwari* along with cadastral surveyors to the River View school site. The land and boundary issues at almost every site were settled this way, usually in one day, by following the step-by-step process described in chapter 5. At River View, and at all other sites, this government survey to ascertain and demarcate land boundaries achieved several things at once. It helped PERRP, the Department of Education, and the Department of Health to determine if encroachment had occurred, to correct it, and to protect school and health facility land from future encroachment. In many cases, it also helped clear up long-standing differences and conflict over unsettled cases. In this process, all records were updated and filed in the government system. PERRP's requiring copies of the mutation or ownership documents to be provided meant that for the first time ever such documents would be kept permanently on site as reference. Settling all these matters, which often had been fomenting for years or even decades, created a celebratory atmosphere that motivated communities to tackle many more challenges in the project.

Note

1. All dollar amounts here and throughout are in US dollars.

CHAPTER 2

Contexts of a Reconstruction Site

Introduction to the Contexts

A construction site has many visible physical elements. For example, its perimeter can be marked off with a purpose-built fence or tape to keep the site secure and control visitors. Materials, vehicles, equipment, temporary structures, and personnel are all visible and moving as work starts and progresses. The site has clearly defined limits.

Outside of that site is the rest of the world. The adage that "context is everything" applies here—"context" being the broader view of factors or conditions in which something exists. The construction site exists in complex contexts that may affect or may be affected by the project; its main context is the surrounding community. The community, in turn, is the manifestation of many influences. In situations of disaster reconstruction, the complexities are almost certain to multiply.

While construction sites exist within innumerable surrounding contexts, many construction and reconstruction projects focus their efforts in the opposite direction: inward. Policy makers, planners, construction engineers, architects, and contractors might see only those contexts directly related to getting shovels in the ground—for example, weather, costs, financing, permits, or the supply of steel, concrete, and laborers. Construction projects sometimes assume themselves to be—or try to be—separate from broader sociocultural contexts, but in reality, such a disconnection is unlikely and can even be self-defeating. While an inward focus is necessary to get a project up and running, to keep it on schedule, and to maintain high-quality work, an intense inward focus creates the risk of losing sight of the other larger contexts that may determine or affect a project's outcomes.

Considering context gives rise to important questions: Will any parts of the context affect how people will relate to the project? Will they help the project? Will they resist or block it in any way? Are there tensions and conflict among them over anything related to the project? Will the project cause any problems or losses for the people? What are the strengths or capacities in the communities that the project could support or build upon? Might the people be interested in participating in or contributing to the work? Could any of these people or project behaviours affect long-term use of the new facility to be constructed?

In postquake Pakistan, even several years after the disaster, much of the reconstruction was either not started or never completed. And Pakistan is not the only country with such problems—slowed or delayed construction appears to be quite common in disaster reconstruction and can even occur on construction sites in nondisaster situations. Why and how does this happen? The reasons are many, but as disasters are expected to increase in the coming years, there will be a growing need for reconstruction and, therefore, a need to identify and understand the causes and solutions of such problems. Some of these lessons can be presented through this book's examination of PERRP.

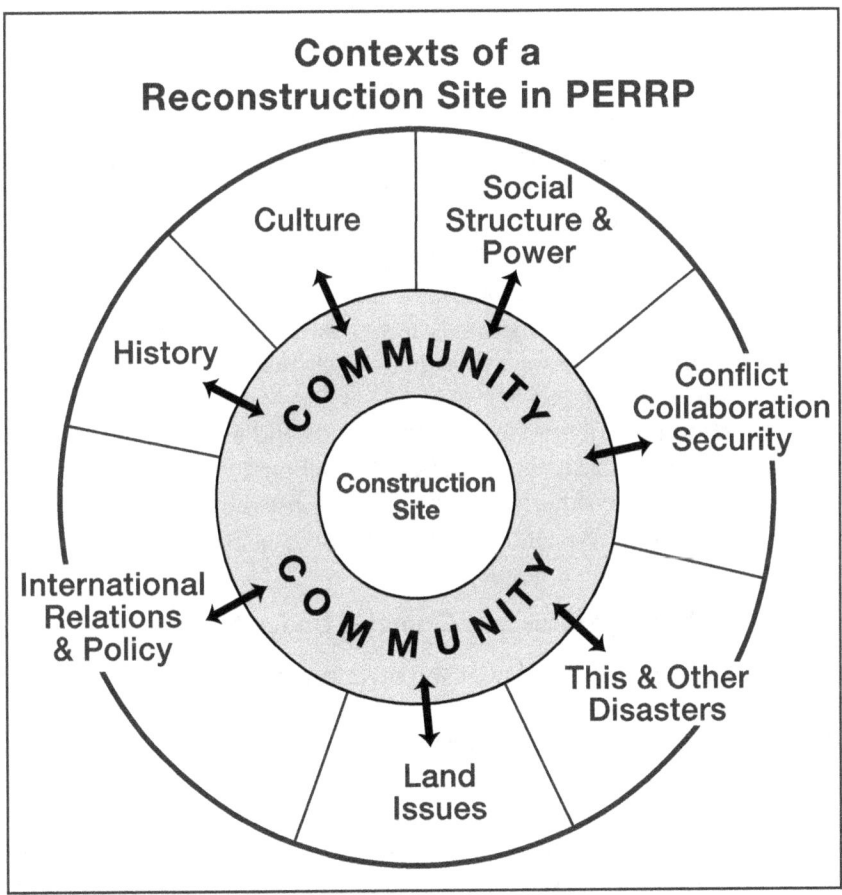

Figure 2.1. Contexts of a Reconstruction Site in PERRP. © Jane Murphy Thomas.

Interventions after disasters have often been criticized for not taking account of local contexts, especially including the affected people's culture (Cannon et al. 2014: 186). One of the main lessons is that the reduction of disaster risk involves many actors at several stages, from preparedness to reconstruction. At every stage there are different perceptions of what is taking place, most notably by the people affected and by the organizations that get involved.

This chapter shows how PERRP took local contexts into consideration. From these contextual analyses, approaches for the social program were then established and implemented; they formed the foundation of the project's community participation and were integrated with the technical aspects of the project, altogether contributing to the success of PERRP.

Context: This Quake and Other Disasters

In the event of substantial disasters like the 2005 earthquake, countries assist one another. Plans, programming, budgets, and agreements have been developed to enable such assistance. In the decades during which these agreements have evolved, countless disasters have occurred around the world: the Chernobyl disaster of 1986; the Bangladesh cyclone of 1991; the European heat wave of 2003; the Indian Ocean earthquake and tsunami in 2004; Hurricane Katrina in 2005; the Tōhoku earthquake and tsunami in Japan in 2011—to name just a few. After each disaster, all entities involved—governments, NGOs, academics, practitioners—gain experience and learn lessons that guide their responses to subsequent catastrophes.

This section takes a brief look at the trends and evolving understandings of hazards and disaster. Specifically, I will outline the changing emphasis from reactive emergency response to preventative approaches, vulnerability assessment, and risk reduction measures.

Trends, Status, and Changing Understanding

Disasters are increasing in number and severity around the world, resulting in more loss of life and destruction of the built and natural environment. In our time, "disaster management paradigms have, arguably, shifted from disaster relief to disaster preparedness, hazard mitigation, and vulnerability reduction" (Hidayat and Egbu 2010: 1269). Relief efforts—providing food, water, sanitation, medical treatment, and shelter immediately after the disaster—have, until recent years, been the main focus in emergencies (Bosher and Dainty 2011). While disaster relief is still in practice and essential to saving lives, disaster management emphasizes better preparation, hazard mitigation, and preventative measures to reduce losses when such events occur.

Understanding of the underlying causes of disaster-related losses has begun to change, and, to reflect these shifts, efforts are being made to update the language used to describe disasters. For example, the expression "natural disaster" is avoided in the research literature. Instead, the critical event—the hurricane, earthquake, flood, or drought—is usually referred to as a "hazard." A hazard is the event, and a disaster is the result: disaster is what happens to people, and those most likely to experience disaster in the wake of a hazard are those who are already vulnerable. As some argue, "Disasters only happen because trigger events (natural hazards) interact with vulnerable people. Hazards are only 'translated' into a disaster if there are vulnerable people to be affected by it. For example, the same hurricane can pass over three different countries in the Caribbean and have very different effects in each" (Cannon et al. 2014: 185). How is it that such events affect some people more than others?

As Chmutina et al. have pointed out, "Hazards cannot be prevented, [but] disasters can be" (2017: 3). Earthquakes, droughts, floods, storms, landslides, and volcanic eruptions are natural hazards. They lead to deaths and damage—that is, disasters—because of human acts of omission and commission, rather than the act of nature: "In effect, the new perspective asserts that disasters do not simply happen; they are caused" (Oliver-Smith 1999: 74). Moreover, as posited by Hoffman, "There is no such thing as a natural disaster. All catastrophes are human-caused at one level or another" (2020: 3).

Human acts of omission or commission are indeed the underlying causes of disaster, as was clearly visible in the 2005 Pakistan earthquake. Over seventy thousand people died and more than half a million homes, health facilities, and schools were destroyed; both common knowledge and formal studies attributed the losses to shoddy construction and unsuitable building materials. Although the applicable building codes for earthquake resistance were known in Pakistan, they were seldom enforced (Durrani et al. 2005). Braine discusses poor construction practices as but one cause of disaster: "Today's disasters stem from a complex mix of factors, including routine climate change, global warming influenced by human behavior, socioeconomic factors causing poor people to live in risky areas with inadequate disaster preparedness, and education on the part of governments as well as the general population" (2006). The underlying cause, however, is poverty. It is "one of the principal reasons why people become vulnerable to natural hazards" (Middleton and O'Keefe 1998: 4).

Vulnerability and Disaster

Vulnerability refers to "the social and economic characteristics of a person, a household, or a group in terms of their capacity to cope with and to recover from the impacts of a disaster" (Zaman 1999: 194). There are many different types of vulnerability: physical, economic, social, educational, attitudinal, and environmental. As Cannon et al. suggest, "People's vulnerability is largely determined by factors of politics (how well government functions and how power is used to benefit all citizens), economics (how income and assets are distributed and taxes used for preparedness) and society (whether some people are suffering discrimination on a gender or ethnic basis" (2014: 185).

To reduce vulnerability and reduce risks, the causes of vulnerability and risks must be overcome. Factors such as local culture, social structure, and the arrangement of power should be put at the center of this undertaking, as these factors can either act as obstacles or support disaster risk reduction.

Disaster Risk Reduction (DRR) and Its Guiding Principles

Although disasters have been a field of study for several decades, recent international attempts for better understanding and practice led to the Hyogo Framework for Action 2005–2015, which was succeeded by the Sendai Framework for Disaster Risk Reduction 2015–2030 under the United Nations Office of Disaster Risk Reduction (UNDRR). It plans to reduce disaster losses and advocates for the "substantial reduction of disaster risk and losses in lives, livelihoods and health and in the economic, physical, social, cultural and environmental assets of persons, businesses, communities and countries" (UNDRR, n.d.a). Although it has its critics, the Sendai Framework is at least a focal point that presents ideals and principles that can be built upon. The UK Department of International Development recognizes the need for this: "Good DRR not only happens well before disasters strike but also continues afterwards, building resilience to future hazards" (Palliyaguru et al. 2010: 278).

Two of the guiding principles in the Sendai Framework are "Build Back Better, for preventing the creation of, and reducing existing disaster risk," and the "empowering of local authorities and communities through resources, incentives, and decision-making responsibilities as appropriate" (UNDRR, n.d.a). These two principles underscore the rationale for technical and sociocultural experts to combine expertise in disaster-resistant reconstruction, as occurred in PERRP. Besides being able to construct new buildings to withstand future disasters, thereby reducing physical risks, reconstruction can also be a process for local institutional building and empowerment.

Context: History, International Relations, Conflict, and Collaboration

While the history, politics, and international relations of Pakistan and the region are an enormous and highly complex subject far beyond the scope of this book, it would be remiss to avoid the subject completely. These factors play a large part in local people's daily lives, shaping their impressions, ideas, outlook, actions, and reactions, including in a postdisaster humanitarian aid project such as PERRP. Significantly, Pakistan's earthquake zone, including AJ&K, is in one of the world's most volatile locations. This section thus gives a brief background on the disaster area's historical, political, and security environment.

Independence and Partitioning

In 1947, the Islamic Republic of Pakistan became an independent country, emerging out of the partitioning of India. It is the world's fifth most populous country with a population of about 220 million, with a 60 percent rural–40 percent urban split. Pakistan is surrounded by Iran to its west, Afghanistan to its west, China to its northeast, India to its east, and the Arabian Sea to its south. Long before becoming a country, the space now known as Pakistan had a tumultuous history due largely to its strategic position between rival superpowers. For centuries, the histories of Afghanistan, India, and Pakistan have been inextricable due to the expansionist practices of Persians and Moghuls, and later the Russian and British empires. Some remnants of these intertwined histories still fester today, notably in the flash point region between India and Pakistan: Kashmir.

The Kashmir Issue

In the partitioning of India and Pakistan, the former princely state of Kashmir was split four ways. India controls both Ladahk and the State of Jammu and Kashmir, with these parts otherwise known as Indian-Administered or Indian-Occupied Kashmir. The parts controlled by Pakistan are AJ&K (also sometimes called Azad Kashmir) and Gilgit-Baltistan, with these parts often referred to as Pakistan-Administered or Pakistan-Occupied Kashmir. In 1962, a fifth division occurred, with Aksai Chin and the Trans Karakoram Tract coming under the control of China. Most critically, both Pakistan and

India claim Kashmir in its entirety and have fought two wars over it. Kashmir remains one of the world's longest unresolved conflicts.

An outgrowth of the animosity between Pakistan and India is the nuclearization of both countries: "Pakistan asserts the origin of its nuclear weapons program lies in its adversarial relationship with India; the two countries have engaged in several conflicts, centered mainly on the state of Jammu and Kashmir" (Nuclear Threat Initiative 2019). Partly due to this scenario, in its short history Pakistan's government has alternated between civilian and military, with about thirty of those years under military rule by General Ayub Khan (1958–1969), General Zia-ul-Haq (1977–1988), and General Pervez Musharraf (1999–2008). It has been noted that "all three of these dictators served as presidents for many years, sometimes using flimsy elections or bizarre constitutional clauses to hide the autocratic nature of their rule" (Development and Cooperation 2018). At the same time, civilian political parties and activities have proliferated.

As shown in the maps on page xviii, PERRP was carried out in KP province's Mansehra district and in AJ&K's Bagh district; the latter having its northern, eastern, and southern borders marked by the Line of Control, which separates India and Pakistan. The earthquake zone and PERRP project area were located in a part of Pakistan where the country is at its narrowest from border to border: only about two hundred miles wide.

Although the 2005 earthquake reached partly into IAK, destruction was concentrated in AJ&K. These two parts of Kashmir are demarcated by what had been the agreed cease-fire line in 1949; in the 1972 Simla Agreement between India and Pakistan it was made the Line of Control and de facto borderline. It is along this line that the Pakistani and Indian militaries are concentrated in what is known as the most heavily militarized zone in the world. Various sources estimate that hundreds of thousands of troops are permanently located there and face occasional skirmishes across the Line of Control. These realities had many implications for the aid programs responding to the disaster, especially for the need for conflict sensitivity.

As described both above and below in the section "War on Terror," this disaster zone was already part of a historic war zone, with long-standing tensions and violence involving adjoining and surrounding countries, and internally as well, with "Pakistan [being] a prime example of a state with significant political marginalization and unequal sovereignty among its political units" (Sökefeld 2015: 174). Additionally, each of the five parts of the former princely state of Kashmir has its own characteristics. Although the majority of the population has religion in common—Islam—each part is culturally, demographically, and linguistically distinct from the other, with different histories, alliances, and politics. While there are little or no antagonistic relations between these five parts, each one has its own internal differences at the district and community levels. Pakistan's more recent decision to make Gilgit-Baltistan a province was seen as a provocation by India and a setback by Kashmiri nationalists. These complex, unresolved historical factors—including the growing issue with major water supplies for both Pakistan and India originating in Kashmir—mean that the simmering conditions could continue indefinitely.

At times, "Kashmir" appears in international news, but only in reference to IAK and to the clashes there between the Indian army, police, and Kashmiri protesters. Excluding the international media response to the 2005 Pakistan earthquake, the international media is silent about AJ&K. In Pakistan, there are distinctions between KP, which is a full-fledged province, and AJ&K, which is an internationally disputed territory. Before this disaster, international NGOs were not allowed to operate in AJ&K, and the government of Pakistan controlled what little UN and multilateral donor funding existed for development programs in AJ&K. As such, AJ&K has remained isolated, with relatively little outside contact and presence there.

Such unresolved conflict and tensions have had many implications for the aid programs responding to this disaster, especially in how they avoid creating or adding to conflict. This necessitated such projects having a high degree of conflict sensitivity and a deep understanding of the contexts in which they operate, as I describe in this chapter. Above all, as discussed in chapter 4, projects need to effectively engage in a peaceful, participatory social process.

The "War on Terror"

By the mid-twentieth century, Pakistan was playing a vital role in Cold War alliances, which was greatly heightened by the USSR's invasion of Afghanistan in 1979 and by the American and international backing of the resistance. The USSR withdrew its forces ten years later, but out of that situation emerged the Afghan Taliban and the Afghanistan-based Al-Qaeda, led by Osama Bin Laden: "The 9/11 terrorist attacks and subsequent US response through the invasion of Afghanistan substantially changed the security environment of South Asia, if not the whole world" (Shafiq 2015: 3). At peak numbers, about one hundred thousand foreign troops from over fifty countries were stationed in Afghanistan, close to the earthquake zone. The overall changed security environment inevitably impacted postquake humanitarian work.

The 2005 earthquake struck in Pakistan's most politically sensitive and insecure locations, at a time of pressures from both outside and inside the country. The years during which PERRP ran, 2006 through 2013, were particularly tense; adding to the tension were the effects of Al-Qaeda and the growth and reach of the Taliban. In 2011, Osama Bin Laden was captured and killed in Abbottabad, the closest city to Mansehra, which was the location of many earthquake reconstruction offices, including PERRP's. The next year in the nearby Swat Valley, Malala Yousafzai was attacked by the Taliban for her promotion of girls' education, while at the same time, PERRP was building schools for girls and boys.

In PERRP's community participation program, there was a strong sense of apprehension and anxiety among local people: would the Taliban influence spread to and take over their communities? There was a quiet worry that they would be punished for accepting help from a country the Taliban considered an enemy. Already traditional and conservative in nature, the inhabitants responded by becoming even more cautious, especially in adhering to the customs of male/female practices.

When asked about the security situation in AJ&K, a prominent community member explained, "We never know what to expect. Trouble can come from different directions. India fires rockets into AJ&K every once in a while, and Pakistan fires back. You don't know if they will retaliate, and what will that lead to? You can't call it war, but it is not peace either."

The Human Rights Situation

Further issues of concern in the disaster response, as observed by national and international human rights organizations, were human rights violations in AJ&K. A range of reports from several sources gave similar observations. Of the reports, the most comprehensive is from Human Rights Watch, entitled *"With Friends Like These ..." Human Rights Violations in Azad Kashmir* (2006). The NGO posits (6–7), "Though 'Azad' means 'free,' the residents of Azad Kashmir are anything but. Azad Kashmir is a land of strict curbs on political pluralism, freedom of expression, and freedom of association; a muzzled press, banned books; arbitrary arrest and detention and torture at the hands of the Pakistan military and the police." A Freedom House report sums it up: "The political rights of the residents of Pakistan Administered Kashmir remain severely limited" (2011: 783). These limitations come from constitutional restrictions and the strong presence of Pakistan's intelligence agency, the Inter-Services Intelligence. There are similar observations and conclusions in reports by the Human Rights Commission of Pakistan, Amnesty International, the Asian Human Rights Commission, and the United Nations Office of the High Commissioner for Human Rights, among others. In sum: at the time of this disaster, the overall political and military environment was tense. With such restrictions in place, the political and security situation could have led to people being either more politicized and outspoken, or more reluctant or intimidated.

How much these factors affected people's participation in any of the reconstruction remained a question throughout the PERRP project.

Security Environment of the Disaster Zone

To recap, the earthquake zone was located in a relatively small geographic space with military presence and pressure on both the west and east sides of it. The zone also had serious internal security risks due to the historic heterogeneity within communities. This combination of security and sociocultural factors made it vital for aid programs to operate with strong conflict sensitivity, with an emphasis on cultural knowledge and sensitivity.

In such a location, where the risk of conflict to any degree is virtually normalized, such realities have implications for aid programs of any kind—but for disaster reconstruction, there can be additional risks. Importantly, construction itself can spark differences and conflict. This is especially the case in postdisaster reconstruction, when so much reconstruction is happening at once and there is extra competition for jobs, money, and precious resources such as land, water, and electricity. Such resources can become flash points, especially in regions where people already have long-standing social, cultural, and political differences.

Construction teams anywhere need to know if there is any amount of disagreement in the community—even if it appears to have little or none. In the last few decades, international sources have recognized that aid programs have special obligations in this matter. One of the main figures in this field, Mary B. Anderson (1999: 1), posed the question, "How can humanitarian or development assistance be given in conflict situations in ways that rather than feeding into and exacerbating the conflict help local people to disengage and establish alternative systems for dealing with the problems that underlie the conflict?"

In the PERRP project area, where tensions bubbled below the surface much of the time, on a day-to-day basis the normal state in communities and villages was one of calm. Therefore, equally as important as understanding the divisions, frictions, and their causes was knowing what helped to keep the peace. Who was responsible for this, and how did they do it? What were the factors that connected people? How did they collaborate? The goal, of course, needed to be to keep what calm already existed. What then could the alternative systems be for preventing or exacerbating the conflict? What could be done to alleviate underlying causes? One of PERRP's challenges was to choose strategies and tools to prevent or deal with conflict if it still happened.

While Pakistan has endured a long history of strife, the same can be said about many locations of the world, especially when examining them closely. This should also raise more questions about disaster reconstruction projects and their operation in different security environments. Hazards and their subsequent disasters occur in countries at peace, where there may be working systems for assistance, protection, security, and justice. Yet they also happen in places with conflict, threats, or restrictions that reduce survivors' access to services and constrain their ability to be proactive or participate in decision-making and problem-solving.

As will be shown in more detail in chapter 4, PERRP's social program set up a conflict-sensitive, do-no-harm approach from the start of the project. This approach had dual benefits: it saved people from trouble and loss, and it enabled construction to proceed uninterrupted by conflict, unlike many of the other reconstruction projects in this disaster response. Our main approach was to be highly participatory, starting community participation by asking rival social groups to come together, form a partnership with PERRP, and then work together throughout the project.

Context: Social Structure, Power, and Culture

When it comes to the contexts of a reconstruction site, possibly no other context can determine more about a project than the social structure and the arrangements of power and culture of the affected people. The content below sets the stage for understanding the kinds of sociocultural contexts and influences that projects should be prepared for. It looks at the importance of developing this understanding and how the project and surrounding people affect each other. It explores social structure, power arrangements, and culture and cultural norms, and it examines what was taken into consideration in PERRP's social program, including beliefs, the norms of language, and the gender roles and customs of *purdah* (separation of the sexes), as well as the local power structures and informal leaders. The first part of chapter 4 delves into detail as to how these realties were then manifested and dealt with at the community level.

To an outsider, social structure, culture, and power in any location, including a construction site, might be invisible. However, as shown in figure 2.1, social structure, culture, and power were among the main contexts that shaped PERRP construction work. Besides the technical, financial, and management challenges that construction projects may encounter, there can also be a wide range of sociocultural challenges. The need for sociocultural expertise is especially important in projects following hazardous events, as the disaster may have compounded social, cultural, and economic factors.

At its simplest, culture is about the traits, values, beliefs, and behaviors of a population, while social structure is about the pattern of relationships and power arrangements among social groups or institutions within or outside of a culture. While separate subjects, social structure and culture are inextricable. Power comes into the picture when talking about status among individuals and groups.

Failure to consider sociocultural and power contexts regularly causes project problems and failures, no matter the location or sector. One particularly apt example comes from a study by Lisa Buggy and Karen McNamara in a situation very different from earthquake reconstruction in the Himalayas: climate change adaptation projects in Vanuatu, an island in the Pacific. The projects studied by Buggy and McNamara focused on issues such as coastal erosion, flooding, and fresh-water scarcity, but the researchers concluded that it was mainly social issues that "contributed to the majority of thirty-four projects breaking down, stalling or being abandoned completely" (2015: 274). Looking at causes of these breakdowns, the researchers observed that "social dynamics, power relations and changing traditional norms at the community level [were] at the epicenter of project failures" (2015: 270). Although Pakistan's mountains and Vanuatu's ocean are very different settings, projects in different sectors can face similar outcomes when such sociocultural contexts are overlooked.

To address contextual sociocultural challenges, construction and reconstruction projects require the expertise of sociocultural specialists. Just as engineers, architects, and other technical specialists first drill down to the physical aspects of a site—to plan if and how to build on that site and predict the behavior of the building once constructed—so too are specialists needed to ascertain social characteristics and how to work with them in construction projects. They are the ones who will be able to bring understanding of the social and cultural environments by foreseeing strengths, vulnerabilities, and behaviors of the people, and by predicting how the project and its surroundings will interact. With this contextual knowledge, these experts can work with construction managers to develop strategies that both respect local realities and work with them to facilitate construction—creating a win-win situation.

Sociocultural experts who have years of experience in one project location will already be highly familiar with the region's social structure, power arrangements, and culture, and so will be able to bring that knowledge to the project. Such region-specific expertise provides invaluable service to the construction project, as being able to draw on existing knowledge saves a great deal of time. In PERRP, our social team comprised about a dozen people, a small fraction of total project staff, who had lived for decades—even their whole lives—in the project area. This collective knowledge was put to use immediately.

An understanding of the communities is especially useful in construction projects, as the projects themselves can spark disputes or conflict among people who may already have long-standing differences over other matters. What manifests as a technical problem for construction managers may be of historical, social, or cultural origin. To alleviate such problems for construction, sociocultural expertise is also needed to handle these underlying problems with sensitivity. As shown in an anecdote, page 68, a serious cultural breach was risky—but with knowledge of the culture, the offense was handled effectively, reducing tensions.

Social Structure and Culture

A construction project is about more than bricks and mortar. Unfortunately, with so much else to consider, construction planners and managers sometimes lose sight of the fact that the purpose of the construction is to serve people.

Social structure has been a central matter in sociology and social anthropology since the emergence of these disciplines in the mid-nineteenth century. While discussed and debated by the founders of the disciplines and figures such as Herbert Spencer, Ferdinand Tönnies, Alfred Radcliffe-Brown, Raymond Firth, S. F. Nadal, Talcott Parsons, Pierre Bourdieu, Max Weber, and Anthony Giddens, there still is no universally accepted definition of "social structure." Notably, in describing a social structure, the social sciences have borrowed vocabulary from building construction: "The Latin source of the word structure is *struere*, which means 'to build.' And the most general notion of this term does, in fact, refer to the framework of elements that constitute and support a building" (Bernardi, Gonzalez, and Requena 2006: 162). One online introductory discussion on social structure expands upon the building metaphor: "A structure can be called a building only when these parts or components are arranged in relationship with the other. In the same manner society has its own structure called a social structure. The components or units of social structure are persons" ("Social Structure," n.d.).

As figure 2.1 suggests, construction builds physical structures, but social structure completely surrounds and permeates the construction site. Social structure refers both to how, in any society, people exist in groups, and also to how these groups relate and interact with each other and their institutions based on factors such as kinship, race, caste, ethnicity, religion, gender, language, age, and sect or denomination. Of further relevance is how such people and groups are arranged in layers of power or stratification—some being at the top or in the highest class, some in the middle, and some in the lowest, who are sometimes marginalized or even eliminated.

It is the stratifications, divisions, hierarchies, and inequalities that give advantages to some and limits to others. For instance, a stratified social structure might restrict human rights, choices of occupations, access to the justice system, and access to resources and public services such as health and education. Being either well-off or the poorest becomes normalized. While such social division may be a universal reality, Shandana Khan Mohmand and Haris Gazdar have argued that, in Pakistan, social stratification ultimately "creates social exclusion, which recreates itself within the community and village, and is usually expressed as an integral part of the social structure—as part of culture and tradition itself" (2007: 3). Such social ordering also involves strong economic ties, as one group may be forced into dependence on another for shelter, land, and livelihood. Some groups are thereby trapped in subservience, unable to break free from the vicious cycle of poverty.

Power Arrangements

Social structure inevitably is about arrangements of power, influence, and control—who has it, and who does not. For project planners and managers, close examination and acknowledgement of these factors—the divisions, connections, and arrangements of power among the people—is essential to formulating approaches that both help meet project goals and respect local realities and culture. This advice is certainly important in the chaos often following disasters, when reconstruction is to be attempted. Accordingly, in each affected community, the PERRP social team identified blocs of power—who had power, what they held power over, and how the project itself was part of the power structure. Such analysis looks at the stratifications, arrangements, or layers of people and groups according to power, then discreetly observes: How are people grouped? Among those individuals and social groups, who has what power, and to what degree? What gives them that power and how do they use it or misuse it? Who is excluded, marginalized, or subject to the power? Who is excluded? Some individuals or groups may hold all the power, or it may vary; some may have all the power to do X, but little to do Y. In such a project, it is necessary to know the arrangements of power—who has it and who does not—so the project, where need be, can influence those who have it and watch out for those who need protection. For further discussion of the power arrangements and blocs of power at the community level, see part 1 of chapter 4, "The Social Component."

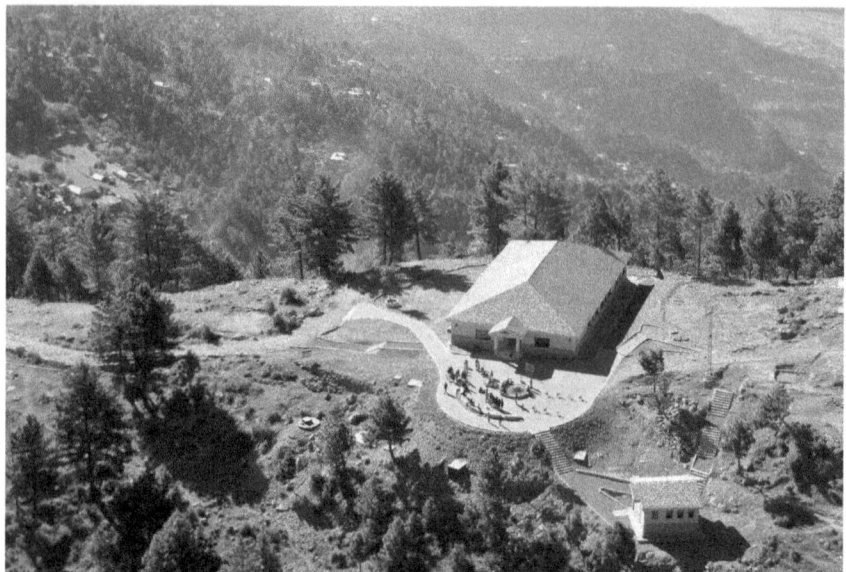

Figure 2.2. The School above the Clouds. Several schools reconstructed were at high elevation, with this one being above the clouds. Here, some students wait outside the newly completed school after a long walk there on mountain footpaths. Government Boys' Primary School Phel, 2009. © Jane Murphy Thomas.

As with the social structures themselves, power is also dynamic. As PERRP witnessed, some people's power changed over time. This was especially visible in this project, because for the first time, each community had a representative committee that was chosen by the community, which worked with the project to meet their urgent need for a new school or clinic. This responsibility gave committee members the confidence and power to get cooperation that they might not normally have had the courage or authority to obtain. Membership on the committee meant the power of some was decreased, and the power of others was increased. For example, early in the project, there were some cases of individuals being domineering and demanding, but they became less so when committee members discouraged that behavior. Sometimes even family members strongly opposed each other, but other family members became the mediators. At the same time, others—especially younger people and those lower in the social hierarchy—had opportunities to speak up for the first time.

In some cases, there can be a fine line between power and influence. As several of the anecdotes included in this book illustrate, power and influence can also be used in positive, productive ways, even in some of the most divided, conflict-prone communities. As experienced in PERRP, such local power and influence can be used by individuals or groups to lead communities to try to achieve things they would not do otherwise. This strong potential for local power to be used in such ways can be nurtured by aid agencies—first by recognizing that such capacities exist, and then by encouraging their use and development.

The question then is: besides designing and constructing new buildings to withstand future hazards—thereby reducing physical risks—what else can such projects do to reduce social, cultural, and economic risks? A construction project is not a social revolution, yet how can such a project avoid inadvertently increasing the power of people who misuse the power they already have? Or avoid making the marginalized more marginalized, or making poor people poorer? At the same time, how can the project encourage and support positive, productive uses of power and influence in a community?

One answer goes back to some of the most basic ideas of community development and poverty alleviation. Essential to both are organized, representative, proactive, empowered communities with strengthened skills, resources, connections, and capacities that they can put to work for their own benefit. Whether or not communities already have groups with such potential, PERRP's social team believed that leading such groups to mobilize the community and to participate in a reconstruction project had the potential to be a major opportunity for institution-building, one of the foundations for development and disaster risk reduction.

Social Structure, Power, Culture, and Norms in the PERRP Project Area

In northern Pakistan—as in the rest of the world—the component parts of social structure and culture interact in complex ways. Understanding these interactions was essential in order for PERRP's social team to plan and develop strategies for our community participation program. The PERRP project area can be described as socially heterogenous, stratified, and hierarchical, and the subsequent inequalities can be "maintained through specific practices and informal institutions, which limit the access of certain groups to livelihood options, social services, and political empowerment" (Mohmand and Gazdar 2007: 33). Specific social structures varied from district to district, and even within districts, villages, and communities.

And while PERRP's two project districts—Mansehra district in KP province and Bagh district in AJ&K—have some significant sociocultural differences, their proximity does mean that they have some things in common. For instance, in both districts, there is a heightened level of tension, both from the region's unstable history and from security pressures on both eastern and western borders. Activity such as construction can easily spark or reignite seemingly unrelated disputes and even violent clashes between people, which then affect both the construction and the whole community.

In the AJ&K and KP project areas, the main elements of social structure and power in the communities are kinship groups, clans, or family (*zaat* or *quom*); castes; ethnicities; tribal groups; religious denominations (mainly Sunni and Shia Islam); fraternity (*biradari*, an Urdu word adopted from the Persian *biradar*, meaning "brother"—hence fraternity, brotherhood, or unity group); and political alignments. "Caste" refers to a people's position in the social stratification, while *biradari* refers more to the wider unity among groups based on kinship ties or religious or political affiliation. The *biradari* "provides security and power for millions of its members. It gives them an identity because *biradari* is not just a matter of being a Jatt or a Rajput[:] it is also a kinship system. The system provides a wider support group than a family" (Ahmed 2009: 91–92). Because many people in these regions use these terms interchangeably, I use the label "social groups" to refer to all such identity groups.

Although Pakistan is a predominantly Muslim country, and caste is considered against Islamic teachings, caste nonetheless remains a strong part of the local power structure and social identity—especially in rural areas, arguably as an inheritance from Hindu culture. The American sociologist Ayesha Jalal (2005) has stated, "Despite its egalitarian principles, Islam in South Asia historically has been unable to avoid the impact of class and caste inequalities." Still, many Pakistanis dismiss or denounce even the idea of castes or classes, claiming that these are problems that exist "next door" in India, but not in their country. This opinion results in there being "little tolerance in the public domain of any serious discussion about caste and caste-based oppression, social hierarchies and discrimination" (Gazdar 2007: 3), which is perhaps indicative of a dominant class or caste. As one PERRP manager explained, "Caste is an explosive issue; it is not discussed in polite mixed-caste company." Aliani describes it another way: "It appears that caste is the elephant in the room. Everyone knows it's there, but no one wants to talk about it, let alone address it" (2009: 12). While some Pakistanis refuse to see caste, few dispute that class is a fact of life, and most are able to cite many examples of class influence in their own lives.

Most, if not all, project communities are heterogeneous. Of community members' many differences, the most common clashes were over politics and class or caste. In this region, people are born into hierarchies or classes of advantage and disadvantage, also inheriting a position of power or a lack thereof. In the PERRP project areas, the population is stratified into over a hundred high, middle, and low castes and subcastes, into which people are born and subsequently spend their lives. These social groups include the Mughals, Sudhans, Jats, Rajputs, Abbasis, Kashmiris, Sayyids, Arians, Gujars, Sawatis, Pashtuns, Tanoli, Awan, Dhund, and Tarkhan. The class or caste of each is often distinguishable by occupation. Low-caste people may be shoemakers, tailors, carpenters, agriculture workers, laborers, or barbers, while high-caste people tend to fill government jobs or become professionals—doctors, lawyers, engineers, and teachers. Almost every community where PERRP worked was multi-clan, multi-caste, multi-*biradari*. Many of the anecdotes and ethnographies included in this book illustrate such differences. For a detailed example, see the ethnography "Government Boys' High School in Flat Land" (chapter 8), which details how long-standing differences between two castes threatened the start of construction.

If any generalization can be made about social structure in Pakistan and the PERRP project area, it would be that people's number one loyalty is to family. As Hazma Alavi has noted, "the pivotal institution in the 'traditional' social structure . . . is . . . the kinship system" (1971: 114). The family is the foundation of Pakistani culture and of all parts of the social structure. Going far outside the nuclear family, members range from immediate to distant relatives. Loyalty and conformity to the family in these collectivist communities is the norm, and individualism is discouraged.

While civil society is sometimes described as weak in parts of the PERRP project area, kinship is a self-representative system: "Leadership of these kinship groups is characterized by the vesting of authority in the hands of a head selected on the basis of virtues prized by the kin network, such as the ability to effectively participate in the business of the kin group" (Mohmand and Gazdar 2007: 5). In other words, people represent their own social groups' interests to the extent of excluding others.

Highly significant in recent times is the intense politicization of social groups, such that they have become voting blocs. About general elections that took place in Mansehra district in the project area, journalist Azam Khan noted, "Here voters don't cast their votes so much as they vote their caste, and it is the clans that rule the roost." Highlighting the complexities, Khan goes on to explain, "the vote bank in these two constituencies is divided among *Swatis, Tanoli, [Sayyid], Gujar* and other smaller clans as well as the [*Pashto-*] speaking population. Language also affects loyalties" (2013). Such politicization also means that "people are already thinking of how to push forward their families and clans in the next election. For a person to win, he had better belong to a dominant '*biradari*'" (Ahmed 2009: 91).

With the *biradari* as the "overriding determinant of identity and power relationships within the [AJ&K] socio-political landscape" (Human Rights

Watch 2006: 12), it is membership in the most powerful *biradaris* and their association with political parties—which are fervidly followed and aggressively promoted—that lead to the key political positions and upper strata government jobs. Holding such key positions enables individuals to create more opportunities for returning favors to fellow *biradari* members, who in turn use that advantage to curry favor with others. In AJ&K, for instance, the most influential social groups are the Mughals, Sudhans, and Rajputs, and almost all AJ&K politicians and leaders come from these groups (Human Rights Watch 2006).

Not surprisingly, the general politicization and discrimination adds to strife and conflict, with tensions simmering much of the time. This reality raises risks for construction projects, which can easily spark conflict among already embittered and competing groups. Real or perceived project favoritism over jobs, income, or opportunities; potential losses of resources such as land and water; and unwanted impositions from outside the community—all can rapidly ignite reactions against the project.

However, in this part of the world, basic social transformation is beginning to occur even while the old guard resists it. Change is occurring "due to capital inflows, globalization, the media boom and trends in women's education" (Zaidi 2008: 3). Other factors include urbanization, rising economic mobility, and the beginning of the breakdown of the feudal system (Hasan 2009). Although the feudal system as it is known in other parts of Pakistan does not exist in the PERRP project area, the caste hierarchy and its coercive power structure are not dissimilar. For the first time in history, poor families in the most remote areas have family members regularly working abroad—mainly in the Gulf States—to send help home; those still at home are hearing about different ways of life and are enabled by remittances to take opportunities they did not have before. The earthquake and its aid programs likewise provided some opportunities that did not previously exist.

One of the main changes occurring in northern Pakistan is through education, although origins are not discounted. As Satti notes, "Caste is (still) defined by birth, even if you change your profession from cobbler to surgeon" (1990: 24). Nowadays, if the son or daughter of a shoemaker or tailor is able to work their way through the education system and become employed or establish their own businesses, they are still rising into more prominent ranks of society, albeit with their low-caste status.

Culture and Cultural Norms

Although culture has been a formal study for well over a century, there is no universally accepted definition of the term. In the late nineteenth century, E. B. Tylor—one of the founders of cultural anthropology—defined "culture" as "that complex whole which includes knowledge, beliefs, arts, morals, law, customs and any other capabilities and habits acquired by [a human] as a member of society" (1871: 1). Roger M. Keesing offered a similar definition, describing culture as the "learned, accumulated experience and socially transmitted patterns for behavior characteristic of a particular social group" (1981: 68). Geert Hofstede posited that culture "is the collective programming of the mind which distinguishes the members of one group or category of people from another" (2011: 3).

Experts in culture and disaster point out the importance of understanding and planning for culture in reconstruction projects; it facilitates work and creates effective results. For instance, it has been argued that

> culture is important—both in the "people's culture" of those who face risk and for the "organizational culture" of those who are trying to help. . . . Culture is not about "residuals" that can be ignored as strange and illogical: it is absolutely crucial to the way that disaster risk reduction and adaptation succeeds or fails. . . . It is foolish to ignore one of the most significant factors affecting success. (Cannon, Kruger, and Bankoff 2014: 27)

While the relevance of culture is obvious to some, putting cultural knowledge into practice is another matter: "Instilling the knowledge of culture in its most profound connotation into much disaster prevention and aid, and most crucially into the policies and practices of international, national, and nongovernmental organizations (NGOs) dealing with disaster, has proven recalcitrant" (Hoffman 2020: 272). This challenge persists even when knowledge of the local culture provides solutions to what may be challenges for the outsider.

Culture is inseparable from social structure and power. How culture manifests itself—even in one location—is highly variable from one time to another. What will work in one culture will not work in another, what is a priority in one culture may not be a priority at all in others, and what is culturally normal and acceptable in one culture may be abnormal and offensive in another. Within cultures there are variations and inconsistencies, and culture is dynamic, especially in times of disaster: "Along with cultural change, researchers can witness cultural conservation and its mechanisms" (Hoffman and Oliver-Smith 2002: 11).

Culture and Cultural Norms in the Project Area

Pakistan is a country of many cultures, even within a small region such as the earthquake zone, but many groups share some of the same cultural norms. For a project like PERRP to proceed effectively in such locations, it was first necessary to build trust with the local people. Without clear signs from the elders and other influential people that they accepted and welcomed the project, others would be reluctant to join in. One way to develop this trust was to show that the project team was culturally respectful and sensitive, knowledgeable of cultural norms and how to work within them. Being culturally sensitive was also an important part of being conflict sensitive, as certain offences could be met with violent reactions. Crucially, being culturally sensitive necessitated knowing cultural norms: what is expected or considered normal, typical, or the right way to behave.

With its many ethnicities, castes, classes, and tribal and kinship groups, the PERRP project area was a complex of many cultures that may appear to blend together to the outsider. Local people, however, can easily distinguish each other's identity groups by physical appearance, clothing, language, names, and other features. The communities' relative isolation maintained their heterogeneity. Both project districts are in the southern lower reaches of the Himalayas, and they are therefore largely covered with mountains—the highest peak being Hari Parbat at eighteen thousand feet above sea level. The rural, conservative populations are spread throughout the mountains and, as there are few roads, most live far from other communities. Their only means of transport is by foot, on paths crossing over or around mountainsides and across valleys, resulting—until recent times—in limited interchanges and communications. At the time of the earthquake, access to information technologies were limited in this region. Across the mountain landscape, television was uncommon while computers and the internet were available only to the better-off in the cities. Cell phone reception was sketchy at best, but access to it increased rapidly as companies providing these services scrambled to increase the number of towers and make owning a phone much easier.

There is a dearth of research and internationally accessible scholarly work on the cultures in this project area, and conducting deep anthropological research was outside the scope of this project. However, from the social team's long-term practical expertise in the local culture and many years of related project experience, certain important factors about the communities were identified as priorities for PERRP to acknowledge and respect. In this regard, despite local differences, the social team's emphasis was on what the people had in common. Besides a common history, similar topography, and a similar communications infrastructure, people in the region shared a religion—Islam—and many related cultural norms.

Religion and Beliefs

Although figures are not available for the project districts, the majority of Pakistan's population—about 96 percent—are Muslim, with the remaining 4 percent being Christian, Sikh, or Hindu. Of the two main Muslim denominations, Sunnis are estimated at 75–95 percent of the population, while Shias are a small minority, with estimates ranging from 5–20 percent, but that percentage may also include the even smaller groups such as Ahmadis, Sufis, and Ismailis. During PERRP, sectarian conflict between Sunni and Shia in some areas—including the project area—was becoming more common; their minority status made the Shia particularly vulnerable.

Beliefs, whether from religion or other sources, are a subject of interest to some disaster analysts. As Terry Cannon, Alexandra Titz, and Fred Kruger note, "people's beliefs (and how people behave in relation to hazards because of those beliefs) can often act as an obstacle to disaster risk reduction." However, they continue, "people's response to any disaster risk reduction initiative is likely to be much greater when their own beliefs are acknowledged and not ignored" (2014: 186–87). Consider, for instance, one example from Nepal: villagers believed flash floods were sent by God, so there was nothing they could do about the floods. However, once these people were shown how to protect their land with sandbags and bamboo, flood consequences were reduced while beliefs were still honored. Since the aid agency had understood and respected the culture, they were able to assist in ways that accommodated both religious beliefs and technical needs (Cannon et al. 2014).

For some, science provides explanations for the causes of disasters, but for others, religious beliefs provide these answers: "Islamic scriptures . . . present an antediluvian view on natural disasters, dubbing them a manifestation of Allah's anger and punishment for sins" (Shahid 2015). Several prominent Pakistanis—humanitarian figures, politicians, and business and religious leaders—drew on this belief and used the 2005 earthquake to draw attention to what they perceived as the sins of many, including those who engaged in immoral behavior, who were corrupt, or who had not paid their taxes or zakat, a tithe.

At the same time, religious beliefs may be used to mediate and support initiatives. Numerous times in PERRP, imams and other religious community members called on Islamic teaching to stop disputes and conflict, strengthen cooperation, and encourage volunteering and contributing to the reconstruction. For example, when obstacles to school construction arose, community members were reminded by members from within their own community that, in Islam, seeking education is obligatory. By calling on their faith and beliefs, quoting the importance of education from the Quran or Hadith (traditions of the Prophet Muhammad), religious leaders successfully reasoned with people to resolve their differences so the new school building could be ready as soon as possible.

Cultural Norms

As part of the earliest assessment, from their in-depth knowledge of the culture, the social team considered the cultural norms and set selection criteria by asking: "Of all the cultural norms, which ones would make the biggest difference in the project? If the project failed to do X, Y or Z, which would cause the biggest trouble for the people or the project? Which would cause the loss of the most opportunities, including opportunities for participation?" We concluded that there were three main intertwined norms: the multilingual nature of the area; gender roles as prescribed by the customs of *purdah*; and the local power structure, including the traditional, informal, nonelected leaders. For the project to work most effectively with local people, we needed to get a wide range of participation from as many of the local language groups as possible, which often included distinct ethnicities, castes, and tribes. We also needed to be able to include both men and women and heavily involve the local informal leaders.

Cultural Norm 1: Language

For the widest diversity of people to be interested in participating in the project to any degree, language had to be a project priority. Between the two project districts, there are significant language differences. While Urdu, the national language of Pakistan, is the official language in both KP's Mansehra district and AJ&K's Bagh district, few people speak it as the mother tongue. Instead, most use one or more of the dozens of other local languages, even within the same district. In Mansehra district, languages include Hindko, Gojri, Kohistani, Pashto, and Potohari, while in Bagh district, people speak Pahari, Gujari, Kashmiri, Punchi, and Punjabi. English, also an official language, is taught in schools and is in fairly common usage, especially in offices and urban areas.

If we had not taken the diversity of the local languages into account, we would have communicated only with the relatively elite, educated, and powerful. While Urdu is normally used in public meetings, and English is common at official levels, both are associated with power, the politics of the dominant castes, and the colonial legacy. To enable people in the project area to participate in their own languages, at least some project staff needed these local language skills. While most project engineers and other technical personnel were from other parts of Pakistan and so did not speak the local languages of the project area, PERRP social mobilizers—in addition to being fluent in Urdu and English—spoke the languages of the villages, meaning they were able to hold discussions and facilitate the participatory process and to settle complex land disputes and issues with construction. For local people, this provided unusual access to information; it also had an empowering effect, encouraged participation, and helped to build trust.

Cultural Norm 2: Gender Roles and *Purdah*
To enable both women and men to participate in the project, we adapted to *purdah* customs that are in strict practice in most of the project area. *Purdah* (literally, "curtain") is a cultural practice or code of conduct in some Muslim cultures that defines the relations and roles of men and women. While *purdah* is possibly one of the most visible parts of culture in the PERRP project area, its practices vary significantly; however, its distinguishing feature is the separation of men and women, with culturally prescribed rules for both genders. With some exceptions, contact with anyone of the opposite gender outside the family is limited or forbidden. The separation also occurs through clothing, with both genders' clothing concealing the body, and women additionally covering their face and hair. Mobility is also prescribed. Women more commonly stay at home or study or work in female-only settings, and, when going outside, are usually accompanied by a male family member or by other women. Men, on the other hand, move about as they desire, except to places deemed for women. *Purdah* is a complex subject, varying in practice even family to family, moment to moment, circumstance to circumstance.

The "curtaining-off" limits visual, spoken, and physical direct contact, and it starts in the home, with separate rooms to receive guests from outside the family: male guests will not see the women of the household, and men of the household will not see the female guests. The separation extends to schools: girls go to girls' schools and boys to boys' schools. Socializing with the opposite gender outside the family is highly frowned upon, and dating (as it is practiced in the West) is not done at all. Most marriages are arranged. In general, where *purdah* is in practice, its rules and norms are observed by both men and women to keep their own honor and family respect.

Purdah also means that girls and women often do not have some of the advantages that boys and men possess. For instance, in Pakistan, while school enrollment of girls varies greatly across the country, generally the enrollment of girls is lower than boys. However, this difference is not due solely to *purdah*. It happens for a combination of reasons: the low value that some put on education; the need to keep girls, and often boys, out of school to help at home or add to the family income; the distance between the school and the home; and a lack of culturally appropriate school facilities (for instance, schools may have no functioning toilets, no female teachers available for girls' schools, or no visual barriers to protect privacy).

In many cases, *purdah* also means that the men dominate community affairs. Women normally do not attend to such matters, and for development projects, having access to local women can be restricted unless the project adapts to what is culturally acceptable. At the professional level, there are some exceptions to the complete separation of the genders—for example, professionals of both genders may hold meetings or workshops together.

In PERRP, about half the beneficiaries were girls and women, so to work within *purdah*, PERRP needed to find ways for both men and women to participate. This need required us to hire both male and female social team members; however, the security conditions emanating from the nearby Taliban sometimes made hiring women to do fieldwork too risky, especially in KP province. In these cases, PERRP used other culturally acceptable ways for men and women to communicate. In KP province, local men formed the boys' school committees and male social mobilizers worked with those men. At girls' schools, the committees were composed of women, while men formed a construction advisory committee. To maintain communication with the women-led SMC, the construction advisory committee appointed a respected community "white beard"—an older man—to act as a bridge between the male construction advisory committee, the women's school committee, and the male social mobilizer.

In AJ&K, however, *purdah* arrangements were different from those in KP, reflecting some cultural and security differences between the two areas. PERRP engaged both female and male social mobilizers in AJ&K, with Kashmiri women mobilizers working both with mixed-gender and all-male committees. In general, these local women social mobilizers were accepted even by the traditionally minded, playing leading roles in some of the toughest conditions, such as the negotiations between all-male committees and contractors.

Sometimes attempts to have women participate were especially challenging, as the norm is for men to look after what they consider community issues. See anecdote "Who Should Attend the Meeting?," page 74.

Cultural Norm 3: Local Power Structures and Informal Leaders

In Pakistan, working within an administrative hierarchy is partly a cultural norm and partly an administrative expectation, as international aid projects are initiated from the top down. The donor and recipient agencies refer the project from the national level to local government officials who, in turn, refer the project to others located in the area where the construction is to occur. Officials at the local level included the District Coordination Officer, the top administrator for the district; the district-level officials of the Departments of Health and Education; the District Reconstruction Unit;

and the Revenue Department. At the community level, head teachers had the most authority, as they represent the government at the school level. Outside the school, each community had traditional informal leaders, including elders, notables, and other well-known, influential people. As the ethnography at the end of this chapter illustrates, complex problems in PERRP regions were handled effectively because the social team knew the local realities and could take a culturally sensitive approach, drawing on sociocultural knowledge and community leaders to solve problems in construction.

The above has been an overview of the cultures, heterogeneity, hierarchies, and diversity of social groups across the general project area; the first part of chapter 4 shows how the social team identified and analyzed the blocs of power at each level, working with them to shift and share the distribution of power.

Context: Land Issues

As in many countries, land issues—notably, disputes over land ownership—are common in Pakistan. When such issues arise, they can result in disputes, violence, and losses to local people, often leading to court cases, long costly delays, or even abandonment of any ongoing construction.

Much of the reconstruction following this earthquake was severely affected by land issues, but in PERRP, we were determined to prevent this by dealing with any such issues long before construction started. The process of settling land issues was one of the first steps in introducing the project's community participation program. With a focus on the Pakistani context, the following section demonstrates the importance of knowing about and dealing early with land issues.

Land Issues Are Serious

Construction, regardless of its context, involves land: construction cannot be done without land, and land often comes with minor or major issues. Pakistan is one of many countries in which the seriousness of land ownership disputes is hard to overstate: these are often matters of life or death. Almost every day, the Pakistani media reports murders committed across the country over land disputes, as individuals, families, and groups try to settle their scores using force. Such disputes often continue over years, even decades, and involve many people. A national TV news outlet reported that an exchange of gunfire between two armed groups of the Jatoi tribe in the southern province of Sindh brought the death toll to nineteen—these people were killed in the same land dispute over the course of five years ("Four Killed" 2018). A USAID report states that in Pakistan "land disputes are the most common form of dispute filed in the formal court system. . . . Between 50 percent and 75 percent of all cases brought before the lower-level civil as well high courts are land-related disputes" (2016: 10).

Such issues are high risk for local people as well as for construction projects, whether for development or disaster reconstruction. In the PERRP project area, the landholdings were not dominated by large feudal landholders as is the case in other parts of Pakistan. With family landholdings being very small—often under two acres—every inch is precious and protected.

In Pakistan, "major causes of land disputes are inaccurate or fraudulent land records, erroneous boundary descriptions that create overlapping claims, and multiple registrations to the same land by different parties. Credible evidence of land rights is often nearly impossible to obtain" (USAID 2016: 10). Land cases are infamous for taking years, decades, or even lifetimes to settle. Innumerable cases are still bogged down in the courts; some cases date back seventy years, for "evacuees" who were displaced in the 1947 partition from India.

Throughout the earthquake zone, the most common issues had to do with land ownership and boundaries. There is a long history of ownership changing without being registered with government. Land is inherited and subdivided among relatives, but ownership often is not formally transferred, resulting in there frequently being no up-to-date land records, titles, or official records of ownership called "mutation documents." Cadastral survey documents are out of date, sometimes even by generations.

Unclear boundary lines are common, whether the land is for residential use, agriculture, or a public building such as a school. For generations, in different parts of the country, it has been the custom for governments to offer to build primary schools on donated land. Primary schools are now dotted throughout the country in vast numbers of small villages, but often the donation of land was never formalized. The ownership was never transferred to the government, and exact boundaries were never surveyed, demarcated, or made known with certainty to adjoining landowners. For a long time, such agreements were common understandings, but when a school was destroyed in the earthquake and reconstruction was planned, suddenly it became apparent there were many different and conflicting ideas about ownership and boundaries. There were land issues at almost every school or health facility built by PERRP.

Pakistan is not alone in land issues being so common—indeed, "land-related issues figure into many violent disputes around the world" (Bruce

2013). In some places, land may be a family's only asset, and each plot has a centuries-old history, inextricable from family history, identity, and social status. Even the potential of losing a few inches or centimeters of land can be a dire threat.

In the developing world, even without a disaster occurring, land issues are one of the main causes and effects of poverty. There, "around four billion people live without the protection of the law. As a result, they can be unfairly driven from their land, denied essential services and intimidated by violence" (Maru 2014). Competition over the land and its resources may also be part of even bigger and potentially much longer-standing differences among individuals or social groups based on such factors as ethnicity, religion, political ties, social power structures, ethnicity, caste, or class. Only in recent years have large-scale efforts by governments and international agencies begun to act on such urgent issues. Some of the international agencies involved in these issues are the United Nations Human Rights Office of the High Commissioner, the International Work Group for Indigenous Affairs, the International Land Coalition, Oxfam, EarthRights International, International Fund for Agriculture Development, and International Development Law Organization.

Disasters such as earthquakes can magnify already severe land issues. New pressures may be added, such as disappearance of land due to fissures, landslides, or floods, and the displacement or absence of owners or users, resulting in occupation of the land by others, reduced agricultural livelihoods, and food insecurity. Historically ineffective land governance can even be made worse with destroyed office buildings and loss of life among government workers. Destruction of government buildings and homes can also result in the loss of what few critical land documents existed. Of these challenges, those that existed predisaster may still be the most entrenched and challenging.

Land Administration, Laws, Police, Court System, and *Patwari* Culture

Overall, Pakistanis tend to have little faith in the police, the slow court system, or the outdated and corrupt land administration system. To get justice, many resort to settling scores themselves—often with violence. Such disputes can result in major losses to local people and are one of the many reasons for frequent delays or abandonment of construction.

Pakistan's land administration and legal systems are often seen as main factors in a vicious cycle that perpetuates land ownership problems: the administration has an antiquated manual record-keeping system, and "numerous federal and provincial laws ... regulate the ownership, transfer, acquisition, taxation, registration, tenancy, etc. of immovable property" (UN HABITAT 2012: 7). The judiciary is beset with low pay, inadequate training, and an overwhelming case load. Despite its well-known problems, the court system is still a common avenue taken for redress. A common cause of long costly delays in construction is complainants pursuing court cases or requesting stay orders to stop construction. While this is a democratic right and there are many legitimate cases, some are considered nuisance cases, while others are motivated more by retribution than justice: the court process is a long, drawn-out affair, a punishment in and of itself for any perceived offenses. Many such court cases involve issues that could have been dealt with more effectively through direct resolution by the parties involved.

In Pakistan, when conflict of any kind erupts, including over land, asking for help from the police is often avoided. When police are called in, it is often an act of revenge by one party against another. As Human Rights Watch has stated, "Public surveys and reports of government accountability and redress institutions show that the police are one of the most widely feared, complained against, and least trusted government institutions in Pakistan, lacking a clear system of accountability and plagued by corruption at the highest levels" (2016: 1). At the district level, police are "often under the control of powerful politicians, wealthy landowners and other members of society" (Human Rights Watch 2006: 15).

There is also a highly diverse body of customary law that governs land rights. These customary laws vary from province to province, and vary as well by local administrative units, tribes, castes, or other social groups, especially around inheritance and division of property.

In the Revenue Department, the blame is usually placed on the *patwaris*, the land record officers, who are notorious for "corruption and misdeeds" (Qadir 2017) and for their "practice of taking bribes[, which is] blamed for kicking off the cycle of violence" (Anwar 2018). In Pakistan, "*patwari* culture" is virtually synonymous with "corruption." For a "fee," *patwaris* are known to tamper with land records or simply reassign ownership. In such an advantageous position as land record keeper, the *patwari* is known to be a powerful person, put in their position by even more powerful people for their own political and financial benefit. There is no transparency. Any number of politicians and governments have vowed to clean up the *patwari* culture and outdated land registration system. As part of the problem is the out-of-date record-keeping practices, the government of Pakistan and World Bank in the Punjab Province have undertaken the digitization of all the records, making them far more accessible. But the realities and root causes of these issues are far more complex, and first require careful, fair settlement of disputes that can then be turned into trusted legal documents.

Eminent Domain, Encroachment, and the Land Grab

Pakistan's Land Acquisition Act of 1894 allows government seizure or acquisition of land. The law of eminent domain "is perhaps the most abused law in most countries and Pakistan is no exception" (Ul Haque 2009). Encroachment and land grabbing, even from official levels, goes practically uncontested. As observed by Pakistan's Supreme Court:

> In our society, the acts of illegal dispossession [of land] are largely committed at the behest of persons who are rich, powerful feudal lords, politicians, builders, government functionaries or persons who head large communities, and on account of their influence and power that place them in domineering positions either over their fellow community members or over less powerful communities living in an area of their influence. (Malik 2016)

In other words, the status and imbalance of power are what underlie many of the land struggles. Land administrators tend to be from dominant social groups, and "[l]and disputes may be the cause or effect of other problems" (Home Office 2017: 4). As found countless times in PERRP, what appeared to be a technical problem for construction—for instance, someone blocking access to a construction site—was, at its root, caused by long-standing problems between groups over unrelated problems or existing land issues.

Understanding the Social Nature of Land Disputes

While land issues are usually considered legal matters, in PERRP they were treated primarily as a social issue. Through a legal perspective, land is a commodity with physical attributes—size, type, location, and value. Land is an asset that can be seized, bought, or sold. However, from a social point of view, all parcels of land have adjoining land that is owned by different people. These people can make decisions about their land, and such decisions may depend on a wide range of factors, not the least of which is the relationship between those who own or use the land. How they deal with each other, as individuals and as groups, may be the most important determining factor about the land.

As long as landowners could come to an agreement and make decisions with each other about their land, they needed the legal system only to formalize what they had already agreed. This was the approach taken in

PERRP: the social team facilitated agreements, and by liaising with government had a cadastral survey conducted and new, legalized mutation documents issued on the spot. These documents were then filed in the land records system. The process often settled disputes that were already years old and meant that court cases were not needed. Details of this process are included in chapter 5.

In PERRP, many lessons were learned about taking care of land issues before proceeding with design and construction. The first lesson was "Do not assume there are no land issues."

Serious Cultural Breach

In any community, what are its cultural norms? What is acceptable behavior and what is not? In these remote conservative project communities, which normally have no outsiders visiting at all, the behavior of such visitors can be very risky.

With construction at a girls' high school well underway, the construction site was the center of attention of the whole community. The site was visible from a long way off across the facing mountains, and the novelty of having something so big happening in such a far-flung place had all eyes on the construction activity and the large number of outsiders: the construction workers brought from other parts of Pakistan by the contractor. Not used to having such strangers in their midst, there was general concern.

Unfortunately, what some feared did take place. Local people noticed something seemed to be happening between a worker and a young woman in the village. He was phoning her, or trying to talk with her in person, then one night he was caught trying to get into her family's house. In such a closed, conservative area where *purdah* is strictly in practice, and only family members may see and speak with each other, this was a very serious offense—an act of disrespect and dishonor to the whole community.

Villagers caught the offender and beat him seriously, and as this was nightfall, committee members intervened and had him locked in the contractor's site office to deal with him in the morning. This was then a village-wide crisis, so serious that elders demanded that construction be stopped and that the contractor be fired; they would rather go without a school than allow such insulting behavior. Over the phone, social mobilizers asked committee members to come to the PERRP project office in the morning to meet, instead of the mobilizers going to the community where emotions were running high. In the morning there was more uproar when it was discovered that the offending worker had escaped, knowing his life could be in danger.

At the meeting, attended by the committee members, social mobilizers, project engineers, and the contractor, the committee still demanded the contractor be fired. They blamed the contractor's senior site manager for this disgrace and not being able to control the laborers, despite already having agreed to such control in the Committee-Contractor Agreement, which had clauses about honoring cultural norms, and in the code of conduct. Committee members predicted more trouble, sure that the remaining laborers on the site would pose an equal risk.

The PERRP engineers explained to the committee members that it was not possible to fire the contractor. For all this, the contractor humbly apologized and offered a solution: he would replace all the workers at this site. He would move them to a second reconstruction site where he was building another PERRP school and bring those workers here. After more discussion about this idea, and a commitment that the new workers would be retrained in the code of conduct and would be better supervised, the committee agreed with this solution. About three days of construction were lost due to this incident.

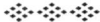

"All It Takes Is One Person"

"All it takes is one person in a community, and the whole project can be stopped. It all depends on how people use or misuse their power. Sometimes in the communities there are individuals who will not listen to anyone, not their own family members or the elders, even when it is customary here to listen, especially to elders. They get an idea—always something in their own self-interest—and they will push so hard for it. They will make threats and take court cases, no matter how much the people closest to them tell them they are being unreasonable. We have certainly had some cases of this in the project. Because of a few individuals' demands, construction would have been stopped for sure. But when it happens, we social mobilizers just wait and let the family and committee work it out. There wasn't a single case where that didn't work."

—Social mobilizer

Who Are the Powerful People? Depends on Whom You Ask and When

Even identifying the powerful people is not necessarily easy. In one village of a few hundred people, all who lived there were from one extended family, but they were split into factions over political differences. In many communities certain castes dominated, even if they were a minority. In another place, two tribal groups each considered itself superior over the other. With such divisions, simply asking who is "on top" could elicit a strongly biased answer, as people tended to identify influential people only from their own group. Issues in identifying the notables or other prominent people made it necessary to triangulate, consulting several sources and making observations in different settings to get the most reliable picture. Even then, over time and in different situations, power arrangements changed. Those who were prominent or powerful in one setting were not necessarily so in another.

Power and the School above the Clouds

There can be fine lines between being influential, prominent or powerful. In one location where a destroyed school was to be rebuilt, the site failed PERRP's technical assessment: it was on a dangerous mountain slope, making it too unsafe to build another school there, and no other land was available. Devastated by this news, the local School Management Committee pleaded with PERRP to reconsider, but the project had to refuse due to the unsafe conditions. The implementation team had only a short amount of time to choose a set of sites and to get approval to build there. The committee was informed, regretfully, that since this site was not suitable, the project had to move on to other communities to find safer, more feasible locations. Again, the committee persisted. If they could find another more suitable piece of land for a new school within reasonable distance, would the project agree to build the school there?

Due to the complex land issues, project management had serious doubts if such land could ever be found, especially in the limited time available to conduct geotechnical testing, environmental assessment, and other preparatory work. Nevertheless, PERRP allowed the committee one month to try. However, as the committee was reminded, PERRP could build only on government-owned land, and had to have the mutation or legal documents to prove its ownership.

One member of the School Management Committee was one of the most influential and powerful people of the area: a retired government official, an education officer. He immediately used his connections and know-how in the government departments to get what the community needed. To everyone's surprise, within only two weeks, from another government ministry he had obtained an almost ideal plot of land on which to build: a large, safe, flat plot beside the road. He and his fellow committee members immediately had the ownership transferred from the forestry department to the department of education, and soon had ownership documents in hand. With the community celebrating this early victory, the technical and environmental assessments could proceed immediately. When construction was completed, the building was dubbed "the school above the clouds." It looks out over the valleys in Kashmir.

Low-Caste Families Pooling Subsidy Funds

At times, members of the lower castes can arrange their own advantages. In a few instances, it was known locally that recipients of government subsidies that had been intended for rebuilding destroyed houses instead pooled their funds for other purposes: to set up businesses or buy land. These were families in the lowest caste who had members abroad sending money home; that money, which was normally used for living expenses, was now somehow stretched to rebuild their houses. At the same time, those at home were able to start generating new income from the land or business.

Low-Caste Son Becomes a Leader

In aid programs, including those in disaster reconstruction, local project staff are part of the area's culture and its social structure, stratifications, and divisions, including those of caste. This adds challenges for the hiring, supervision, direction, and promotion of staff, especially in basing this on merit and not repeating the normal societal hierarchy.

One PERRP staff member was from a project community and of the lowest caste, but he joined the project as a recent university graduate with a Master's' degree. Usually left out of higher education due to low status and poverty, his father, a tailor, had borrowed money to send his son to school. Although he had very little work experience, with his aptitude, dedication, and experience in leadership and conflict sensitivity in his own community, he soon became a respected, admired PERRP leader and a manager in the multicaste staff, partly by knowing how to handle delicate situations.

Landowner Suddenly Claims Encroachment; Shunning Threatened

Internal influences can pressure community members to conform to the cultural norms or wishes of the larger community. These pressures can take such forms as coercion, demanding reciprocity, threats, or punishment in various forms, including what may be considered the worst by many: shunning.

In one project community, without warning even to his own community, a man applied for a court order to stop construction to protect land that he claimed as his own. Some months earlier, the social team had the community—including this man—attend a day-long event to identify and settle any issues related to land ownership. The social team also had the government land official—the *patwari*—survey the land and put pegs in the ground to demarcate the school's boundary line. This man had attended the survey and he had raised no objections at that time. Now, several months later, he was claiming that the school boundary wall would be built on his adjoining land.

Community members were aghast and angry with the man for making this unfounded claim while construction was already underway. If a stay order was granted, it would stop construction. First, they tried reasoning with him based on his attendance at and agreement with the *patwari* survey. Committee members used all their knowledge about the history of this land, its ownership, and the exact locations of boundaries. They argued that, on behalf of the community, he should honor their request to not interfere with construction as the school was needed by every family. When after such pressure he would still not relent, the committee gave him their most severe warning: if he did anything that would stop construction, they would organize a community shunning against him. No one would talk with him or his family. Shopkeepers would not deal with him and the whole community would be officially against him. As this is possibly the most serious cultural punishment, he withdrew the court application, which would have caused delays and been less effective anyway. Instead, construction continued unhindered.

"What? Now I Have to Learn the Folk Songs and Wear Traditional Clothes?"

An engineer came from Europe to visit the project and some construction sites to see how the work was being done. After meetings with engineers and architects, during which he heard the project had a social team, he asked to join social mobilizers to attend community meetings. Genuinely interested and wanting to be considerate of the culture, he asked lightheartedly, "But does this mean I now have to learn folk songs and dress in traditional clothes?" This was a deliberate exaggeration coming from a definition of culture that includes the arts. He further wondered, "Is that what you mean as culture? How on earth does culture fit in a construction project?"

As he did then go along to some meetings, his comments gave rise to discussion in the social team about culture per se, a topic that hadn't been discussed until then. Members of the social team explained to the visitor that we hardly ever used the word "culture" in this project as many people—especially those from other work disciplines—misunderstand it as a high-level, extraneous, abstract thing.

As one social mobilizer put it, "the word 'culture' seems to bother or threaten some. Among other project staff, we just talk about and explain things about the communities that might make a difference to some decisions about design or construction. Although the community people speak for themselves in this project, we social mobilizers often act as cultural interpreters. That means talking to designers, engineers, and managers about what is important to the community people—the way they do things, what they think is right or wrong, what they want. You know, those are the ways culture is defined, but it's not necessary for us to use that high-class word, 'culture'."

"Why Didn't You Just Tell Them They Had to Change the Culture?"

Some disaster reconstruction planners, policy makers, organizations, project teams, and frontline workers show little or no respect for the local culture and have difficulties accepting it the way it is—regardless of whether they share the same culture, come from another part of the same country, or come from abroad. Although the theory of being respectful may be common, there can be large gaps in putting it into practice.

At two separate educational gatherings, I was asked the same question about the people of the PERRP project communities: "Why didn't you just tell them to change their culture?" In one case, I was asked this question at a workshop in the USA with engineers from different international agencies who focused on development and disaster reconstruction. The second time was in a Canadian university class in a peace and development studies program. In both instances, I was presenting the advantages for sociocultural considerations and community participation in construction projects, giving PERRP as an example.

In the American workshop, I explained that to have community women participate in PERRP, we needed to be sensitive to the cultural protocol of the place where we were working—which meant working with men and women separately, according to the customs of *purdah*. The situation also required us to start with the men. After hearing some detail about how the project accommodated these factors, a few attendees were flummoxed. One male engineer blurted out, "That seems like a lot of trouble to go to. Why bother with all that? Why didn't you just tell the elders they should allow women to participate? Tell them to change their culture!"

A man in the audience of engineers, himself from Pakistan, spoke up:

This is reality in my country. Government programs, NGOs, and development programs that want to help women—especially in our villages—have to develop a relationship of trust with the men first. Once they know that you can be trusted, you will be enthusiastically welcomed. Keep in mind we are talking about traditional communities, in an area with a long history of trouble from outside, making people skeptical of outsiders, whether Pakistanis or others. The earthquake and influx of aid agencies also made them cautious.

In the Canadian university class, where students knew each other quite well, one student was not so polite. Her response to those who had asked this question was, "Did you miss our classes on cultural sensitivity? What kind of colonialist question is that? Do you really think we should expect people to change their culture? Why should they change their culture for us?"

To the above remarks on both occasions, I added that PERRP worked by creating an entirely new experience for both women and men so that both were able to be involved with a school construction project—and could do so within their own cultural norms. With this new experience, many built skills that could be applied to other situations, including new expectations for how construction should be managed and how they should be treated by government or other reconstruction projects. This in itself was a big cultural change.

Who Should Attend the Meeting?

At one place, where a Basic Health Unit (BHU) was to be built, the all-male committee was informed that meetings would be held to discuss the design of the BHU. According to *purdah* customs, there would be separate meetings for men and women. Attendance of women was especially encouraged, as they and their children would make up the vast majority of the BHU users. Meeting dates were set, and committee members were asked to make sure men and women were invited to their respective meetings. The men's meeting was held successfully as planned, but when the women's meeting was to occur the next week, only men arrived! When we inquired about the women, some men explained there was no need for women to attend, because they could answer all our questions. The social team was stuck in a quandary, worried that canceling the meeting would be a cultural offense, as dozens of men had arrived. Still, social team members proceeded to insist on talking with women. Convincing reasoning had to be given.

The BHU was to include a birthing center, and the Department of Health was encouraging women to deliver at the BHU with trained birth attendants instead of at home. Because of the inclusion of this birthing center, the social mobilizers explained that it was important to talk with women to get their ideas and generate interest in the BHU, and out of respect for customs of modesty only women should attend that discussion. The social team asked the men to choose another date, assuring them there would be culturally appropriate arrangements. PERRP's women social mobilizers would attend, accompanied by some of PERRP's women architects. Acceding to that agenda, the men chose another meeting date and dispersed satisfied. A week later, about a hundred women, many with their children, sat on the ground under the trees. A female social mobilizer facilitated the meeting, thanking the women for attending and explaining why their ideas were needed. The four female architects explained preliminary designs, showed photos of other BHUs, and explained the basic labor and delivery rooms. In this case, few ideas were generated from the audience, as most had no birthing center experience to compare it to. It could have been the beginning of dialogue as the conversation generated much interest, and the women liked the novel idea of getting together for discussion.

Unfortunately this BHU was never built, as the community was split into two rival factions. Despite extensive efforts by the social team, the two factions would not come to a firm agreement over location for the new building. One faction wanted it on the same footprint as the old BHU that had been destroyed, while the other wanted it moved to another location. As a result, the Department of Health canceled building there altogether and had PERRP assigned to another location for reconstruction there instead.

Land Issues? Perspective Matters

While almost all construction in PERRP was completed on or ahead of schedule, outside PERRP, much of the Pakistan earthquake reconstruction was slow, delayed, or abandoned. One of the many reasons for this was the failure to prepare for issues related to land ownership. Many of the aid agency decision makers were new to the scene and were either unfamiliar with Pakistani realities or simply did not know how to proceed. Mistakenly, they simply assumed there were no issues that would hinder their reconstruction. They assumed that the necessary land would fall in place, or that somebody else would take care of any such possible complications, and that all they had to do was build. This was not so.

In the early stages of PERRP, some Pakistani government officials erroneously advised the project team that we would encounter no land issues. It appears that issues related to land ownership are often overlooked in construction planning for a range of reasons: lack of awareness, officials' unwillingness to disclose possible complications, dismissal of the seriousness of such issues, and a refusal to deal with them altogether.

Case in point: after the PERRP project ended, I was recruited by an international engineering firm to help prepare a proposal for a construction project in a country that I had never visited and was not familiar with. However, I was put in online contact with the people who did know the country and project region; my role was to work with them to establish a process and, from their input, write a proposal for community participation. Given my experience with issues of land ownership, my first questions were about this topic. Local government officials and the prospective project engineers all said, "No problem, land issues are not a big deal here." However, when I asked the same question of NGO personnel working in the communities where the construction project was to occur, they replied, "Here, fighting about land is so common."

Ethnography: Government Girls' School Sabaz Zameen*

Sabaz Zameen is a pseudonym. To maintain confidentiality, the names of all schools, villages, and castes in this example have been changed.

Sabaz Zameen village in KP province was one of the school reconstruction sites assigned to PERRP. The school was to accommodate 450 girls from primary to secondary grades. The site was almost ideal technically: most of the land was flat, it was near the road, and it was not surrounded by other buildings, making access to the site easy for construction. Our technical team thought construction could proceed without hinderance, but the social feasibility of construction was another matter. Problems between local groups presented high risks for construction.

For an outsider visiting Sabaz Zameen, there were no visible signs of its complex social makeup. It is a village surrounded by the lush green of well-tended agricultural fields and stands of trees. Just below this verdant surface was the tension of deep divisions among the people. Such a volatile social context significantly increased risks for the community, the imminent reconstruction process, and the long-term use of the new school.

At Sabaz Zameen there are two castes—here called the Balla and Demani—and virtually all local people belong to one of these two social groups. Historically, the Ballas had been the higher caste—wealthy landowners or landlords—while Demani have been their subjects, the tenant farmers stuck in the vicious cycle of poverty. Unable to afford their own land, Demani have been stuck leasing land from the Ballas and then having to pay rent in the form of most of their crop, leaving them with little for all their hard work.

When PERRP first arrived at Sabaz Zameen, the social mobilizers needed to deal with the strained relationship: their differences were so serious that people would not even sit down with each other to talk about the potential new school. They had a long history of quarreling, opposing each other on just about everything; even when something good happened, each tried to take credit for it. If an achievement was clearly due to the efforts of one caste, the other tried to downplay it or put obstacles in its path. Their differences were so great that even though the people of both castes are Muslim, they had defiantly built separate mosques only three hundred feet apart. Normally the mosque is considered a point of unity, a way to come together because of the common beliefs, but not in this case—the Balla and Demani would never even pray together.

School staff were also split. The head teacher had been transferred here from a long distance, and as the Demani gave her accommodations and other help, she sided with the Demani, while all her government-appointed teachers were from another even higher caste, the same caste as authorities in the Department of Education. With so many divisions, it was difficult to see how they would ever be able to solve the community-related problems for construction or carry out any of the roles that the project would assign to them. Serious discussions ensued within the social team and with project management and engineers. We considered not even building in this location at all; however, the social team decided to push ahead to next steps, to give it a try and somehow form a local committee.

As Sabaz Zameen school was a girls' school in KP province, the government required that the committee—here a parent teacher council (PTC)—be composed of women only. PERRP's social team therefore decided to strike two committees: the women-only PTC was formed to work with teachers and help with school functions, while a separate committee of men was struck to act as the PTC advisory committee, since construction-related matters—land, water, electricity—in this culture fall into the male domain. The main purpose of the PTC advisory committee was to prevent or solve community-related problems for construction. Both Demanis and Ballas eagerly joined the committee, motivated by their rivalry and not by any sense of cooperation; nonetheless, they met many times together with social mobilizers to form the partnership with the PERRP project, to learn the design and construction schedule, the procedures, and many other details, including the social program's processes for grievance and conflict resolution.

In these early months, while the buildings were being designed and construction was being tendered, the social team built up strong working relations with district officials; the District Coordination Officer, Department of Education administrators, and the local District Reconstruction Unit, as well as local notables, community members, and committee members. By the time the construction contractors arrived, these relations were well established, and it had been agreed by all that if there were differences or disputes, the committee and the social mobilizers would have people sit down together to resolve the issues in friendly ways. At each meeting, social mobilizers explained the PERRP communication protocol and its grievance procedures, noting that these would mean there would be no need to fight over anything. This was repeated frequently at regular and special meetings attended by the advisory committee, contractor, and PERRP, as well as at meetings with government people. Everyone agreed that this collaborative process was much preferred over the more frequent violent clashes, calling in the police, or pursuing court cases that go on for years. This kind of third-party facilitation was a new experience. The Demanis and Ballas, as well as government officials, welcomed these ideas.

This process of establishing community participation before construction started meant that when the construction contractor arrived, social mobilizers worked with the committee and contractor as they made a detailed Committee-Contractor Agreement on all the points that would often cause conflict. This agreement answered a range of questions: What land outside the construction site would be needed by the contractor? Where was it, and for what purpose was it needed? Would it be needed, for example, for a site office, laborers' camp, or to store materials? Would this land be rented? If so, then from whom and under what terms? Point by point, each item was put into a written agreement, to which the advisory committee members—both Balla and Demani—and contractors were signatories.

But even with all this preparation and these agreements, things started to go wrong only a few weeks later, just as the construction contractor was ready to put shovels in the ground. With no previous information or warning that this was happening, the PERRP office received a letter from the District Coordination Officer demanding an explanation in response to a letter of complaint he had received from the Demani, which accused the project of favoring the Ballas. The letter had been written by the local leader of the Demani without the community's knowledge. This leader had himself attended all the project meetings and knew all about the established grievance procedures, but he saw an opportunity to get advantages for his own caste. He had previously worked in local government, and so he used his connections to the local politician whom the Demanis had backed, asking him to use his influence with the District Coordination Officer to stop this alleged favoritism.

With such accusations flying and construction due to start any day, the project's social mobilizer team knew an immediate, assertive response had to be made. The Ballas took this inflammatory letter as an affront and the situation could have easily escalated into caste conflict, lawsuits, countersuits, revenge, blockades, damage to property, construction stoppages, and even loss of life. Social mobilizers asked for an emergency meeting of the PTC Advisory Council, construction contractor, and PERRP engineers. To lead this mediation, the social team had the PTC advisory committee choose a respected local man. He happened to be the chairman of the PTC advisory committee and a Balla, but he was well respected by both Ballas and Demanis, as he was also a retired teacher from this village. He was admired for being pious, honest, impartial, and well aware of the caste differences.

It was agreed that the meeting would be held at the Demani mosque, since they were the complainants and would never go to the Balla mosque. Meeting in the mosque to settle disputes is also common as, despite caste differences, it is considered neutral and sacred ground where people are less likely to tell lies. By custom, agreements made in the mosque are considered similar to oaths. The meeting was attended by all Balla and Demani PTC advisory committee members, the *kateeb* (religious leader), the contractor, PERRP engineers, the social team, and former (but still influential) elected officials, who were both Demani and Balla.

At first the whole audience was split and arguing, but the retired teacher reminded them of what they had all agreed to months earlier through PERRP—that differences would be settled face-to-face in open discussion. So, with this respected man leading, discussion was brought under control. The offending letter was then read aloud to the audience. It accused the construction contractor of giving jobs to only the Ballas, but the audience of both Ballas and Demani pointed out this was not true, identifying men from both castes who had been hired. Next, the letter accused the contractor of doing business only with the Ballas, renting land from them and giving them other advantages. Participants concluded, yes, the land rented by the contractor was Balla land, but this was logical, as all the land surrounding the school was owned by Ballas, and the nearby land was needed by the contractor to put his equipment and supplies. The third and final accusation was that the contractor had given special help to the Ballas by improving the water well on their land, but this issue was immediately dismissed by the *kateeb* who acknowledged, yes, the well was on the Balla land, but an improved well would be a new benefit for everyone, not just the school. He said that the well's improvement would not only increase the supply of water for construction, but that all the students and the school's neighbors would benefit from this improved source for a long time to come. And, as he pointed out, there was no other source of water. With his firm stance, this complaint was also dismissed as not valid.

Finally, everyone—Ballas and Demanis—agreed that the letter to the District Coordination Officer and District Reconstruction Unit should be withdrawn. They wrote and cosigned a formal resolution to this effect, stating that the issues were resolved, and sent it to the District Coordination Officer. In the resolution, they also renewed their support for the school, saying there was no further dispute and restating their gratitude for being given a new school.

Although the Demanis came to the meeting still backing the man who had written the letter, by the end of the meeting, they were deeply dismayed with him. His fellow caste members in attendance now told this man he should be playing a more positive role and putting his energy into more productive things, starting by using his political connections to upgrade the school from a high school to a higher secondary school. Surprisingly, he took on this challenge, and by the following year, was successful in getting the upgrade. This upgrade was considered a big achievement for girls' education, as the added grades and time in school would prepare the female students for university. To build his political favors even more, he had the minister responsible for the upgrading attend the official inauguration of the new building, during which he announced that due to his own efforts, the minister had agreed to the upgrade.

Only five days passed between the day PERRP received the surprise letter of complaint to the day that the dispute was resolved. During that time, the construction contractor continued working with no time lost.

Over the next three to four years, until the project ended, some visible changes happened in the relationship between the two castes. Although they were still in competition with each other, this competition was a little more balanced and not exclusively hostile. A Balla family donated land for the school toilet block to be built, and not to be outdone, a Demani family that owned a little land donated a piece of it for a retaining wall. When the school was upgraded, two new teachers were provided—one a Demani, one a Balla—even though such inclusiveness had never been a priority before.

Also following the resolution of the dispute, the PTC advisory committee, with social mobilizers facilitating, came to an agreement, assigning responsibility to each caste for certain tasks for the school, construction, and other community development. After many years of nothing but disputes, they finally sat together and made plans for their community. In those meetings, social team members observed that both sides in this split would have liked to settle their differences and unite earlier, but only now had agreed on ways to do it.

Although there was still no love lost between these two castes, the above process broke some ice. There were no further incidents about school construction and, when the building was completed, they rallied around it. Furthermore, both castes developed skills in seeking other help for the village. The Demanis had the road paved by going to the Member of Provincial Assembly, who was known to support Demanis, while the Ballas used their opposing political connections to get a tractor, a thresher, and financing for a fifteen-mile link road.

This case study shows that even with good sociocultural knowledge and established, agreed-upon procedures, anomalies can still arise. Without the initiative of the social team, the trouble caused by this man's letter could have remained unresolved indefinitely, only adding fuel to the fire. The only other option for resolution—a court case—could have taken months or years, and still might not have solved the problem.

The strategy used by the social team provided a different approach. Rather than waiting and hoping for a solution, with the knowledge that such a wait would risk a construction stoppage, the social team acted as a catalyst to find a solution, immediately seeking out the person in the community who was most likely to be able to mediate, choosing a suitable venue, and asking representatives from the two factions to attend. As was the strategy in all conflicts in this project, the social team did not act as the mediator, as doing so could have turned disputes around to being between "them" (insiders) and "us" (outsiders). Instead, knowing it could have more long-term beneficial effects, the strategy put the responsibility of dispute resolution entirely on the people. It also helped emphasize that the construction of their new school depended entirely on their reaching agreement.

This example is important as it illustrates several main points—most notably, that the social context of a construction project can have a strong effect on construction. Alleviating such problems takes an understanding of the social structure and culture, which suggests that construction projects can benefit from having a team of sociocultural experts. With a well-thought-out strategy for community participation, a social team can both help a project save time, and help communities develop their own capacities.

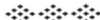

CHAPTER 3

Community Participation
What Has Happened to It?

Introduction

A former colleague called me just to say hello and catch up after a long time—twenty years, to be exact. He had been my boss on a construction project in Bangladesh in the late 1990s. As the project officer, he stayed at the company's head office in Canada and visited the construction site twice a year, while I was the on-site project manager. We were working for an international engineering and construction firm: he was a civil engineer, while I was the community participation specialist. This was the first time that particular company had hired a non-engineer to head a construction project, but the Government of Bangladesh and the donor agency had stipulated this was to be an experiment: would having a social expert as the head of a construction project instead of an engineer make a difference to the sustainability of a new flood control embankment?

After the twenty years, my former boss wanted to know what I was up to. Since our Bangladesh days, he had gone on to higher executive work, which had put him out of touch with what was happening in construction at the community level. When I told him I was writing a book about community participation and construction, he was surprised. "You're writing a whole book about that? Is that kind of thing still needed? Community participation has been around forever: even long before the Bangladesh project. Back then, even the biggest international aid donors and financial institutions like the World Bank required it. Surely, participation must be everywhere by now!" See anecdote, page 104.

Yes, I replied, probably all aid donors have had that policy for decades, and yes, there probably is not a project or project report in any sector in the whole world that doesn't claim community participation was involved. But there is a big difference between words and action, theory and practice. The rhetoric is everywhere, but having actual, meaningful participation has never been the norm. I told him that community participation, and the ineffective ways in which it is implemented, are heavily criticized in the literature on international development. It has become a much watered-down idea.

My former boss had seen what a difference community participation made on our project in Bangladesh, so he was curious to know what this book would say about community participation in earthquake reconstruction in Pakistan. I told him that, in fact, one of the chapters in the book would bring him up to date on this very question: so what has happened to community participation?

This chapter explores the concepts of participation and community, reviewing the background and critical perspective of both. Included here are six anecdotes from various countries, which show how participation and community mean many different things to different people for different reasons.

Background: Emergence of "Community Participation"

In the international development field, the concept of community participation has at least a fifty-year history. It first grew out of dissatisfaction with the way international aid was being handled in developing countries. Following World War II, United Nations and early international aid programs began emerging on all continents: "By the nineteen-sixties, virtually all the nations of the Western industrialized world and Japan had joined in efforts to assist the developing countries both through their own bilateral programs, and support for a variety of multinational programs" (Herbert and Strong 1980: 121). When the United Nations designated the 1960s and 1970s as the First and Second Development Decades, public interest and awareness in international development—and the number of NGOs and aid programs involved in it—grew exponentially.

Thus began the gargantuan growth of so-called "developed" countries providing assistance to the "Third World" in the form of transfers of technology, skills, person power, ideas, and goods. While there were some successes, it did not take long to see the faults in such a top-down approach: bulldozers that were provided to build roads sat idle when there was no supply of spare parts; schools were built in regions with no teachers; modern bakery ovens were supplied to places that had no fuel; "improved" seeds were introduced to farmers who had no money to buy the inputs required to make them grow; water wells were drilled where there is environmental contamination—the list of failures goes on and on.

By the 1970s, analysts—especially from NGOs within recipient countries and aid workers returning home to Western countries from Asia, Africa, and Latin America—questioned why so many of the aid programs were weak or failed. Why was it that so much money, care, and interest was being poured into helping the poor, yet hardly anything improved? What was happening, many realized, was that well-intentioned people in Western aid agencies only transferred what they thought was needed by the poor—ideas and material things. Worse, some observed that this kind of aid was creating dependency. As Barbara Harrell-Bond put it at the time, "Given the body of literature which evaluates the impact of aid, few practitioners in the development field (who think about such matters) still retain unquestioned confidence that their interventions are always beneficial to the recipients" (1986: xii). In many ways, aid had simply failed.

Until the 1970s, aid was largely a top-down enterprise. What was missing were the views of the people themselves. There had been little to no effort to understand the intended beneficiaries—not their cultures and contexts, not their views on their problems and needs, and certainly not their preferences and priorities. Various types of "help" had simply been chosen and handed out.

From this understanding emerged a paradigm shift. Aid agencies began realizing the importance of community participation and began making changes in their field: from raising awareness about community participation to developing methodologies and tools that could more effectively engage local people and successfully include them in the analytical and decision-making processes. The new thinking was this: how a decision was made could be just as important, if not more important, than the decision itself.

As the participatory approaches took off on a wide scale, so too did a new style and new policies and vehicles for aid delivery. Until that time, aid programs acted as service providers, dispersing their help across a population, or in some cases, to highly targeted sub-groups: the poorest of the poor, women, people with disabilities, people from minority groups, and other marginalized populations. Recipients were treated as aid receivers; they were not involved in decision-making, little or nothing was expected of them, and the underlying causes of poverty were not addressed.

The change toward participatory development meant mobilizing communities or initiating group formation so that members, especially the poor and marginalized, could become more proactive. In Asia, this grew out of the 1960s cooperative movement in Bangladesh; and it grew into success stories, such as the 1970s community forestry program in Nepal and the Grameen Bank in Bangladesh. From that model followed the rapid expansion of microcredit around the world.

The idea of community mobilization was to draw together people who had been isolated by the factors that perpetuated their poverty. While causes of their poverty could very well have come from the community, the community could also some provide ways to help alleviate the poverty. In any case, the targeted groups were inextricable from the community context. Instead of isolating them to help them, it was more effective to encourage people to organize and work together; to be proactive while identifying problems, needs, priorities, goals, and ideas; and to make, implement, and monitor plans. The idea was, as participants developed skills and resources, they would be better prepared to deal with livelihood development in the mainstream: for example, they would be able to cut out middlemen and loan sharks and learn to how to use microcredit, and they would be able to deal with banks, credit, and savings. Such programs also typically became more holistic, dealing with education, healthcare, and other capacity development, whether in agriculture, forestry, water management, environment, sanitation, fisheries, or crafts and trades. Similar proactive problem-solving attitudes were promoted, with the community or group becoming the vehicle for change and aid delivery.

A goal of working with such groups was the empowerment of individuals and of communities and their constituent parts. Empowerment is a result of participation in decision-making. "An empowered person is one who can take initiative, exert leadership, display confidence, solve new problems, mobilize resources and undertake new actions" (Saxena 2011: 32). At its heart, the idea of community participation and empowerment is the reduction of vulnerabilities. However, those may be identified and prioritized by the people themselves, who may set goals such as making more income, being able to grow enough food, having better health care, escaping exploitation by the landowner, making it easier for children to go to school, settling disputes over land, or preventing the farmland from washing away in floods. Participating in decision-making and working together to reach common goals, with any amount of success, can be empowering.

As the NGOs led the way in implementing participatory approaches, governments and international donor agencies started to incorporate them in their programs. Participation then became a condition for the financing of projects. In the 1990s, participation no longer represented a threat, and it acquired its place in the then-dominant institutional practices and discourses—in other words, it became mainstream (Sliwinski 2010: 179). The United Nations and other donor agencies, governments, and NGOs took on more lateral strategies, including participation in their own policies and programming.

Over the same decades, community participation has become a wide field of study for academics and practitioners. It is now a worldwide discipline in countless university departments and among researchers, field workers, and NGOs on the ground. There are masters and doctoral programs; organizations, workshops, and conferences; and countless books, journals, and online resources solely on the subject of participation and its uses and applications in all sectors. However, there is no standardized blueprint for a community participation program. It needs to be specific to every place, time, and circumstance.

While there still is no blueprint for or standardized definition of "community participation," many ideas have been put forward. Cernea has described community participation as "empowering people to mobilize their own capacities, be social actors rather than be passive subjects, manage the resources, make decisions, and control the activities that affect their lives" (1985: 10). Another early source suggested that community "participation is a process through which stakeholders influence and share control over development initiatives and the decisions and resources which affect them" (World Bank 1996b: xi). As Cohen and Uphoff have pointed out, "Participation is not just an end in itself, but it is more than a means" (1980: 213–35). It is, at least, the process of developing local people's voices and engaging in joint analysis, decision-making, and action.

In postdisaster situations, community participation is possibly even more important, as it also functions as part of the social recovery.

Experience is increasingly demonstrating that an emergency is the time to expand, rather than reduce, participation, even if there is no formal policy framework for participation in place. By including properly structured community participation mechanisms, physical outcomes and the quality of oversight can actually be improved, especially when large sums of money are involved (Jha et al. 2010: 184).

Well-organized participation achieves several important things at once. It is not only about social justice, humanitarianism, and altruism; as Peter Oakley observes, "Greater participation is important to increase project efficiency and effectiveness, to encourage self-reliance among participants and to increase the numbers of people who potentially can benefit from development" (1991: 115).

Influencers

Influential Thinkers

Since the 1960s, change in development approaches has been influenced by innumerable experts on all continents. But two key thinkers in the community participation field stand out.

The first is the late Paulo Freire, a Brazilian educator specializing in adult learning and motivation. His philosophy of education and teaching was based on the concept of *conscientização* ("conscientization"), the process of raising people's awareness of power through participatory analysis of their problems and subsequent problem-solving. This transformative process treats the learner as a cocreator of the knowledge; "hence participation is both a means and an end" and a transfer of power, becoming an empowering process (Okui 2004: 3). Internationally, Freire still has significant influence on the theory of adult learning, development, and participation, with his 1970 book, *Pedagogy of the Oppressed*, continuing to be regarded as one of pedagogy's foundational texts. Freireian ideas underlie the whole participatory movement.

The second key thinker is Robert Chambers, professor and research associate in the Institute of Development Studies at the University of Sussex, and still one of the most widely published and well-known participation experts. Chambers's early publications *Rural Development: Putting the Last First* (1983) and *Whose Reality Counts? Putting the First Last* (1997) were revolutionary, prodding scientists and other professionals to improve their own understanding and areas of expertise by listening first to farmers and other local people, then handing the pointer stick over to them, devolving their own power. From Chambers came the term participatory rural appraisal (PRA), a "family of approaches and methods to enable local people to share, enhance and analyze their knowledge of life and conditions, to plan and to act" (Chambers 1974: 953). From PRA came numerous other tools and approaches with similar purposes, including Participatory Learning and Action (PLA), popular theater, action reflection, and appreciative inquiry. Chambers has been described as "development's best friend" (Cornwall and Scoones 2011: 13).

Influential Case Studies

Pakistan has produced at least two models of community participation that are held in high esteem and replicated around the world: the Aga Khan Rural Support Program (AKRSP) and the Camilla Cooperative Movement. The AKRSP was pioneered in 1982 in the Northern Areas (now Gilgit-Baltistan) by Shoaib Sultan Khan. Khan credited the AKRSP approach to the German Raiffeisen model for cooperatives, which had begun in the early 1800s in response to crop failure and famine. The AKRSP used the same principles—namely "establishing a partnership, making collaboration and assistance dependent on villagers, first fulfilling obligations and their entering into a series of dialogues through village organizations to identify their needs" (Khan 1990: 2). In this way, the AKRSP established a partnership in which both partners had demanding roles and responsibilities. The AKRSP went on to establish over two thousand village organizations in the Hindu Kush, Karakorum, and Himalayan mountain ranges. As partners, villagers improved their agriculture, health, education, and livelihood development. Khan explained: "While building an irrigation channel, road or reclaiming land, etc., the villagers are also building their own local institution" (Murphy Thomas 1994: 4).

In the 1960s, Shoaib Sultan Khan's mentor, the late Ahktar Hameed Khan (no relation), founded the Camilla Cooperative Movement among the poor in what was then East Pakistan, now Bangladesh. After the separation of East Pakistan, Khan returned to Pakistan and, in 1980, founded the Orangi Pilot Project (OPP) in a Karachi slum. The OPP went on to become a model for urban slum and unplanned settlement development around the world.

In *Personal Reminiscences of Change*, Khan explained how he started his work: "I first wandered around in the Orangi slums, educating myself. Gradually, I learnt what sort of people were living there, their problems, what they thought of these problems, what was being done about them, and what they were doing for themselves" (Murphy Thomas 1995: 71). Through participatory processes, the OPP mobilized Orangi's one million residents to solve their own problems. The OPP introduced self-financed, self-built sanitation facilities, low-cost housing, basic health services, women's work centers, family enterprise, and credit. Years later, it was observed by an OPP proponent that "this transformation has happened because we believed there is tremendous potential within the poor" (AHKRC 2010: 207).

Influential Books

Two ground-breaking and oft-cited books set off two related movements, but extended and applied their ideas in different contexts—one to disaster situations, and the other to situations with conflict:

Rising From the Ashes: Development Strategies in Times of Disaster (1989), by Mary B. Anderson and Peter J. Woodrow, shows how to gain a balanced understanding of locations, situations, and communities in all contexts, with or without a disaster. Anderson and Woodrow present a framework for identifying capacities—skills, attitudes, and resources that can be put to use when designing or evaluating projects. Anderson and Woodrow also urge aid agencies to gain knowledge of the local people's vulnerabilities, problems, and weaknesses, so that capacities can be used to reduce these vulnerabilities: "Development is the process by which vulnerabilities are reduced and capacities increased" (1989: 12).

Do No Harm: How Aid Can Support Peace or War (1999), also by Mary B. Anderson, transfers and applies main ideas from *Rising from the Ashes*. In *Do No Harm*, Anderson encourages aid agencies to see both the "dividers" that separate people and the "connectors" that bring them together. As her title suggests, Anderson argues that assistance can maintain or strengthen existing unity. But she also warns that, if handled inappropriately, aid can spark or add to frictions, disputes, hostilities, or open conflict: "Aid workers should try to identify local capacities for peace and connectors and design their aid programs to support and reinforce them" (146). Adopted from the field of medical ethics, "do no harm" can be applied in poverty alleviation or for disaster assistance in any sector. As we found in PERRP, the principle works equally well in disaster reconstruction. For example, despite being heterogeneous and conflict-prone, communities almost always had strong capacities or connectors, and they had local elders or other influential people with reputations for conflict prevention and resolution.

In short, it is recognized that community participation in a structured, well-organized program creates better decisions that get better results: "Local people are all too familiar with their community needs and problems. They have the greatest stake in what happens" (Murphy Thomas 2013a: 1). Participating in projects can build skills and create opportunities, and both the involved agencies and beneficiaries can gain knowledge and understanding.

Participation Issues

Almost as soon as participation caught on in the development field, criticism about its use started. As early as 1974, Chambers was already writing about "the gap between rhetoric and reality" that needed to be narrowed (85). The word "participation" was being used to mean just about any sort of activity and was losing its original intent. By the mid-1980s, "participation ascended to the pantheon of development buzzwords, catchphrases, [and] ... euphemisms" (Leal 2011: 70). Others suggest that "community participation" has become a contaminated term (Stiefel and Wolfe 2011: 29).

Now, more than fifty years after it entered the development lexicon, it could be virtually impossible to find a policy, program, plan, proposal, report, or project that does not claim to include participation, regardless of sector. And while participation is still widely promoted, so too is the literature criticizing its use and misuse.

Along the way, it has been recognized that there are different types and degrees of participation. Different sources (Shapan 1992; Pretty et al. 1995; Satterthwaite 1995; Murphy Thomas 2012a) have presented typologies of participation, which identify ways that participation occurs, the effects these can have, and to what degree. There are instances where groups mobilize and undertake their own initiatives or are mobilized by others to make decisions and act together. However, there are many other examples where communities are said to have participated, but it is in name only. These include situations when only representatives talk with each other; when local people are only listening or present when something is announced; or when local people are only asked to give information, time, labor, or other resources, but they are otherwise not involved in analysis or decision-making.

Use and Misuse of the Phrase "Community Participation"

To illustrate some of the ways in which the term "community participation" is used and misused, I include below examples from general earthquake reconstruction in Pakistan. These examples show how "participation" is sometimes used as a colloquial or generic label, even when the community did not participate at all.

A donor agency having earthquake-destroyed schools rebuilt by contractors stated that these schools were being constructed with "community participation." Upon inquiry in some of those project villages, it was found that villagers knew very little about the school that was being built, had no knowledge about who the donor and construction contractor were, and had no community group to help it happen. If a problem arose, a contractor's representative would go to somebody living nearby—an influential person or Department of Education official—but local individuals or officials often could not solve the problem for many reasons. In most of the reconstruction, this was the extent of participation, and often resulted in unresolved problems that led to conflict, stalled construction, or produced court cases. As PERRP went on to show, many of the stoppages were unnecessary: a structured program of community participation could have prevented many potential problems.

There are times when the word "participation" is considered simply fashionable, or when the value of community participation is known but is still scorned. One government agency official in earthquake reconstruction facetiously claimed to have community participation in his programing. He remarked, "Whenever we have any problems with those [community] people, we just send in the police." Unfortunately, this was true. This approach invariably involved violence and coercion, causing many more problems and losses for the local people. The official then mocked PERRP's community participation, adding, "Why are you bothering with all these community meetings and talking with villagers? It's such a waste of time."

Some sources use the word "participation" to validate what they have already decided. One NGO planned to provide communities with livestock to replace those lost or killed in the earthquake. They claimed to have reached their recommendations based on what they called "community participation"—but what they actually did was take their own questionnaire into the project area and have individuals answer the questions. They then took the answers away, analyzed the data themselves, and presented the results to donors and others as if they had come from the community.

In some participation efforts, individuals may benefit, but not the community. For the first years following the earthquake, countless projects gave away a cow, a shelter, a water tank, a small grant, seeds and fertilizer, or fruit trees, with nothing expected of the community. Since a community leader might have called a meeting or helped identify recipients, and people in the vicinity accepted these gifts, some called this "community participation." At best, the gifts may have had good results for individuals, but nothing was improved for the community as a whole.

Sometimes the idea was just to give away donor money and hope for the best. One donor agency's idea of community participation was to grant a block of money to people in a village and, giving them few criteria, let them figure out how to spend it. Elite capture was practically the norm, with enthusiastic participation mistaken as community-building. Decision-making was based on the most persuasive people's ideas, and sometimes these people had the block grant money spent on their favorite projects. In one place, a powerful man had a road built to his house. In another, a water storage tank was built on private property, limiting water access for others. In a few cases, the money was disbursed among the people, but there was nothing to show for it.

Some organizations have it the wrong way around. If participation doesn't happen at the beginning, it is highly unlikely to happen at the end. One organization, without knowing any community priorities or consulting with any local people, decided they could contribute by building a short link road to a certain community. The project hired and paid local people to do the labor, which the agency called "community participation." However, the organization made all the decisions, and no local group was consulted or included. After construction was complete, the agency asked the people to form a committee to maintain the road. To comply, influential people in the community just put a few names—their own family members—on paper, but did no maintenance at all.

What Went Wrong and Why?

The main controversies and issues regarding "participation" can be grouped into a few causes: simple lack of awareness, lack of know-how and support, lack of clarity and specificity, and deliberate obstacles.

- **Lack of awareness:** In many cases, it simply is not known that participation is an actual field of study and practice, a movement with a history, expectations, attitudes, and many accompanying tools. There is just no awareness of this as a discipline in itself; the word "participation" is only used in a generic or colloquial manner of speaking.
- **Lack of know-how and support:** In other cases, people may have a little knowledge about what should or could be done to facilitate community participation, but they either do not know how to go about it or are in a situation where there is little or no support for it. It is quite common for projects to be designed without the insights and input of local people, and the resulting plans, schedules, budgets, and processes don't leave room for participation, so it doesn't happen. Decision makers may see no reason for incorporating participation, and they might fail to see the benefits of doing so.
- **Lack of clarity and specificity:** Some participation efforts suffer from what scholars called "lack of specificity": that is, while participation is implemented, the specifics are missing (Cohen and Uphoff 1980: 213). It is not clear who is participating or what they are doing, what approaches or activities are involved, where and when participation is happening, what leadership or facilitation is involved, or what its purposes are. Too often, the expression is used in vague and generalized ways.
- **Deliberate obstacles:** The reality, Somesh Kumar states, is that "people's participation takes place in a socio-political context. A host of factors have been identified as obstacles to participation." Some of the obstacles may come from administrative systems that rigidly maintain their top-down, blueprint-style processes, while others may come from within a social structure in which marginalization is the norm. Kumar adds: "Most of participatory development fails to take into account the large obstacles and hence the impact is hardly sustainable and pervasive" (2002: 29).

People's participation does not happen only due to lack of know-how: it is not uncommon for community participation to face opposition, especially by those who are more powerful. The opposers can either be subtle or forthright in refusing participation. Depending on their own area of expertise, their refusal is rationalized by statements such as "those [poor, uneducated] people don't know anything about [health, science, education, engineering, building design, economics, management, etc.]; only we professionals have the education and skill needed." Such an attitude can come from a lack of sensitization through their own education, limited exposure to actual participation, or earlier exposure to something called "participation" that they considered a failure or threat. After so many decades of at least the rhetoric of participation, a growing number of officials or other decision makers have already experienced earlier participatory projects that they perceive as failed—although the "failure" may have been a case of organized communities using newly gained voices and a sense of power that threatened the same decision makers' authority. As these decision makers see it, now it is participation that has been imposed on them top-down, and they reject it. In PERRP, this was the case with the Department of Health, which refused to allow a full community participation program to go along with the reconstruction of health facilities (see the anecdote "No to Community Participation!").

Sometimes, it is the donor and implementing agencies themselves who fail to seek out participation; they have a misplaced notion that people won't or can't participate—that they have no time, skills, or interest in participating. Harvey, Baghri, and Reed discuss this mistreatment: "Agencies sometimes even create disincentives for participation, simply by their treatment of community members. If people are treated as being helpless they are more likely to act as if they are" (2005: 178).

Opposition to people's participation can come from different kinds of reasoning. In some cases, it is a matter of power—and refusal to relinquish or share it. Some reasons include: "We don't want them [community people] because they will just interfere and tell us what to do." "You don't need to ask the people. I know everything you need to know." "Don't bother trying, the powerful will just dominate anyway." "It will just raise people's expectations and they will start demanding everything from us." Other opposition comes from the mistaken belief that participation costs extra time and money: "It will take too much time and bother, and will just slow us down. We just want to get on with the job, to get construction done!" "Getting the people involved will just open cans of worms, a Pandora's box of problems." All such concerns and complaints were made by a few people at the beginning of PERRP.

However, as the PERRP social component demonstrated, these critiques were countered through structured, systematic, clear, and inclusive participation. Our work demonstrated how, if appropriately planned and implemented, community participation can save time, prevent situations that can slow or stop reconstruction projects, and also save local people from a lot of trouble that happens on construction sites. With the project completed in six years, community participation in PERRP took no extra time and was only a small fraction of total project costs.

As stated above, sociopolitical contexts can create obstacles for participation. In parts of the world, participation is akin to revolution. At times, participation is seen as inciting people and is a threat to the status quo (see the anecdote Myanmar—"What is This?!").

Still, there is criticism of participation from different angles. A book by Bill Cooke and Uma Kothari called *Participation: The New Tyranny?* (2001) spawned a wave of such criticism. As suggested by the title, a few have questioned if participation has become just another form of tyranny: local people may be involved, but who controls the methodologies, agenda, and decision-making? And do these methodologies, agendas, and decisions reinforce existing divisions and inequalities, so that the better-off still benefit more than others?

In response to Cooke and Kothari, Samuel Hickey and Giles Mohan wrote an essay called "Towards Participation as Transformation: Critical Themes and Challenges" (2004). This text too made waves in the literature. Sarah C. White states: "The idea of participation as empowerment is that the practical experience of being involved in considering options, making decisions, and taking collective action . . . is itself transformative" (2011: 60). Despite doubts expressed by some, there are many others who are witness to the changes that occur when community participation is in practice. They are optimistic and argue that the transformation process is still happening—even maturing: "the evidence so far in the new millennium suggests that participation has actually deepened and extended its role in development, with a new range of approaches to participation emerging across theory, policy and practice (however, although characterized as tyrannical, this mainstreaming and spread are highly uneven)" (Hickey Mohan 2004: 3).

Why Does Participation Matter?

"As most donors support local-level work with the most vulnerable and poorest people, 'community' has become the badge of honor that enables the organizations which receive the funds to claim that they are doing the right thing" (Cannon, Titz, and Kruger 2014: 93). Agency projects with community participation also imply a certain level of authenticity or quality—their results can be trusted because the people have had their say.

However, when community participation is claimed but is not actually implemented, or is implemented to such a small extent it hardly counts, there are two significant consequences: one, huge opportunities are missed for actual participation; two, it may simply be misleading to those who want actual participation to happen. It is like claiming to have made an investment in something when, in fact, no such investment was made. Perhaps more critical is that, without broader participation by community members, the most vocal members—who often belong to the majority group—tend to get their say, perpetuating the hierarchies and power arrangements that contribute to poverty. Participation at least allows a broader representation of the community, which is the first step in making those fundamental changes.

Critical Perspectives on Community and Participation

In discussing community participation, one of the most essential questions is: what does "community" mean? Ironically, this question may be one of the least-considered parts of the participation movement, yet communities are the reason for this practice. At the same time, in sociology, "community" has been a long-debated subject—one that is still not settled.

This section looks at the background, definitions, and ideas of community, then tackles recent challenges and critical perspectives, as well as what these suggest for community participation. So, what does "community" mean? A fundamental concept in sociology, the English word "community" emerges out of the Latin *communitas*—the notion of something being common or things having some things in common. The concept of community was central to the work of sociologists in the late nineteenth and early twentieth centuries, including Ferdinand Tönnies, Max Weber, Karl Mannheim, and Talcott Parsons: they emphasized collectivity, belonging, and the grouping of people who have traits or factors in common. Over time, dictionary definitions have reflected the idea of community as a form of unity. For instance, Merriam-Webster defines "community" as a "unified body of individuals" (n.d.), while the Cambridge Dictionary defines it as "the people living in one particular area or people who are considered as a unit" (n.d.). Community, of course, can refer both to people with a common location or to people with interests in common: for example, the Muslim community, the apple growers' community, the online community, or the academic community. However, "social scientists have actually never agreed on a definition of the concept of community" (Mulligan 2015: 342). As for me, I will simply quote from Oliver-Smith: "I have no intention here to become entangled in the long complex debate regarding the definition of community. For my purposes, the word community designates a group of interacting people who have something in common with one another, sharing similar understandings, values, life practices, histories and identities, within a certain framework of variation" (2005: 53).

Some literature on development, participation, and disaster risk reduction is bringing new challenges to the dictionary definition of community: "The first criticism of the idea of community is that it falsely implies unity, collaboration, cooperation and sharing" (Cannon et al. 2014: 101). As argued by Oliver-Smith, community "does not connote homogeneity and certainly does admit differences within and among communities. More than anything else, community is an outcome, a result of a shared past of varying lengths" (2014: 98). The most experienced organizations and individuals working with communities on the ground are well aware of the complexities.

In a definition that is much closer to reality in many parts of the world, especially in relation to development, disaster reconstruction, and recovery, communities are far more complex and variable:

> "Community" can be described as a group of people that recognizes itself or is recognized by outsiders as sharing common cultural, religious or other social features, backgrounds and interests, and that forms a collective identity with shared goals. However, what is externally perceived as a community might in fact be an entity with many sub-groups or communities. It might be divided into clans or castes or by social class, language or religion. A community might be inclusive and protective of its members; but it might also be socially controlling, making it difficult for subgroups, particularly minorities and marginalized groups, to express their opinions and claim their rights. (UNHCR 2008: 14)

The concept of a community comprising many subgroups describes many parts of the world, including the PERRP project area. It implies the need for agencies and projects to recognize not just communities but their subgroups, the arrangements of power, and the actors involved so that options and strategies can be chosen.

Definitions, Meaning, Language

What needs to be emphasized here is that this is a debate about one word in the English language. What does "community" mean to other cultures in other languages, as opposed to what sociologists interpret it to mean? One must also ask if understanding of the term is biased by the English language. For example, there is no one word in the Urdu language that directly translates as community in English. However, the Urdu vocabulary does contain similar concepts. There are words for the traits and factors that people have in common, including geographic location, and for the groups or networks that people belong to, such as castes, tribes, clans, religions, religious denominations, political affiliations, or *biradari* ("unity group"). The Urdu word *loge* (meaning "the people") then is attached to these words: meaning, for example, the people of the Raja caste, or the people of Swati tribe, or the Abbasi *biradari*. In any case, the English word community has crept into Urdu, perhaps due to its frequent use by donors, governments, and NGOs. In written Urdu material such as reports and newspaper articles, the word "community" is sometimes spelled out phonetically using the Urdu alphabet. It is still understood as an English word.

However, even without a translatable word, and even with the known divisions, differences, and conflicts in these communities, the local people involved with PERRP still showed strong characteristics of what is known in English as "community." They shared cultural norms, collectivist norms, religion, a sense of social and geographical belonging, and common values, goals, and priorities.

In this case, all groups also shared a strong desire to rebuild their health facilities or schools—a condition for their children to continue their schooling and for health services to be available in a safe environment. Even adversaries could find ways to come together for this purpose. In the project, there were several critical instances where community members who were long-standing rivals or enemies had to come together to settle related disputes, especially around land issues, before the project would proceed with design or construction. In such cases, when rivals risked losing the one thing they both wanted, ways were found to cooperate, revealing the few but strong—or strong enough—goals they had in common.

Critical Perspective: "Community Is a Myth"

Although debate about community has existed for a long time, in recent years, a limited but influential literature has taken a more radical look at the concept. Cannon et al., who argued that the word "community" falsely implies unity, collaboration, cooperation, and sharing, also posit that community is so widely misunderstood, misapplied, and misused that "much about the concept is a myth" (2014: 100).

According to Cannon, aid programs are too often stuck in the romanticized, idealized, dictionary-type definitions of community. He argues that "we must ditch the idea that it [community] is fluffy, warm and cuddly and can cure all ills" (2014: 1). But then this argument is taken much further: not only is the romanticized, idealized, warm-and-fluffy dictionary definition to be ditched, the word "community" should also discarded. As some would argue, this is throwing the baby out with the bathwater.

The "community as myth" literature discusses community in the general development scene, as well as in climate change and disaster reconstruction and recovery. While Titz, Cannon, and Kruger do state at one point that "we are not entirely against 'community' concepts as such" (2018: 3), the attention-getting titles of such publications do not reflect that opinion. Some sections in the World Disasters Report 2014 are titled "The Myth of Community?" and "What Is Wrong with Using 'Community'?" (Cannon et al. 2014: 93, 99), while the title of another paper is "Why Do We Pretend There Is 'Community'?" (Cannon 2014).

The community-is-a-myth argument is based on a few main points. The first point has already been discussed: that the warm-and-fluffy dictionary definitions of community are only idealized, romanticized notions. The second point is that, in reality, communities are hierarchical, with arrangements of power based on factors such as race, ethnicity, gender, class, caste, or age. These arrangements place some people in highly advantageous positions, while others have no power at all. And this power, or lack thereof, is related to underlying causes of poverty and vulnerability. In these ways, the elite continue to dominate, often capturing benefits for themselves and their own social groups, while the vulnerable are left out. And where communities are divided by such factors, "conflict, friction, intra-community exploitation and sub-groups are the norm," perpetuating the cycle (Cannon et al. 2014: 103).

The same scholars argue that these realities too often are not considered in the design or execution of projects. As Cannon et al. put it, "a great deal of 'community-based' activity (by NGOs, supported by donors, international development banks, etc.) fails to take into account the power relations that lead to division and conflict within the communities, and are often precisely the cause of the problems that the outside organization is trying to address" (1). They also argue that the terms "community" and "community-based" have become entrenched in local, national, and international aid planning and programming. Researchers, donors, NGOs, and others all claim to be working with communities or in a way that is community based. The authors point out that aid programs assume that these labels somehow legitimize whatever actions or activities are involved.

The trouble, they claim, is that the label "community" distracts from understanding the actual causes of problems: "A significant part of why some people are poor and vulnerable are the processes of exploitation and oppression that are going on in the so-called community. In other words, using the terminology itself is in danger of diverting attention from the causes of the very problems being addressed, and instead substituting a framing of problems that avoids looking at their causation" (Titz, Cannon, and Kruger 2018: 3).

In essence, the message is that the hierarchical power structure is so entrenched that it overwhelms the possibility of "community," at least in the idealized, warm-and-fluffy sense.

Not surprisingly, the validity of "community participation" is also questioned. Who in the community will participate? Cannon et al. state that "because of internal divisions and power relations, participation is almost likely to be distorted" (100). The importance of careful targeting is also emphasized: "If clarifying whom one is working with is a prerequisite of any serious participatory approach, then why not use a more precise vocabulary, be specific about the group one is working with and skip the term 'community' entirely" (Titz, Cannon, and Kruger 2018: 21).

Critical Perspective: Communities Are Real but Highly Complex

As someone with decades of community-based work in different countries, and as head of the community participation program in PERRP, I want to respond to the community-is-myth argument. To proceed, it is highly relevant to restate that all communities in the case of PERRP were in some of the most challenging conditions that exist anywhere: they were conservative, complex, heterogenous, conflict-prone, hierarchical communities with layers of power, wealth, and poverty. They were also squeezed in between neighboring countries with a long history of war, in a location with a long history of war and security and political tensions. Even so, as the rest of this book indicates, it was still possible for a project to facilitate unprecedented, representative participation to meet project goals and build local capacities for further development. I do not claim that PERRP broke up the layers of power, but for a few years at least, communities got experience in how power can be shifted and shared. As discussed in chapter 2, the PERRP social team first worked on understanding the social structure in each location, then it identified the blocs of power (see table 4.1) and how the project could feasibly influence power sharing, at least on a temporary basis. The experience of PERRP is suggestive of the potential impact that such power sharing could have if temporary projects were to be supported with long-term follow-through. PERRP was an example of how communities are not myths: they are real, just very complex.

However, it needs to be emphasized that the community-is-myth argument does raise many vital points for understanding the realities and complexities of communities. That content is of high value and is a long-overdue addition to the literature in development and disaster reconstruction and recovery, and it is frequently referenced herein. Examples include Cannon's appeal to "make [a] clear distinction between economic and social groups and not pretend that they do not exist" (2014:

2). Cannon et al. point out the importance of identifying and analyzing a community and its differences, conflicts, and power structures and how these could be "bridged whenever they constitute barriers to vulnerability reduction and disaster relief efforts" (2014: 113). At the heart of the issue is this: "Unless the inherent and integral power relations involved in the 'community' are actively understood and incorporated into the required process of transformation, then it is highly unlikely that . . . activities will have any significant impact" (Cannon, Titz, and Kruger 2014: 112).

The trouble is that, while these scholars provide detailed and accurate analyses of the problems, the solutions they provide are counterproductive. These scholars focus only on what is wrong with the word "community" and what to do about it, when the same soapbox could be used for a strong appeal for improved education, training, and understanding of the realities of communities, as this subject matter is so well presented in the same writing. The appeal could extend to improving policies, research, funding, practice, and everything else it takes to help the vulnerable. Instead, the main focus is simply on the term community and why it is wrong or misleading to use it.

In response, I contend that arguing for the dismissal of community as a concept is not at all warranted. The perception of communities being only harmonious, homogenous, and "warm and fluffy" may very well be a myth, but communities, as highly complex entities, are real. My perspective aligns with that of Faas and Marino: "Abandoning community altogether would not only create a gaping and nearly untraversable chasm in the idiomatic vernacular but also we fear too strong a language in opposition to the community concept metaphor telegraphs a hostility, however inadvertently, toward those who use it to mobilize scarce social, political and material resources to confront power and contest structural violence. As we see it, 'community' can be a beacon signaling pathways to the good and uncharted routes to the otherwise" (2020: 483).

Discussed in more detail below are the main reasons for my stance. The other authors' definitions of "community" and "power" are too limited, and the few alternatives suggested are weak and subject to the same power structures. If the word community were to be thrown out, it would be a setback in decades of efforts to reverse the top-down trends; talk of discarding community may already be creating a vacuum, or even intimidation, in the field of community work.

Power and Capacity

In the community-is-myth literature, only the negative side of "community" is considered, and power is discussed only as something oppressive, exploitive, and destructive. In reality, there are many types and degrees of power, and that power is dynamic. This oversight presents a distorted or partial view of a community. It makes no allowance for local ideas of community or people's understanding of their own community, and it speaks as if communities are not already very aware of—and dealing with—their own complex power structures. Perhaps many agencies do not even imagine that communities have their own informal peacekeepers or power moderators. And certainly far more effort is needed to understand power: the types and degrees of power, the variety of power structures, and how even the latter can work to alleviate some of the problems they cause.

The extremely important view missing is that within communities—even in some of the most highly stratified, conflict-ridden communities such as in PERRP—there are capacities and potential for cooperation. One especially valuable resource are the local people who are known and respected for their moderating influence. These are the people who are not only well aware of the community's power structure but are able to use their own power and know-how to work within those structures, and even to bring a balance of power into conflict resolution. They use their skills in negotiation, mediation, and conflict prevention to call on history, customs, beliefs, or other arguments to influence others; they also act as an important role model for others. In PERRP there were countless examples of these respected moderators. See ethnographies, pages 33, 76, 172, 248.

Projects planning to work with communities need to recognize these moderators and encourage their leadership and influence in such roles, with the project providing support and a neutral platform, at least on a temporary basis. From this platform, local mediators and community members can work together to solve problems and achieve something new. In providing the neutral platform, the project can provide structure and a transparent process, and it can prompt participants to make and agree to the "rules of the game." While they may also pick up new skills from the project, such moderators will remain long after the project has been finished. After playing this leadership role on a more public platform than normal, not only may their prominence as influencers have grown, but others may have learned from their example as well.

In PERRP's six-year time frame, local power structures could not be changed and the underlying causes of vulnerability could not be wholly alleviated—but presenting new possibilities and strengthening new skills and resources in the community could prompt other changes. The likelihood of lasting change also depended on long-term follow-through with a supporting group—an NGO, government agency, or umbrella group—that could continue to provide a neutral facilitating platform, which did not happen in the case of PERRP, as explained in chapter 4.

As the community-is-myth argument points out, and as discussed in chapter 4, elite capture is a fact of life in many kinds of projects. Elite capture can be especially prevalent in disaster reconstruction, as such projects involve large amounts of money and valuable construction materials, equipment, jobs, and services. In these situations, the better-off can to try divert advantages to themselves or their own social groups. Projects can control this by looking ahead and preparing appropriately.

In PERRP, forms of attempted elite capture included instances in which head teachers insisted only they—without community members—be the decision makers in the construction of their new school; times when local "big men" demanded the construction contractor divert project resources for repairs or construction on their private property; and occasions in which local people made organized efforts to demand jobs. But analyses conducted by the social and technical teams at the beginning of the project helped foresee such problems (see the "What Could Go Wrong?" analysis in chapter 4). With this information, we built in measures to prevent or manage such problems. Other measures to prevent elite capture were implemented in communication protocols, in the responsibilities assigned to local committees, and in the field with social team presence in the communities and on construction sites.

Arguments about Semantics Don't Change Power Structures

While a few scholars make the case for dropping the word community, they suggest very few alternatives, and those that are offered lack specificity and would therefore add confusion. It is difficult to imagine how the sorts of alternative words suggested would improve understanding of the subject. A main source states, "It would be more honest and more helpful to speak of 'people-centered' rather than 'community-based' approaches or better still, to state exactly with whom and where one works. Examples given are 'why not target individuals or groups with specific characteristics rather than 'community,' such as 'school children and their parents when implementing a school feeding program'; 'all women in a given village,' or 'all immediate neighbors in a block of streets'?" (Titz, Cannon, and Kruger 2018: 22–23).

Why not target such groups? This approach would not improve the situation as any such sub-groups would still be subject to the same power structures that exist in the community. As demonstrated in PERRP, even a single school can be divided into blocs of power: all the women in a given village may be just as representative of blocs of power as the men, or neighbors in close proximity may still be divided. When choosing sub-groups, how could one avoid selecting people or places based on race, ethnicity, kinship, or any other factors that divide communities and reinforce the hierarchy? This reality highlights the priority need to understand the power structure and develop strategies to have it shifted and shared. Effective community participation still depends on understanding and dealing with these arrangements of power.

Dropping the word community—and, in effect, going back to referring to targeted groups—would take us back decades, back to when targeting was the modus operandi in aid work. Back then, it was thought that the best way to help was to strictly target women, the landless, the poorest of the poor, people with disabilities, and so on. But the results such targeted efforts achieved were less than desired, which was one of the main reasons for shifting to a community emphasis. Many learned that you cannot effectively help people by separating them into target groups, or isolating them from contexts, as many causes of and solutions to their problems may lie in that same community. Such targeting also overlooks the many opportunities and resources there can be in any community and would go back to the top-down approach.

Given that so much of the local and international donor aid policy, planning, and programming is directed at the community level—at least in rhetoric—and that there is an influential call to drop the word community without providing realistic alternatives, there could be counterproductive results—namely, a vacuum. Many, including communities and the governments and NGOs that work at the community level, would be left to ask, "What now?" Getting rid of community could already be tying decision makers' hands, causing hesitation or even intimidation as they wonder: "If we keep using the words community and community-based and some such vocabulary, will we be misunderstood as being uninformed, or out of touch? What will we do?"

In any case, "community" is forever in English speakers' minds as an everyday word, a kind of shorthand or catchall phrase to refer to groups of people, however they may be constituted. Rest assured, the word community—and its equivalent in other languages—will not go away. As a word, it is an important placeholder between individuals, families, and all outside forces, whether it refers to harmonious units or those ridden with divisions and differences.

More Suggestions and Recommendations

For more detailed, practical direction on implementing community participation in a disaster reconstruction project, see this book's conclusion. It combines the lessons learned from many experiences, including from

PERRP's own field-based social mobilizers, engineers, and construction managers.

An Embankment Alignment in Bangladesh

Despite decades of donor agencies, government agencies, NGOs, and other groups promoting community participation and consultation with stakeholders, these processes frequently are not included at all.

In 1999, the Canadian International Development Agency (CIDA)—acting as a donor agency—and the Government of Bangladesh's Water Development Board (BWDB) decided to construct a new twenty-mile flood control embankment. The country was already crisscrossed by flood control embankments, but they were so poorly maintained that they had to be continually replaced. With this in mind, the BWDB and CIDA had decided they did not want this to be just another embankment construction project: they wanted to do an experiment. What they wanted to find out was if a construction project took participatory approaches with the local people, could that participation lead to better maintenance of flood embankments? Through a competitive tendering process, they contracted a large Canadian engineering company, but stipulated that the work had to be headed by a social expert, not an engineer. I was hired as the project manager.

What CIDA and the engineering company did not know—and what the BWDB had ignored—was that there was a far bigger and more immediate problem than long-term maintenance: extreme opposition to the embankment alignment that had been chosen. This opposition was so serious that, upon our first visit to the project area, my deputy manager (chief engineer) and I were met with armed opposition. Traveling by boat up the Dampara River, we were met by several dozen men carrying weapons, who were waiting on shore and warning us not to land. If we stepped foot onto the land, they said, they would shoot. Standing in the boat facing the crowd onshore, it was up to me to figure out what to do next.

I was curious to know why they were so upset. What exactly was wrong? I wanted to hear from these people, but as the river current was strong, the roar of our boat motor made it difficult to hear their words. I explained over the roar that we wanted to talk and understand their opposition and determine if anything could be done about their complaints. The men relented and invited us to come ashore, where we sat down together, joined by dozens of other villagers to listen.

Over the next few hours, we heard the details about how the BWDB surveyors had arrived two years previously, surveyed the land, and decided where the embankment would go without any local consultation. They did this even though over a hundred thousand people would be affected by the project. Few opposed a new embankment as it would stop the frequent destructive flooding. Their problem was with the alignment that the BWDB had imposed: it would go right through the middle of prime crop land, destroying it. We also heard their ideas about an alternative route for the embankment which would take it off the prime crop land and be closer to the river. Additionally, they pointed out extensive, complex land ownership issues. Land records had not been kept up to date, and with the division of land due to inheritances, earlier land boundaries no longer applied. Further discussion resulted in a long list of specific complaints, and for each complaint, we also collected their proposed solutions. Departing, I emphasized that we were making no promises but would be back to talk again.

Back at the office in Dhaka, we were immediately at loggerheads. All of the villagers' complaints and requested solutions seemed reasonable to me, but it was practically unheard of to make changes once the BWDB had made its decisions. After all, the project had already been designed to meet BWDB specifications, and BWDB, CIDA, and the engineering firm had no experience with getting villagers to participate in such decision-making. At first, the chief engineer flatly rejected all the requests. At a meeting attended by him and CIDA representatives, I pointed out there were three options. The first option would be to proceed as planned; however, due to the likelihood of violent opposition, that option was discounted. The second option would be to abandon construction completely, which would be the more likely choice for BWDB. The third option was to listen to the people and try to find alternative solutions. CIDA said, "Look at those options. Are there any feasible solutions?"

As no one wanted to walk away from the project, I then worked intensely with the engineering team to understand their refusal to accept the complaints and ideas of the villagers. They were mostly concerned that the villagers' preference would put the earthen embankment too close to the water. Due to river behavior, they said, an embankment in the villagers' proposed location would be eaten away by the current. Ceding that some compromise would be needed for the project to go ahead, the engineers then offered two criteria for a new alignment to be acceptable: 1) it would have to be certain distances from the river, as would be identified in each location by the engineers, and 2) everyone had to come to an agreement about the choice. To get this common agreement, an engineer's assessment would need to determine that the embankment was far enough from the river to avoid risk, and the area's complex land ownership issues would need to be settled in a timely manner between monsoon seasons, with the embankment being built on land with free and clear title. If villagers agreed to these two criteria, the project would go ahead.

We took this offer back to the original location, and to eight other locations along the line of the proposed embankment, to start negotiation for a new alignment based on the engineers' criteria. With the help of a retired local deputy commissioner—who was both an expert in land acquisition and a member of the community—the project was able to reduce or eliminate many of the local people's concerns by introducing several innovations.

Following the engineer's criteria and facilitated by the social mobilizers, we asked the hundreds of landowners to negotiate the alignment of the new flood embankment among themselves, as that would also determine the land that needed to be acquired. After coming to an agreement involving 322 plots with 1,200 owners and co-owners, their proposed alignment and plots of land were resurveyed by the government, and new land ownership documents were issued on the spot. An assessment of potential asset loss was conducted and villagers were compensated for these losses on the spot, before construction started—an occurrence that was unprecedented in Bangladesh.

In the end, the new alignment suited everyone. The engineers deemed it technically sound. Almost no crop land was lost, no resettlement was needed, and owners received cash payment right away, before construction started. Land records were updated on the spot, saving years of costly court battles. The project facilitated both community participation and government cooperation. Over ten thousand people had their first major flood protection; the embankment saved their homesteads and crops and provided them with the first road in the area. The project was completed within the budget and within the three-year schedule.

This is an example of two sets of knowledge that could have clashed in practice. The engineers had technical knowledge and enacted top-down practices of standard operating procedures: they worked according to predetermined orders from higher levels. In contrast, the sociocultural specialists' primary concerns were bottom-up: they focused on respect, social justice, and the protection of the people, their land, and their wishes. In this case, the gap between the two disciplines was closed when each party recognized that cooperation could lead to the fulfillment of everyone's objectives.

In community projects, the subject of power and how it is used or shared is an important consideration. Being the project manager put me in the most powerful position on the team, giving me the authority to ask the project engineers to reconsider their choices. Had an engineer been the project manager, as is far more common, it is highly questionable how much influence a sociocultural specialist would have had—if one would have been involved in the project at all. It was the power of the donor and cooperation within the project that made this management arrangement possible.

My experience in this project, especially in land issues, strongly informed my work to settle land issues in the PERRP. Although there was no land acquisition in PERRP, the Bangladesh project's land acquisition expert demonstrated that it was possible to get cooperation from government officials to make things happen swiftly, especially if community members could come to agreement among themselves first.

As the project ended, the chief engineer and I went to the communities along the embankment to say goodbye. One of the men, who had first met us on the riverbank brandishing an old rifle in his hands, now apologized to us for greeting us that way. He said, "We just never imagined anybody would listen to us back then. But you did."

Syria—"We're Not Too Happy You're Here"

Though the rise of participation in the development field was heralded by many as the solution to countless existing problems, it was not seen that way by others.

In the late 1990s, I was contracted as a consultant by two Rome-based UN agencies: the Food and Agriculture Organization (FAO) and the World Food Program. I was asked to go to Syria to train the Syrian department of agriculture's rural extension workers to more effectively engage farmers. I was told by staff in Rome that, on visits to their Syrian field offices and agriculture projects, they had observed that extension workers had minimal contact with farmers—and when they did, they acted as if they were issuing orders to the farmers. It was a case of the educated, city-based extension workers simply telling the poor farmers what to do. The UN staff who had arranged for my consultancy had seen how the FAO and other agencies were playing a leading role in some countries in introducing participatory approaches, and they wanted their Syrian program to adopt similar approaches. But this view was not shared by all.

Upon arrival at the Damascus International Airport, I was met by the local FAO representative, who said, "Don't take this personally, but we are not very happy you are here. This community participation stuff is crazy and just the latest fad dumped on us from head office."

Despite his reluctance and doubt, we proceeded, setting up a workshop with around twenty key extension workers from across the country. In the workshop, after a couple of days of introductory exercises and discussions to break the ice, I demonstrated what I would be encouraging them to do with farmers—a participatory analysis. I had the extension workers analyze their professional situations, to think of problems, priorities, and resources; I asked them what needed to be done and how it could be done. Eager to talk, and apparently enthusiastic about taking new directions with farmers, they spoke openly about their own work problems. Despite the political conditions—this being in the days of the brutal dictator and president, Hafez al-Assad—they shared their perspectives, and such talk could have been dangerous, especially since all their problems as described stemmed from a lack of government support. As they said, their main problem was that they had practically no funding or resources to go to the rural areas for any work with the farmers.

Knowing that continuing to talk about solutions would be too political and thus too risky for employees of the regime, we instead went ahead with plans to visit a few rural communities. To avoid taking a crowd of extension workers to tiny villages, I would take multiple trips, with three or four different extension workers each time, to four or five places. The trips would be both a demonstration and an opportunity for practical experience: the plan was to sit down with a few farmers in each place, and have the newly trained extension workers talk with the farmers in a conversational style, explaining to them that this was only the start of a process. There would then be follow-up meetings in which farmers could talk more about their problems and work toward solutions. That was the plan with these extension workers, but soon that plan went far off the rails.

Despite the plan to go to the villages as discreetly as possible, several UN vehicles showed up to take all trainees all at once, and soon we were in several large, white UN vehicles traveling in a presidential-looking convoy up the highway out of Damascus. Not only did the trip turn out very differently than had been agreed, so too did its result.

About an hour north, in the hills, we arrived at a community hall building and were ushered inside to be greeted by an audience of a few hundred poor men, women, and children, and then I myself and a translator were taken directly to a podium at the front to give a speech. Unprepared for this, I talked to the audience about why I was in Syria, describing the new training program and the process that extension workers would be following. Soon there was a rumbling in the audience, and people were angrily talking among themselves, clearly disturbed. As this talk escalated, one of the senior extension workers came to me at the podium and suggested that we leave the building quickly, which we did. Outside, it was explained to me that whoever arranged this meeting had enticed people to attend by giving them the false story that a foreigner was coming from Damascus to give each family a cow. The rumble was people starting to demand the gifts they'd been promised. We returned to Damascus immediately.

I never found an explanation for what had happened. While the UN vehicles reportedly had been provided due to a miscommunication, clearly someone had decided that no community-based participation would happen. Unfortunately, this turned out to be another case of rural communities being misled and manipulated.

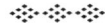

Ontario, Canada—The Potato Patch

Two of the most fundamental skills in community participation are how to listen to and talk with people. One summer, when I was a teenager, I convinced my father to let me take over the family's half-acre vegetable plot for one summer. I wanted to grow potatoes so that I could be a member of 4-H, an agriculture club—one of the few youth activities in our far-flung, rural, forested area. He agreed, but on the condition that I look after the potatoes, including all the necessary weeding. As the potato plants grew, so did the weeds. Despite his many reminders, I never got around to removing them.

One day—unannounced, and out of the ordinary for our region—a government agriculture officer showed up, making it his business to view any agriculture in sight. Assuming my father was responsible for the vegetable plot, his reaction was instant: "What have you let happen here? This is terrible! You've just let weeds grow like this!" Walking among the greenery, he proceeded to criticize my father for the mess, and demanded of him, "Well, do you at least know the names for these weeds? What about that one, and that one?" My father did not answer, and discreetly gestured for me not to say anything. Finally, the agriculture officer decided he'd had enough of such irresponsible people, and headed back to his car, adding another insult: "This is really a shame. You should not let your crop go like that."

As the agriculture officer left, I asked my dad why he hadn't said anything to him. "Doesn't matter," my dad said. "Just let the city people have their say." A young recent university graduate—who may never have grown anything himself—had talked down so disparagingly to my father, who had been growing potatoes his whole life. Neither my father nor I had mentioned that the lack of weeding was my fault.

We never saw that agriculture officer again. It wasn't until about fifteen years later when I first discovered Chambers's writing that I felt vindicated for being so upset by the agriculture officer's behavior. As Chambers wrote:

> Agriculture scientists, medical staff, teachers, officials, extension agents and others have believed that their knowledge was superior and that the knowledge of farmers and other local people was inferior; and that they could appraise and analyze but poor people could not. Many outsiders then either lectured, holding sticks and wagging fingers, or interviewed impatiently . . . not listening to more than immediate replies, if that. (1994a: 963)

I had seen city people treat us like this before. Chambers' book had been meant for workers exactly like our visitor, but it obviously had not been part of his education.

No to Community Participation!

Refusal by officials to allow community participation can come for different reasons: they may already have experience with "participation" being imposed on them, or they simply are not willing to share power.

Besides having many schools to reconstruct, PERRP was also assigned sixteen health facilities, which included fifteen Basic Health Units (BHUs) and one fifty-bed hospital. While the area had already been drastically underserviced by health facilities before the quake, the destruction of those facilities had greatly complicated overall medical and health conditions and added many more demands. When PERRP arrived a year after the quake, virtually all hospitals and clinics were operating either in what remained of heavily damaged buildings or in tents or the open air, struggling to provide the services needed. These services were in far higher demand following the quake.

PERRP had the same assignment for both schools and health facilities: both types of buildings were to include substantive community participation, which would facilitate construction and involve the community in improving local health and education. While the School Management Committees became highly active in helping with construction and hosting community activities with teachers, parents, and students (sometimes in the school building itself), such broad participation was not allowed for health facilities. PERRP had proposed to the Department of Health that committees at each health facility could help with construction, and that, with Department of Health training and leadership, the committees could become community promoters in preventative health—creating a new role in the area.

While another project did train the committees in health, and the Department of Health did allow the formation of temporary construction committees, Department of Health officials refused to allow community participation in health matters. One health official stated, "What do those village people know about health? They know nothing. We [doctors] are educated and know all about health, so there is no use for villagers to be involved."

The same official further explained the refusal of community participation. He and the others in charge had worked in the field long enough to have experienced the first wave of donor agency community participation efforts in the 1990s, and our efforts were now seen as an imposition. He explained how, at that time, another donor project had required community participation, but it was "nothing but trouble." All of a sudden, villagers had started showing up at the clinic demanding to know where the health worker was or why certain medicines were not in stock. "They started thinking they were the bosses. So, we just stopped all this participation idea," he explained.

Unfortunately, while the School Management Committees contributed greatly to school construction and thrived in including the community and parents in the improvement of education, no such activity or benefits occurred for the health facilities. PERRP could not trace the 1990s project that had been brought up by the district official, but it appeared to be one that led the people to raise their voices, but this backfired. This change may have come about too fast and too hard, to the extent that those in power could not accept it. The prior project simply had not dealt with the realities of local culture and its power, nor the ways in which the power structures could support, not compete with, each other.

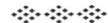

Myanmar—"What Is This?!"

In some parts of the world, the concept of participation is still considered revolutionary and so is associated with inciting populations and threatening the status quo—the reason I had a bit of trouble getting a visa for Myanmar. At the Myanmar embassy in Bangkok where I was applying for the visa, it was necessary to complete a detailed questionnaire, which included providing details of my work for the previous ten years. I dutifully filled it in, listing several short- and long-term assignments in Afghanistan, Pakistan, and Bangladesh, and presented it at the embassy's visa department, along with my passport and requisite photos.

From where I waited, I could see the visa officer talking about my application with another official, both bent over side by side at a desk in an adjoining office, carefully perusing what I'd written. When the visa officer came back to the counter, he called me up to the front of the line, and pointed at my application in his hand—now marked with many yellow highlighter slashes where I'd written the words "community participation." "What's this?" he demanded. I explained, "That's what I do as work: I show people how to organize and participate in projects together." As soon as I said it, I regretted it, as the look in his eyes seemed to confirm something with him—that I might be a threat—and he again told me to wait and returned to the same official, both of them turning to look at me silently. I was told to come back in three days.

Three days later, I was met by the same officer and two more officials. Although I'd applied for a tourist visa, they demanded to know what I planned to do in the country, should I get a visa. I told them my plans, showing them my itinerary, reservations and tickets for the boat trip planned on the Irrawaddy River. And no, positively not, I was not planning to do any work in communities; I was there only for a holiday.

This was in 2009, when the military government was still holding the Nobel Laureate Aung San Suu Kyi under house arrest. Given the intense pressure Myanmar was under due to the international sympathy for Aung San Suu Kyi, these officials seemed to think I might be one of those foreigners coming to organize the Burmese, to incite or mobilize people against the government. I was told to return the next day. It was not looking good as they still looked nervous about me, but I was relieved to be granted a visa. Keeping my promise, I spent most of my time on the water and only ventured onto land to visit exquisite temples.

Afghanistan—Afghan NGOs Start Up in Refugee Camps in Pakistan

No matter how dire circumstances may be, concentrating on capacities and participation can bring many benefits.

In the late 80s, I worked for an international NGO in the Afghan refugee camps in Pakistan, where over three million people had fled from war in Afghanistan. Like all the other NGOs, the one in which I worked provided help and services to the refugees. In our case, we provided schools, clinics, and water wells on the remote desert land where the camps had been established. Although I lived outside of the camps with a large extended family of Afghans, I worked in the camps, where I watched daily how the people coped with the crisis. Even before the war, most of the people who were now refugees were among the world's poorest, and some had already been in the camps for years. Despite these hardships, most still were self-assured and hospitable, with the strong sense of purpose and determination for which Afghans have been historically recognized.

One day, driving out of the vast camp, which was spread across the desert in all directions as far as the eye could see, a European colleague and I stopped the car and got out to look over the sand-colored view. Gesturing to the expanse of crude mud houses, he said, "If this happened in my country, I think we'd just lay down and die. We simply could not survive the misery of living in such a situation."

To put it into the development lexicon, the Afghans' positive attitude was one of their main capacities. They put this positive attitude to use in different ways to cope with or reduce their many vulnerabilities—the camp's living conditions, their treatment by camp authorities and police, and the poor supply of food and water, among other severe hardships.

As I worked with the NGO, I started encouraging the Afghans I met to put their strengths to work: to speak up about the problems they were facing in their camp neighborhoods, to get together with others, and to use the NGO as a platform to get solutions from the Pakistani administration of the camps, while also offering to help the administration however they could. A few took the suggestion, made their requests known to the administration, and offered to identify where help was most needed, mainly in the widows' section of the camp. These actions got results—notably, there was a visible improvement to the camp administration's food ration and water distribution.

In the NGO, and later for the UN Office for the Coordination of Humanitarian Affairs, I began training the refugees in related subjects: project design and management, proposal writing, monitoring and evaluation, and especially in how to form their own NGOs. The idea was to encourage Afghans to organize this way while they were still refugees, but especially to think ahead to when there would be peace in Afghanistan and they could go home. How then would they work in their own communities? How would they influence their fellow community members to work together for the good of the community?

This was at the time that the USSR was planning to withdraw their troops from Afghanistan, and the international aid community wanted Afghans to be prepared to take over the aid programming—a process of "Afghanization." Also, by then some leading Afghans were pleading with the aid community to "now let Afghans make the decisions for Afghanistan." Most of the staff of the international NGOs were Afghans, but more Afghan involvement was needed in the form of their own NGOs. To start, I was assigned to train and facilitate the first six Afghan groups who expressed an interest in organizing. However, even after months of work with each group, they still refused to meet one another. Reasons for the refusal were partly over historical differences such as ethnicity or sect, but even more significant was each refugee's war history. As the communist Afghan government was still at war with the resistance, it was a dangerous time for all. Refugees feared each other based on political alliances and what reputation those alliances had.

When the groups finally agreed to get together for the first time, about fifty people arrived, many bringing their bodyguards and their Kalashnikov rifles, which they leaned against the meeting room wall as they took their seats at the table. That first meeting was tense but productive, and from that day, the number of groups grew rapidly. Within a few months they did the unthinkable and formed their own community of NGOs: an umbrella group.

Within a few years, there were hundreds, and later thousands, of Afghan NGOs. A few of the Afghans involved then went on to become cabinet members in the post-Taliban government. They identified the NGO training they had as refugees as their main education for mobilizing and landing these top jobs. One of those individuals was the minister of Rural Reconstruction and Development, who located me nearly fifteen years later to help him set up the country's first Afghan rural development training center, which is where I was working when the Pakistan earthquake struck in 2005.

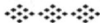

CHAPTER 4

The Social Component

Introduction

This chapter, on PERRP's social component, is presented in three parts. Part 1, "At the Community Level," looks at realities on the ground when PERRP arrived a year after the quake, including the necessary process of building and maintaining trust within the communities and figuring out with whom exactly the project should work.

As discussed in the previous chapter, the literature in international development and related fields has for decades been highlighting weaknesses in the practice of community participation. While its original intents and goals are still highly valid and pursued by many, much of what is claimed to be "participation" is implemented in rhetoric only. One reason for the resulting failures is the common misunderstanding of the word "community." In PERRP's community participation program, the sociocultural team placed emphasis on working with a clear concept of "community" and developing specific knowledge and understanding of each community that we worked in, including its broad contexts. We asked: who were each community's people, what was their social structure, how could they be motivated, and what would they do to participate? This chapter introduces the people and communities who were involved in PERRP and defines the communities in terms of geography, social composition, and arrangements of power.

This first part of the chapter, therefore, refers to the emphasis in chapter 2 on understanding the social structure, the community, and its subgroups—including how they function and relate to each other, especially in terms of power. While the literature often raises the subject of power structures, there is a dearth of case studies on recognizing and dealing with these structures. Part 1 provides a detailed example: it dissects how power arrangements were identified, describing each bloc of power and PERRP's process in helping to shift and share this power.

Part 2, "The Social Team and Process," details how the social component and community participation were organized, managed, and implemented; the social team's composition and duties; the participation process; and our facilitation of decision-making within the program. This part includes exercises that were conducted to develop understanding of the communities:

- a stakeholder analysis (table 4.3) identified those with a stake in the project, and responsibility for that consultation or participation
- a capacities/vulnerability and conflict sensitivity analysis (table 4.4) identified strengths, weaknesses, and opportunities; especially, to prevent or manage conflict
- a "What Could Go Wrong?" analysis (table 4.5) was conducted from several perspectives and was invaluable in foreseeing, preventing, and mitigating problems

Part 3, "How Communities Participated and Contributed—Monitoring," discusses community participation in different forms, including monitoring, giving time, making decisions, problem-solving, organizing school events, providing gifts in kind and cash, and preventing and resolving conflicts. It also looks at benefits to the committee members and what happened to the committees once the project was completed.

Part 1: At the Community Level

What PERRP Found on Arrival

Due to the time that it takes for a donor agency to prepare for a large project and then tender contracts, the PERRP project arrived on the ground thirteen months after the earthquake struck. The implementing agency was new to working in Pakistan but had engaged a local firm to assist in start-up. In November 2006, a small senior management team—myself included—arrived in Pakistan. In some ways, this late arrival was unfortunate; in other ways, it was a distinct advantage, as PERRP was able to learn from the many lessons this disaster response already had to teach. While PERRP was setting up basic project administration such as acquiring office space in Islamabad, setting up field offices, recruiting staff, and performing all the other needs to fast-track a construction project, the social program also was being established.

By the time PERRP started, the early emergency phase was over, but the general organizational response was still chaotic. Hundreds of NGOs and donor agencies were present, as were many United Nations agencies, and all were providing relief assistance in different sectors such as food, shelter, health, livelihoods, water, and sanitation. Of the hundreds of agencies, over fifty were carrying out hundreds of projects to help reconstruct houses and public buildings, but there was little coordination. Public mistrust was widespread, as much of the reconstruction had already stalled—if it had started at all. Even so, there was pressure to start construction, to get shovels in the ground and to complete the facilities. Several technical challenges complicated the construction work, including escalated prices and the region's difficult topography, altitude, and climate, as well as shortages of water, electricity, reliable construction contractors, skilled laborers, and materials.

As is common in disasters of this size, when large numbers of aid agencies arrived, prices skyrocketed for most needs—for example, office rentals, equipment, and construction supplies—and there was stiff competition for staff and construction contractors. There was an especially severe shortage of contractors who had experience managing construction to improved international industry standards. Skilled laborers were also in short supply in the project area due to the quantity of reconstruction underway, and there was a significant absence of skilled Pakistani laborers, as many were working in the Gulf States and elsewhere.

But there were additional challenges in simply implementing the project. One disadvantage of their late arrival was the immediate challenge of identifying which of the thousands of destroyed schools and health facilities PERRP would reconstruct. There had been a breakdown in data sharing, leaving government lists of the sites unreliable. Before PERRP arrived, many of the destroyed sites had already been assigned to other donor projects for reconstruction. Some of those had gone ahead with reconstruction, but in many instances, those sites had not been started and their plans were unknown. Agencies often did not inform Pakistan's Earthquake Reconstruction and Rehabilitation Authority (ERRA) of their intentions to go ahead or not, leaving lists of sites outdated. Using the ERRA lists, it took several months and innumerable visits to potential sites for PERRP to finalize the list of places—mainly schools—that the project would construct. In the meantime, PERRP staff concentrated on designing and constructing sixteen health facilities, which had been much easier to identify.

The problems with identifying potential sites were a symptom of a general lack of coordination. Coordination of reconstruction work was important due to the sheer number of agencies who were running hundreds of projects, but, as was widely acknowledged at the time, efforts to coordinate were not effective (Haiplik 2007). Still, for PERRP, the few coordination meetings that were held—roughly once a month for about six months—gave us a major advantage. At the meetings, NGO and donor agency representatives complained that most of their construction had serious problems and that many of their sites were already stalled, unable to proceed. Attending the meetings on behalf of PERRP, I found that the experiences of the other agencies could teach us many lessons; out of these meetings grew a long list of problems for PERRP to prevent and mitigate.

Some of the problems were simply a matter of agencies not doing their homework. One donor representative spoke in exasperation about communities fighting over land issues. However, when he was questioned about addressing the problems, his projects had no way to deal with them or with the people who were in conflict. He had never even heard of the government's Revenue Department or the *patwari*, who are the locally based government officials responsible for land matters. He had not done even this basic research.

In these meetings, there was practically no evidence that the agencies had considered the social side of construction. At this early formative stage, despite all these agencies and projects involved, PERRP was the only one with a dedicated social team that had a structured program specifically to deal with the communities during the design and construction phases. All in attendance at those meetings were administrators, engineers, architects, or construction managers. No doubt well versed in the technical aspects of design and construction, most were well-intentioned newcomers who were not at all familiar with the realities of Pakistani communities. Others were Pakistani professionals who were familiar with the social and cultural realities but were unable to adjust a project accordingly.

Many agency representatives expressed surprise and frustration over problems with local contractors and people in communities—yet, in many cases it seemed that their own agencies' lack of preparation that led to such problems. At each meeting, the same complaints were repeated. Many voiced exasperation with "inept" construction contractors, attempts to manipulate prices, cost overruns, contractors who did not follow designs, an inability to keep workers, and so on. But most of their complaints were of a social nature. There were major land issues, encroachment, violence, sabotage, fights among people in the community, conflicts between community people and the contractor that resulted in blocked access to the construction site, and court stay orders that halted construction. If these agencies sought solutions, they often left these attempts to construction workers, who did not have the skills needed to deal with such matters, or to the respective government departments, who were notorious for inaction.

From attendance at these early agency meetings, PERRP made its first checklist of potential problems, prevention strategies, and solutions. While starting work in the communities with the engineers, the social team also consulted a wide range of perspectives on other potential problems and what others advised as solutions (see table 4.5, "What Could Go Wrong?").

Relationships and Trust Building

For projects in these locations, trust is a crucial matter. When PERRP first visited communities at potential sites, one of the main challenges encountered was the mistrust from local people, which was expressed in public meetings. In almost every case, people said they doubted what PERRP representatives were saying. Over the months since the earthquake had happened, we were told, they had had many visitors from NGOs and government agencies. "Those visitors," they said, "like you, asked a lot of questions and said they would help us—but then they went away and never came back. So why should we believe you? How do we know if you actually plan to rebuild our school here?"

To this skepticism, PERRP representatives would explain that the government of Pakistan and the United States Agency for International Development (USAID), as the donor agency, had asked PERRP to come to this community and figure out if reconstruction was feasible. The people were informed that now that the technical and social assessments had been completed, it had been determined that this was a good place for reconstruction—but nothing required PERRP to build here. It was completely up to the community to decide to accept this project or not. The PERRP representatives would then explain the project and what would be expected of the community in terms of participation.

Once communities gave their official willingness to proceed, relations between community members and PERRP staff began to be established as community members watched on, wondering: "Will they do what they said they would do?" Confidence in the project grew once a rhythm was established—a plan was announced, then it was carried out and completed, and that cycle repeated itself many times. Staff members were in the communities daily, senior management and donor officials visited to meet the people, large public meetings were held, plans were shared, and rapport was established. Soon, community members responded with enthusiastic participation, as they saw PERRP doing what it said it would do.

For these kinds of relationships to become established, PERRP staff needed to show themselves to be credible and trustworthy. For both men and women from a range of social groups to trust the social team—whose members also came from multiple social groups—the project needed to consider a wide range of factors. These factors included, as discussed in chapter 2, the languages of the area; the cultural norms, especially those that define gender roles (*purdah*); and the roles of traditional informal leaders. Not only would these leaders bring important conflict resolution capacities to the project, but getting their buy-in would be a precondition for local people feeling comfortable with participating and authorized to do so. This also necessitated understanding the power structure and if there were ways to shift and share any of the power—as well as understanding the existing frictions and their underlying causes, and what the project would need to do, or not do, to avoid causing or increasing problems between local people. It was also essential for the project to have specific, structured conflict prevention and resolution approaches. Had PERRP not proceeded so cautiously in this unstable and politically charged environment, we could have caused significant security problems for the local people, and the project could have become another one of the many stalled or abandoned reconstruction efforts.

Whom to Work With

Any project with community participation needs to identify: With whom will the project work to initiate and facilitate participation? Who exactly will carry out the work on the ground? There can be many options to consider.

Whether long-term or short-term, disaster related or not, in sectors such as agriculture, water management, communications, housing, or health, it is common to subcontract some of the work to others, especially to locally based companies or NGOs. In projects implemented by NGOs or companies that have been contracted by donor agencies, the implementing agency's policy or contract will require, allow, or forbid subcontracting. In PERRP's contract, it was required that all design and construction work be subcontracted to Pakistani companies. For the PERRP social component, there was no requirement to subcontract the community mobilization, leaving the senior management team to decide.

Hiring locally is an important step in recognizing that capacities already exist in disaster-struck areas—and that these capacities can benefit the project and can be strengthened over the course of the project timeline. However, as one analyst points out, "More often than not . . . implementing agencies and NGOs are apparently either not aware of already existing institutions, organizations, orders, and arrangements at the local level, and of internal factions and power structures, or these are intentionally not taken into account in favor of a smooth realization or fading-out of their projects" (Titz, Cannon, and Kruger 2018: 18). In PERRP, we sought to tap into existing institutions to determine who would do the work on the ground—but what would be the best choice? Would the project hire NGOs or create an in-house team from its own staff? The advantages of the former choice would be the existing NGOs' local knowledge and their continued presence after the project was completed. However, there would be the risk of them not working at the pace and precision desired by PERRP. If we had our own in-house social team, we would be able to direct and manage work at the intensity needed. The disadvantage would be that, at the project's end, the highly trained and skilled staff would disperse—a benefit to development or reconstruction efforts elsewhere, but not as a direct follow-up to this project.

Ultimately, the choice was made by local NGOs themselves. When PERRP social specialists visited and interviewed Pakistani and international NGOs working in the earthquake zone, most indicated they were already too overstretched in other earthquake reconstruction projects and could not take on any more work. The only existing community-based organizations were ones formed by the NGOs, and they were already busy in other NGO activities. The only option left was for PERRP to set up its own social mobilization team to work at the community level. But who would we work with there? In these locations, there were no organized, available, or ongoing representative community-based groups that existed to lead the community for disaster or development work. The only other existing groups were noninclusive. They were for religious or political purposes, based on kinship, caste, denomination, unions, or other factors that were symptomatic of the social divisions and arrangements of power.

There were, however, informal leaders whom locals relied on to address specific problems or resolve conflicts in their community. From time to time in various matters, they would be collectively consulted by government officials or community members, but these informal leaders had no official group. With no other suitable, available community-based organizations present, the social team saw that these informal leaders, if they would assist, had great potential. One other important consideration was that new groups could not be formed out of thin air. To increase the acceptance of such groups and to increase the likelihood of recognition and facilitation by the government or other agencies in the future, the groups needed to fit in with the government's legal framework and have an existing legal identity.

Such considerations pointed to the legal but long-dormant School Management Committees (SMCs) and Parent Teacher Councils (PTCs)—entities that could be reactivated. This potential, however, had to be explored diplomatically, as it also represented some of the tensions that existed around the schools as discussed below.

PERRP's Approach to "Communities"

In PERRP, we recognized that a community is not just a place, but that communities exist in highly complex sociocultural and political contexts. From decades of previous experience in the project area, PERRP's social team members made no assumptions that communities were harmonious. Rather, we knew that the social structure in the project region meant there were many subgroups with long-established reputations as diverse, hierarchical, and prone to conflict. For a project to initiate participation and operate effectively, it was important to know the subgroups in each community and their places in the hierarchy as seen through local eyes.

At the same time, where there are strong differences, it is easy to overlook factors and traits that groups and people do have in common. While this was the case of communities in the PERRP project area, PERRP proved that there were outstanding capacities and a willingness to contribute, especially when the people were challenged to do so. To get a more balanced understanding of communities early in the project, the social team conducted capacity and vulnerability analyses as discussed below.

PERRP's participation strategy was problem based and capacity driven. That is, instead of picking ideas out of the air for activities that community members could do, the program had stakeholders foresee needs and problems, and then put community capacities to work in meeting these needs and preventing and solving these problems. As the committees succeeded in many such tasks, it had empowering effects.

Who Were the People and Communities?

In KP province's Mansehra District and AJ&K's Bagh district, the communities lived in the areas surrounding the seventy-seven facilities that PERRP built. Beneficiaries numbered over one million: the sixteen new health facilities served a population of about 300,000, while the sixty-one new schools had an enrollment of 17,000 students from 556 villages with a combined population of approximately 800,000.

Community by Geography

In each case, PERRP's communities were defined first by geography. The project had been assigned to construct facilities that served large catchment areas, as defined by government and the local people. Each school catchment area—varying in size from six to thirty square miles—included several villages and subcommunities that were spread across the area. The health facilities, which were far fewer in number, had much larger catchment areas. Each catchment area was defined by distance and time:

how far people came to access school or health facilities, and how much time it took to reach them—usually by foot, as roads and transport are scarce. A few of the facilities were in congested urban areas, but most were in remote rural communities in the mountains. By local common understanding, the PERRP communities had at least a rough geographic outline; the facilities were focal points, as they were usually the only facilities of their kind in that catchment area.

Community by Social Composition
Each of the catchment areas had a diverse mixture of social groups, with different castes, kinship groups, *biradaris*, groups with political affiliations, sects or denominations, and tribal and ethnic groups.

Types or Degrees of Participation

Across the many communities served by PERRP, there were different forms of participation, and participation was carried out to varying degrees. By far the most direct and thorough type of participation came from committee members, who numbered over six hundred. They were heavily involved in decision-making; problem-solving; conflict resolution; the detailed procedures for working before, during, and after construction; and all the planning and volunteer coordination that this work necessitated. Especially during the construction phase, which lasted many months, most members were involved on a daily basis. Another form of participation was in the way of contributions: committee members encouraged others to donate and lend property or to contribute resources needed for construction. Details of the forms of participation and contributions are provided in part 3 of this chapter.

There was also widespread participation by committee members and other volunteers who organized and attended events in which they listened and gave input. At public events organized by the committees, it was common for hundreds of people to attend, with public figures, head teachers, and students giving speeches. When architects presented the designs of the new facilities for community feedback, some teachers invited senior students to attend the committee meetings so that they could present their own opinions and ideas. Parents started visiting their children's schools for the first time and children got to take part in new school activities, including sports days, public speaking, and performances with songs, skits, poetry, and art making.

The construction site itself provided opportunities for sharing information, another form of participation. PERRP encouraged the committees to invite visitors to serve as observers. Outside the safety perimeter at each site, construction engineers regularly answered questions about the construction and features that made the new buildings earthquake resistant. With many other reconstruction sites progressing slowly or being stalled, this kind of information sharing by PERRP sites drew attention. With this construction speeding along unhindered, members of the public came to watch for fun and out of curiosity, as these schools were often the largest building in the vicinity, were situated in prominent locations, and were being built with construction methods and materials—reinforced concrete—that were rarely seen in these rural areas. To such observers, those sites became touchstones.

Even community people who had no connection to or direct benefit from the reconstruction efforts often attended and assisted just to know what was happening, or because someone in the community asked them to help. Better-off people sent their children to private schools or went further afield for private medical care, but many still were motivated to contribute to the new community facility.

Power and Participation

Analyzing the Power Structure: Why and How

In the research literature on community participation, power is a main issue, as it can determine who participates and who may be left out. Yet there is little practical information in the literature on how community participation can be handled. The following is provided as a detailed account of how, in this project, analyses were conducted to identify the blocs of power, the results of which were then used to shift and share that power.

Working in a community with many subgroups within a geographically defined area, the project's social mobilizers set about to develop their understanding. As full-time participant observers in the communities—in the market, at tea stalls, at prayers at the mosque, at social occasions, and in meetings with officials—they observed each community's social structure, determining who had the most power, who had the least, and who was in between.

At the community level, it was a matter of listening, observing, and having a mental checklist of questions. Social mobilizers asked themselves: To whom would government officials refer the project? If asked, who would people say are the most prominent or "in-charge" people? Who has a reputation for making things happen? Who did the in-charge people identify as prominent? In this culture, for whom did the hosts of meetings or gatherings reserve seats of honor? What is the social identity (ethnicity, clan, tribal group, etc.) of each prominent person? From whence does each person derive their power? How do they use or misuse it? Who and what are the "dividers" and "connectors"? Whom do people listen to, show respect for, and admire or fear? Who is involved in settling disputes or conflicts or taking other initiatives for the community? Who has a reputation for acting more in the interests of the community, and less in self-interest?

Because social mobilizers came from the same districts that PERRP worked in, they were easily able to recognize social groups by people's names, occupations, education, economic status, and physical appearance—including racial characteristics, clothing, and stature. By such observations, the social team members could identify which castes, clans, religious denominations, and ethnic or tribal groups were present in any location. As this is a sensitive subject, social mobilizers then discretely observed and researched relations between the groups, including frictions, conflicts, and the ways in which collaboration did occur. This kind of information was necessary to help the project be conflict sensitive: the social mobilizers needed to know who could play leading roles in conflict prevention, resolution, and collaboration.

As the above kinds of observations were being made, social group membership—the stratifications, hierarchy, or layers of social power, as well as the frictions, conflicts, and their causes—became apparent. The PERRP social team discerned the blocs of power. In some communities this hierarchy was immediately visible, while in others it emerged over time. With this profile of each community, the individual social mobilizers developed a clear picture of the social group actors, including their roles and their power. They then used this knowledge to know who to encourage and support, who to protect, who to depend on, and who to turn to for solutions. In general, this knowledge was used by social mobilizers to watch over and guide participation.

Knowledge of the power structure in each community was also important in the ongoing discussion by the social team, and it was shared with engineer counterparts to help with decision-making in different situations—especially in regard to the project's communication protocol, which included grievance procedures. None of this research was formal or in written form, but some formal survey methodologies were adapted—notably triangulation. Due to the divisions among people, it was essential to have information from multiple sources and to use different methods. What resulted was a relatively clear understanding of the power structure in each community.

Arrangements of Power at the PERRP Community Level

The social team identified the blocs of power in the communities around schools. At the top of the hierarchy were head teachers and their immediate circle of advisers or confidants. Then came the community's influential

Table 4.1. Power Structure—The Blocs of Power in PERRP Communities.

Power within the community:
- At the government school: head teacher with circle of friends and advisers
- In the community outside the school: powerful, influential community members, including elders, notables, religious leaders, and elites
- Owners of land surrounding the school or granting access to it
- Parents and students—women, men, girls, and boys from the poorest families

Power in the community from outside sources:
- The PERRP project
- Design and construction contractors

community members, followed by owners and users of land that either surrounded the school or granted access to it. At the bottom of the hierarchy were the parents and students. As shown in table 4.1, coming from outside the community were two other significant parts of the power structure: the PERRP team itself and the contractors who were engaged to do the construction.

The Blocs of Power

Power of the Head Teacher

In their position, head teachers were the official representatives of the Department of Education. They held this role based on their own education, experience, caste, or tribal or ethnic identity, or—as is the case with most government jobs in this highly politicized environment—due to attachment to a political figure or party. Often head teachers are not working in their own villages; instead, they are transferred elsewhere as a reward, warning, or punishment, resulting in frequent changes in school administration. Head teachers then have their own unofficial circle of people whom they trust and whom they call on for advice or support: people from their kinship groups, relatives and friends, other teachers, people from their department, or connections from a political party.

Some head teachers are strong, respected educators who are dedicated to their profession and who put substantial effort into promoting quality education, while still remaining part of the sociopolitical hierarchy. Many others, however, are not so motivated, and they often have weak teaching skills and get little training and low pay. There is widespread teacher absenteeism.

In this position, head teachers often maintain the conventional idea of authority, and they see parental involvement as not needed or even unwelcome. Historically, parents are not involved at the school at all; there are no parent-teacher meetings, and schools often don't even issue report cards. While the head teachers are still accorded respect, the school is the head teacher's domain.

Over the years, many education development projects have attempted to bring change along the lines of what foreign donors considered the "modernization" of education, but these efforts have sometimes had limited effect. Some attempted changes—and the ways in which they were implemented—led to failure. In the 1990s in different parts of Pakistan, there was a shift toward introducing more bottom-up approaches in education, health, and other fields. At that time, School Management Committees (SMCs), Parent Teacher Councils (PTCs), and their respective guidelines were introduced to Pakistani communities by various international donor projects. These committees were later legally mandated and obliged to operate at each school. However, in bringing in these committees, the internationally funded projects did not consider the highly complex social hierarchy and power structures in these locations. For such committees to work, it would require a shift or sharing of power that was not welcomed by the head teacher or the other teachers. This well-intended but externally imposed idea meant that, at least in the project area, such committees had existed in theory only. Worse, the earlier failures with "community participation" in education had created a strongly adversarial relationship between educators and members of their communities.

With the design and construction of a new school pending, and many problems being anticipated—especially over land issues, which a head teacher would likely have little inclination or ability to solve—the local prominent people and landowners were especially important to include in the reconstruction work. These people were best positioned to solve related problems and could do so quickly. Without their participation and buy-in to the project, we faced increased risk that such problems would interfere with construction, delaying the completion of the badly needed new school.

Not surprisingly, when PERRP first talked with the head teachers and their allies, the idea of any community participation was commonly resisted. A few flatly rejected the idea, saying it was not needed: "Since this is a government building and I represent the government, I know everything you'll need to know." According to some head teachers, nobody else in the community would be needed; this was a type of elite capture in which the powerful would try to control all the decision-making. The PERRP social team offered friendly encouragement, explained that their workload would be increased if they tried to deal with construction alone, and implemented other ways of reducing friction. Without these strategies, community participation may not have happened at all.

Much of the resistance to community participation came from having to involve community members who would be from rival castes, political affiliations, ethnic groups, or sects. These people with differences were easily dismissed by the head teachers, who held powerful positions. Among those who at first resisted or were dismissed were the informal leaders, who were other prominent people with their own power.

Power of the Informal Leaders, Notables, Elders, and Elites
Within the school, the head teacher is the authority, but the wider community has its own leaders. Each district had elected government representatives, although these people tended to be distant and were involved only in unusual circumstances. Yet each community also had an informal, non-elected power structure that was present and active, although it was normally not involved with the school at all. This leadership included elders, notables, and other respected, well-known, and influential people; however, a few in this traditional structure occasionally misused their power to get benefits for themselves, their families, and their social groups. These people may have been influential only within their own social group, or they may have had influence among others as well. Almost invariably, these leaders were men who came from a range of occupations: they were shopkeepers, farmers, transporters, bakers, informal social workers, political party representatives, union leaders, journalists, and religious leaders; they could also be retired or active government employees such as head teachers, teachers, and military, health, education, agriculture, or forestry officers. They were not a fixed, organized, or traditional group—they were simply well-known people in the community and were involved from time to time in different matters.

The power or influence of such figures determines much about the community. While it is sometimes an informal leader who causes or contributes to the divisions, this same person can also be seen as a problem-solver who has the power or influence to bring people together, to keep the pot from boiling over, to prevent or settle disputes. In both KP province and AJ&K, these informal leaders are known for their conflict resolution abilities, influence, and authority. In KP province and Afghanistan, the jirga—a community-based decision-making body or gathering of the elders and other influential people—hears all sides in a dispute, and by consensus renders decisions that are customarily binding. Jirgas are sometimes controversial and face accusations about their fairness. They tend to be held only when disputes are prolonged and have reached a critical state; they are not used in early conflict prevention or resolution. AJ&K has similar customs in which the elders and influential people come together to settle a dispute, but there is no particular name for it. Having such capacities in a community was invaluable to PERRP, as we found that, once some of the informal leaders became members of the committees, their skills in conflict resolution and problem-solving, combined with the PERRP social processes, worked exceptionally well.

At the same time, as these leaders would remain in the community and in their roles long after the project was completed, it was important the project did not usurp or interfere with their influence. We knew, therefore, that we would need to respect the leaders and be seen in the community doing so. We also knew that we needed to harness their skills, resources, and enthusiasm, and to offer new skills and strengthen their already extensive capacities, which could be put to use in future community development efforts. As an external group, meeting with these informal leaders was a courtesy, and we acknowledged the leadership, influence, and traditional authority they had. Gaining their acceptance was an essential first step in developing a needed long-term working relationship. Without their buy-in, the wider community would not have felt authorized to participate.

With power, of course, comes the risk of elite capture. While there were some attempts by individual elites to grab project favors from PERRP—as introduced in chapter 3—the likelihood of this happening had been foreseen early on (see the analysis in table 4.5, "What Could Go Wrong?"), and preventative measures were included in the project approaches. Dealing with elites and elite capture was a responsibility of the committees. As such, demands by elites were easily quashed by their peers. In early community-wide meetings, PERRP's construction engineers provided details about what kinds of work and services the project would provide and what would not be provided or allowed, stating that only the work already specified in a contractor's contract would be undertaken. When elite capture was nonetheless attempted, committee members could, when needed, find people of even higher status or more influence—for example, a certain relative or political party leader—to discourage the elites, or use other reasoning or pressure to dissuade them of their attempted demands, as in the anecdote "Landowner Suddenly Claims . . . ," page 71.

Power of the Landowners Outside School Land

At the schools to be built by PERRP, the land was owned by the government, but there was potential for issues with each site's boundary lines. If there were disputes, they would most likely come from those adjoining landowners who could exercise their power to stop construction through court stay orders or from refusing access to the site. Well before construction began, PERRP took steps to include these landowners in the project process, settling land disputes and establishing and respecting boundary lines.

Power of the End Users, the Parents and Students in the Poorest Families

While the head teacher was at the top in the power structure in the school community, parents were at its bottom due to their positions at the lowest levels in the social hierarchy. These were the men, women, boys, and girls who are normally excluded or marginalized.

As part of the government-to-government assistance, the government of Pakistan and USAID had agreed that PERRP was to build only government schools, which had a reputation for providing low-quality education. Better-off people sent their children to the mushrooming private schools, meaning attendance at the no-fee government schools was from the poorer families. Poverty pushes these families further down the social hierarchy, leaving them with no voice and no ability to participate—so it was normalized that the head teacher was in charge of education and the school, and that parents never visited the school or received reports about their children's progress. Customarily, these parents were intimidated: they lacked confidence and believed education to be the teachers' and government's responsibility. The PERRP-activated committees gave many parents their first experience at their children's schools.

Power of the Project

Realistically, any donor project arriving in a community has significant power. Wise, respectful use of this power can bring about many other developments. Besides providing the funds, services, and planned benefits, a project can become a strong neutral platform and a catalyst in a community. To lay the groundwork for community participation, PERRP's social program used its position of power and influence to have power shared among the beneficiaries of the project, even if that power sharing was only temporary.

Approaches chosen by the project sometimes brought people together who, until then, may have resisted or opposed each other. This opposition was so strong that, in some cases, it was unacceptable for them, their family, or fellow group members to reach out to the other or even sit in the same room as the other. See ethnography, page 76. But since PERRP had asked them to work together to help get a new school or health center built, most agreed to do so because of their desire for a new facility. Realistically, the project had the power to ask people to do things that they would not normally do, and to do them together; this also gave the communities a platform that they could use to deal with each other, whereas normally there is no such platform. Being connected to the project provided an explanation and justification for different behavior. The project became a safe, friendly place to come together.

Power of the Construction Contractors

Although contracted and under the supervision of the project, PERRP contractors were used to working alone in communities, without any help from a social team or organization that would host them, as is the norm for construction in Pakistan. Such contractors have a reputation for taking independent actions, often with an attitude of eminent domain, similar to a takeover or invasion. In construction projects, contractors either are given or assume the most powerful position, as they are the ones whom the client has sent to get the job done. Contractors with this mindset have a reputation for ignoring local requests, and so contractors and community members frequently blame each other for any problems.

Power Shifting and Sharing

Participation by the wider community required a shifting and sharing of power—a delicate matter in communities with a strong, established hierarchy. In the study and practice of community participation, such arrangements of power need to be clear. Projects should ask: "Do powerful people have an effect on your ability to work with the people?" (Cannon, Titz, and Kruger 2014: 113). Or, more pertinently, in such circumstances in which the power structure is strong and will not disappear in the short time frame of a project, how can a project work within a given power structure while still helping the people? In PERRP's case, getting participation by the community was set up as a three-step process. As the first step, the social team started at the top, getting buy-in to the project by the head teacher, which then made the second step possible—bringing in the community's informal leaders or influential people. This in turn facilitated the third step, which was participation by the wider community.

A main reason why there had not been community participation or functioning SMCs or PTCs at the schools before was because the government had issued counterproductive committee guidelines. Those guidelines put the head teacher in control, but they also gave committee members—whom the head teacher chose—the responsibility to monitor and report on the head teacher and other teachers, creating a contradictory and adversarial relationship. Not surprisingly, the head teachers then rejected any committee activity, maintaining their sole position of power.

To have the committee acceptable to each head teacher, the social team suggested to them that, for the duration of the project, those guidelines that created friction would be suspended, and new ones would be introduced—starting by removing the monitoring role. Table 4.2 shows the first proposed change—that, for the duration of PERRP, committee members would not be monitoring the teachers for any reason. Instead, they would offer only friendly support and help.

The social team, again stressing the temporary nature of the proposed changes—PERRP had no authority for what would happen after the project—also convinced the head teacher of the benefits of other changes shown in table 4.2, starting with a new committee member selection process and the requirement that members be representative of the catchment area and its social groups. Additionally, while the head teacher would remain in the committee's top position as general secretary, a new position for a community representative would be created: the chairperson, the committee's second-in-charge. The chairperson and all other members would be chosen by the community, a major change that shifted and shared power. Head teachers accepted the suggested changes, likely due to the clear advantages of having extra help, plus the emphasis on these being only temporary arrangements. With this buy-in, the social team then recommended that the head teacher, as the authority, call a meeting of these local leaders to discuss construction of their community's school and what they could do to help.

The PERRP team then moved on to the second step of the process, in which dozens of elders, notables, and other influential people attended a meeting chaired by the head teacher. By this point in time, having their school rebuilt had become urgent to all. As community members witnessed the slow progress of other reconstruction projects and saw signs that international funds for reconstruction were already drying up, it was commonly understood this might be their community's last chance to have their school rebuilt. The agenda of these meetings began with the social team again presenting the project ideas and plans, including how

Table 4.2. PTC/SMC Guideline Changes to Shift and Share Power.

Government guidelines:	Temporary changes introduced in PERRP:
Committee to monitor and report on teachers, including their attendance	Committee not to monitor teachers, instead to offer only support and help
Committee members prescribed by government, to be chosen internally	Committee members to be selected by community members in a public process
Head teacher maintained permanent leader as committee general secretary	Added community member as second-in-charge, the chairperson
Members restricted mainly to parents of children attending same school	Membership opened to parents and influential people in the community as chosen by the community
No social or geographic representativeness required	Required geographic and social group representativeness

the community was needed to make it all happen. Invariably there was interest among the informal leaders to be involved, but they also were sensitive to the authority of the head teacher. Purposes for these new committees were agreed upon:

- prevent or solve community problems related to design or construction
- support the school and help improve education
- share responsibility with government for building maintenance

Membership criteria for committees were also decided:

- be representative of local sects, castes, and ethnic, tribal, or other social groups
- have geographic representation from the catchment area and user communities
- be known as respectful and respected
- be willing to volunteer, as there would be no pay, honorariums, or allowances from the project
- act without promoting any political affiliations
- live in the community
- be known as an education promoter and problem solver who is interested to help the community
- have no vested interests in the project, and not be in a position to make money from the construction

With this much decided, the third step—to get community participation underway—was initiated by the head teacher and informal leaders, who jointly called the first public meetings in which the project was formally introduced and the committees were formed. This much alone was a significant change in power sharing.

Some power was also extended to the local landowners. While landowners in these locations can wield power that can severely affect construction, the rights of such owners are frequently ignored. PERRP, however, chose the opposite tactic. Rather than wait and hope that no such issues arose, the social team invited the landowner stakeholders into the project process to draw attention to potential land issues, to address these issues, and to ensure that their rights were honored before construction started. While the process acknowledged their rights, it also brought them under community scrutiny for encroachment or any other practices the committee deemed unwarranted. While the project still dealt with many land issues, this strategy proved to be the main reason that there were no court stay orders to stop construction.

A significant rearrangement of power also occurred between the communities and construction contractors. Since the committees had been well organized and active months before the arrival of the contractors, this gave the committees an unusual and prominent footing. Along with the management tools such as the Committee-Contractor Agreement, the presence of this new community voice gave the committees power in ways that they had not experienced before.

Parents and students also shared in this power, and were brought into the scene much more than usual. Once the committees were formed, they instituted some of the activities that nonfunctioning school committees were supposed to do all along, especially facilitating parent-teacher interaction. The social team also had the committees work with teachers to introduce student activities, many of which occurred for the first time: sports field days, public-speaking competitions, and school maintenance. There were also a few instances of parents, for the first time ever, making complaints about the teaching, as related in the first of the following anecdotes. Teachers frequently reported how local involvement with the construction had also generated far more community interest in education than they had experienced previously, as described in the anecdote "Community Helping . . . ," page 169. Another anecdote, "Brother Who . . . ," page 170, illustrates how complex it can be, despite all the processes used, to have community or family agreements maintained or honored.

Part 2: The Social Team and Process

The Social Team

Normally, a construction project does not have a dedicated social component with specialized staff to prepare and implement a structured community participation program. In the case of PERRP, the social program started with the USAID request for proposals: along with all the many required details for design, construction, subcontracting, supervision, management, budget, and the like, bidding companies were required to propose how they would liaise with communities. This unusual requirement was backed up by another innovative requirement: that the head of the liaison or social program was to be part of the project's four-member senior management team, along with the chief of party, deputy chief of party, and chief financial officer.

The social element in this project was not part of a broad USAID policy; instead, it came from the personnel that were responsible for conceptualizing USAID's reconstruction program for Pakistan. From their experience working for USAID, other donor agencies, and NGOs in other countries, they had observed that some mistakes made in school construction projects were due to local people not being consulted or involved in any way, and they wanted to avoid this. To make the social side of construction an integral part of the project—not to have it be placed in a subdepartment, or outsourced, where it could be treated as less important—matters of community participation were placed at the senior management level. This was important especially when this level of authority was needed to carry out the social program. For policy makers and planners for other projects in which serious thought is being given to the shifting and sharing of power at the bottom levels, serious consideration needs to be given to the composition of the management team at the top level.

PERRP was the only reconstruction project with a team of social specialists whose sole job was to work with communities and construction management. Normally contractors work alone, without a community committee or anyone local to take responsibility for sociocultural integration. If a problem arose from the community, a member of the technical team would try to deal with it, but they often were not successful. Sometimes contractors tried to get government to solve a dispute or to pay people to settle it.

Among both contracted and subcontracted NGOs and agencies with hundreds of projects in postquake reconstruction, most had little or no experience in construction per se. Their expertise was in early emergency response or long-term development in a range of sectors including medical assistance, preventative health programming, water and sanitation, shelter, food, livelihoods, agriculture, forestry, and education, but then they were engaged by donor agencies to also carry out a range of small-scale reconstruction such as rebuilding destroyed primary schools, usually one-room structures. To do so, the NGOs hired their own engineers to oversee light construction or the installation of prefabricated buildings. While these NGOs' field workers or social mobilizers continued their normal main programming, they would be also called upon to react to problems related to interactions between community members and construction workers, or they would take the problem to the responsible government departments. This frequently resulted in delayed responses, no response, or no resolution—main reasons for many stalled reconstruction projects. While the phrase "community participation" was frequently used, upon further inquiry or observation, it usually meant what was done on an ad hoc basis between individuals, without organized community responsibility or other involvement. Whether handled by a construction contractor or NGO, the approach was reactive, not proactive. For the six years that they worked in the earthquake zone, PERRP's social mobilizers listened for, watched for, and made inquiries to find other construction projects with any kind of structured, participatory program similar to their own, but we were unable to identify any. However, later, while PERRP was underway, our implementing agency did carry out a second reconstruction project, which was modeled on PERRP, for another donor agency. (See the section in chapter 3 titled "Use and Misuse of the Phrase 'Community Participation.'")

In PERRP, the design of the social program was based on theories and principles that drew on a number of my own influences, as discussed in chapter 3. These included Freireian ideas of encouraging people to analyze their own situations and to become proactive, to participate, and to take action to transform things. Then, as urged by Chambers, was the need to sit down with people, get to know them, listen to and respect them, and be ready to hand over the metaphorical pointer stick and use the participatory methodologies developed by Chambers and countless others. Also adopted was Mary B. Anderson and Peter J. Woodrow's emphasis on seeing the strengths or capacities—not just the problems or vulnerabilities—of communities, as well as Anderson's idea of looking for what connects people, even in conflict-prone situations. An especially strong idea came from the Aga Khan Rural Support Program, which suggested that projects make structured, demanding partnerships with poor communities: this idea was heavily influenced by the work of Akhter Hameed Khan, and his confidence in the "tremendous potential within the poor" (AHKRC 2010: 207). In general, the primary purpose of this social program was not as an ongoing, stand-alone community development program; instead, its purpose was to support design and reconstruction in a short-term project. Potential results from this approach were foreseen: if well designed and well executed, a social program could also result in strong local institution building.

To determine the number of social team members needed, I took a number of factors into consideration: what was the travel time from the field office to the construction site? If the mobilizer then needed to spend two or three hours at each site, how many sites could they reasonably visit in one day? How many construction sites or communities could each one serve in a four-day week, keeping the fifth day for office work, meetings, and reporting? Ultimately, I chose to hire eleven people from earthquake-affected areas to work as social mobilizers. As the twelfth member of the social team, I was in charge of the design and management of the social component in the communities, and also coordinated this work with design and construction through senior management.

The social team was a small percentage of PERRP's staff. Out of the total of about two hundred project staff members, the social team was made of twelve people: I myself and eleven local women and men who were survivors of the earthquake and who came from the same districts as the project. Most social team members were recent university graduates with master's degrees in various disciplines—political science, economics, law, education, international relations, and physics—but none had anthropology or rural sociology degrees, as such degrees were either available only at universities in faraway cities or not pursued because, as students, they were interested in other subjects. Three of the PERRP social mobilizers had several years of experience in this kind of work; two others had been primary school teachers before the quake, while the others got their first jobs straight out of university when the NGOs arrived for emergency relief operations.

In KP province and AJ&K, the prequake community-level jobs reflected the political situation. In KP province, local, national, and international NGOs had been operating for decades, providing jobs and valuable work experience. The people we hired to work as PERRP social mobilizers in KP province had worked for a few years in these NGOs in various community development projects: in water supply, livelihood development, education, agriculture, forestry, biodiversity, wildlife conservation, and other sectors. As AJ&K is a disputed territory, Pakistan had never allowed international NGOs to operate there until the earthquake happened—afterward, however, they were allowed in freely. Until then, there were few opportunities for community development jobs in AJ&K.

With little or no social mobilization experience, we hired social mobilizers based on what they had already been doing in their own communities, considering this experience to be the best indicator of their interest, suitability for the job, and depth of understanding. While many dozens of candidates were interviewed, all those selected had been involved at home as informal volunteer social workers or activists. Their activities included leading or helping in different emergencies such as floods, accidents, or landslides; organizing services for the disabled; getting friends together to tutor poor students or give classes to street children; working in campaigns to promote vaccinations, school attendance, and sanitation practices; participating in charitable work at the mosque; starting organizations at university; and demonstrating for various causes. It was this kind of practical experience that counted most, as from that experience, they could also articulate the complexities and challenges of a project, and could demonstrate their analytical and problem-solving abilities. All were fluent in English, Urdu, and local languages, and all had come through government schools, not through a private education system. All members of this highly dedicated team are named in the acknowledgements to this book.

As discussed in chapter 2, of all the skills needed by social mobilizers, what stood out was the need to be respectful and adept with cultural norms, specifically in regard to language, gender roles, the customs of *purdah*, and the local power structure and informal leaders. Of immediate importance for the project was the social mobilizers' distinct multilingual abilities. The project engineers and other PERRP staff had been recruited from Islamabad, the capital city, and from other parts of Pakistan, and so the mobilizers—who came from the project districts—were the only project staff who spoke the many local languages prevalent at the PERRP sites. Their knowledge of communities before, during, and following the disaster was invaluable.

The social mobilizer's role was to know and help steer the project through the social and cultural context of the immediate area, while also working side by side with their counterpart engineer (discussed below in chapter 5). The mobilizers were the project's eyes and ears in each community: they listened to what people were saying, solved problems, met with local officials, contributed to the ongoing iteration of approaches, assessed risks, and generally helped to shape the social process over the duration of the project. The social process was revised and refined through ongoing discussion, frequent meetings, and self-assessment. The social mobilizers developed skills in facilitation, group formation, performance monitoring, social assessment, report writing, participatory methodologies and approaches, data collection and analysis, and event planning and management. The duties and responsibilities of the social mobilizers were to:

- work with project engineers as counterparts, to understand the technical needs and plans, and to work jointly with them to introduce measures in the community to help construction start, continue, and finish on schedule
- work with the community to identify people's needs, help them to organize, and follow through to help prevent or solve problems
- contribute to ongoing analysis and iterative processes in order to develop the participation program and carry it out at the community level
- act as a project representative to local officials and organizations
- contribute to ongoing performance monitoring
- contribute to monthly reports, annual reports, and others

To emphasize community priorities and encourage the development of community leaders' capacity, the relationship between social mobilizers and committees was delineated: each committee was in charge and responsible for their community, while the social mobilizer was only the facilitator or adviser and acted as a bridge with the project. To avoid undue local pressures, the only proviso about the social team was that mobilizers could not work in their home communities.

To prepare for daily joint work at construction sites, social mobilizers and site engineers were trained together to understand their respective roles, as discussed in chapter 5. After a few days of orientation, social mobilizer training drew on the experience of each mobilizer, and consisted of a combination of learning-by-doing, action research, and iterative development. This style of training particularly suited the quick start-up of the project, and it enabled new staff to become familiar with two subjects at once: the communities and the needs of construction. For each school or health facility that would be built, a social mobilizer and project engineer were matched to work together, with their responsibilities clearly divided into social and technical areas as outlined in the communication protocols. The social mobilizer and project engineer needed to support each other's work—a complimentary partnership that proved vital.

The social mobilizers' daily activities varied according to the stages of construction. When construction of a site was completed, the social mobilizers also completed their duties; they then moved to the next sites to start the process again. Social mobilizers often worked in pairs to support each other. Each social mobilizer was responsible for an average of five or six sites. Social mobilizers, along with committee members, handled a wide variety of matters on a daily basis.

Examples of Social Mobilizer Work from One Month

In Bagh District, AJ&K:

- Government Girls' High School Chatter #2 inaugurated by senior deputy mission director of USAID along with program manager of District Reconstruction Unit, district education officer, PERRP staff, members of School Management Committee, and hundreds of community members and students.
- Library management training for twenty-five volunteer teachers and head teachers was planned but postponed at eleventh hour due to trainer's involvement in a road accident.
- Final inspection was carried out at Government Boys' High School Dherray, BHU (Basic Health Unit) Thub, BHU Sohawa, and BHU Sahlian Dhundan, along with program engineer, District Reconstruction Unit, School Management Committees, and Health Management Committees.
- Urgent operation and maintenance training given at newly inaugurated Government Girls' High School Chatter #2.

- Boundary line demarcation facilitated by School Management Committee at Government Boys' Primary School Pehl regarding the construction of a boundary wall.

In Mansehra District, KP:

- In May, events were celebrated at schools. The social team gave some school bags to Parent Teacher Committee, which they awarded to the students who had the top marks. Such events were held in twenty-six project schools in Mansehra District.
- One head teacher reported that, due to the quality of the constructed schools, demands for enrollment were increasing. At each school under construction, several students were refused admission as the students were still in the tents and there was no room for new students; even so, the demand for enrollment was increasing, in anticipation of when the construction of new schools would be completed.
- The executive district officer visited schools under construction in Khawari and expressed his satisfaction over the quality. He said in public a number of times that he wished all schools in Mansehra District were built like this.

Social mobilizers' skills were tested early on. As reconstruction and its slow pace had become highly politicized, local political party representatives sometimes spoke at public meetings, trying to take credit for the arrival of PERRP. With the public already informed that the project was a humanitarian gesture from one country to another, social mobilizers and committee members diplomatically reminded audiences that this project had nothing to do with political parties. While such political maneuvering was common and expected in other public gatherings, direct political gesturing ceased within the first few months of PERRP, as committee members and political figures learned to self-regulate.

Social Process and Community Analyses

Given that this reconstruction project arrived in Pakistan over a year after the quake, the pressure was on to get shovels in the ground as quickly as possible. With project engineers and designers fast-tracking their work, the social team did likewise. Under such time limits and pressures, this was not the situation for a conventional, in-depth, time-consuming social and cultural analysis; rather, a pragmatic approach was required.

When choosing potential reconstruction sites, the work of the social team and engineers began on the same day in the same communities. This on-site work began only ten days after the project first arrived in Pakistan and, within one month, the first three communities had formed their committees to work with the project. While engineers conducted technical feasibility-testing assessments, the social team members went to work almost immediately to conduct social analyses that helped to increase their knowledge of the communities in a number of subjects. The first was a basic rapid social assessment. Over the next few weeks, the social team carried out a more detailed social analysis, which can be used as "a tool for project planners to understand how people will affect and be affected by development interventions" (Rietbergen-McCracken and Narayan 1998: 20).

Unlike conventional research that relies on questionnaires and surveys, in which an outside researcher collects data and then takes it away to be analyzed according to their own understanding, PERRP used participatory methods. These included participatory action research methods, rapid assessment, participant observation, key informant interviews, focus group discussion, mapping, and an iterative approach. However, some formal data collection was still conducted; community members were trained to do so in their own committees for monitoring purposes. Often, these methods were applied while on the move, as the social team observed, listened, and discussed in a range of situations: in groups standing along the road; at construction sites; in vehicles; in meetings with community members, officials, or engineers; in briefings and debriefings; in workshops and facilitated discussions; and in visits to the schools or health facilities to talk with staff, parents, and students.

To start the social program's process—described in more detail in chapter 2—the social team members synthesized the project's contexts and took next steps to apply that knowledge at the community level. Historically, the project area had been complex. PERRP took place in a region with a long history of tension, which was now experiencing additional strain from Pakistan-India conflict—mainly over Kashmir—and "war on terror" activity close by. These risks of insecurity and conflicts of varying degrees were present throughout the project. The general area, including the two project districts, also had a complex social structure. It was a multicultural, multilingual, heterogeneous, stratified, hierarchical, and politicized environment, in which people lived traditional, conservative lifestyles. Most people in the project area were among the country's poorest and were living below the poverty line. Given the negative reputation of reconstruction projects already, PERRP would need to be especially both culturally and conflict sensitive.

The PERRP social team conducted three main sets of analyses to develop understanding of the communities: a Stakeholder Analysis, a Capacities/Vulnerabilities and Conflict Sensitivity Analysis, and a "What Could Go Wrong?" Analysis.

Exercise 1: Stakeholder Analysis

Purpose

A Stakeholder Analysis was one of the earliest exercises needed. This quick exercise compiled a comprehensive list of the people and organizations that had a stake in the project, including those who would be needed to provide input from time to time. Not recognizing who stakeholders are and failing to prepare for how the project will relate to them can lead to oversights and missed opportunities. A Stakeholder Analysis identifies the specific organizations, departments, groups, and individuals who have a stake in the project and with whom the project needs to work. It is a framework of information that assists in coordination.

Conducting the Exercise

Compiled with input from senior management, the social team, community leaders, and government line agencies, the stakeholder analysis served as a reminder among project staff of the many parties involved—parties they would need to work with.

The PERRP social team defined "stakeholder" as any individual or organization of any kind that had a stake in the construction work and the reconstructed facility. Who would benefit from the construction? Who would be interested in and support the work? Who could be negatively affected by it? Who could hinder, block, or damage the project or construction? Who else would have responsibility for aspects of the project? Whose help might be needed by the project? Who would the new facility need in order to be able to function effectively in future? In discussion with social mobilizers, engineers, and others in project management, these questions were posed and a list of stakeholders was drawn up. We questioned what roles each stakeholder would play and what roles they might expect from the project. Among project staff, agreements were made about which team members would be responsible for each bloc of stakeholders, as well as what types or degrees of consultation or participation would be used. From the earliest days of the project, particular efforts were made to start building relationships with these stakeholders, through holding introductory meetings and discussions.

The Findings

As table 4.3 shows, the stakeholders were clustered into groups: international- and national-level government, provincial or state government, district government, private sector, and community. Depending on contract requirements, the roles of these stakeholders may have already been specified, especially regarding who reported to whom. Table 4.3

Table 4.3. Stakeholder Analysis.

Organizations and Individual Stakeholders	Who is responsible in PERRP? Types and degrees of consultation or participation:
International-Level Government: United States Agency for International Development (USAID) Government of Pakistan	**Senior management:** Report to these stakeholders and keep them informed; take directions, consult, obtain required approvals, and request assistance; host representatives visiting PERRP project offices, construction sites, and communities.
National-Level Government: Government of Pakistan's Earthquake Reconstruction and Rehabilitation Authority (ERRA) National Engineering Services Pakistan (NESPAK) Ministry of Interior	
Province- or State-Level Government: For KP: Provincial Earthquake Reconstruction and Rehabilitation Authority (PERRA); Ministry of Education For AJ&K: State Earthquake Reconstruction and Rehabilitation Authority (SERRA); Ministries of Education and Health	**Social team,** with senior management as needed: Hold meetings with stakeholders, provide and request information, get input, request assistance, seek approvals, invite stakeholders to attend events, etc.
District-Level Government: Deputy Commissioners (head administrators) Departments of Education Department of Health (AJ&K only) Land Revenue Departments (responsible for land) Road Maintenance Department Water and Power Development Authority (WAPDA)	**Social team,** with senior management as needed: Consult, provide and request information, seek approvals, get input, request assistance, solve problem, invite to events, etc.
Contractors and Suppliers: Design and construction companies, suppliers, workers Local subcontractors, suppliers, workers	**Senior management team:** Prequalify, contract, monitor, supervise, provide information, build capacity of these stakeholders.
Community Level: Community members: elders, elites, notables, religious leaders Head teachers and teachers Parents Students Health facility staff and users Neighboring landowners People along routes to facilities to be constructed Elected officials	**The social team:** Carry out all work daily with the community, including communications. Social mobilizers facilitated the community participation. For design and construction at each site, a social mobilizer and site engineer worked together as counterparts.
Implementing Agency: CDM Smith company and PERRP management and teams: technical, social, and administrative	**All PERRP staff**
Other organizations and projects doing reconstruction	**Social team,** with senior management as needed

also indicates the type and degree of participation or consultation that would occur. In PERRP, senior management personnel were responsible for working with the government of Pakistan, the Earthquake Reconstruction and Rehabilitation Authority (ERRA), and USAID. This work was in the form of reporting, meeting, planning, joint decision-making, and hosting the donor and recipient agency personnel to visit project sites at any time. Senior management and project engineers at the regional level and at each construction site were responsible for collaborating with design and construction contractors.

At the provincial (KP) and state (AJ&K) government levels, the social team was mainly responsible for consulting with government personnel to carry out tasks in the field. For example, provincial and state support might be needed to invite representatives to meetings or to get advice, permits, cadastral surveys, or documents. In addition to liaising with government and communities, the social mobilizers also connected with other organizations and projects doing reconstruction. In this postdisaster scenario, there were many NGOs and projects present in the same districts also working in reconstruction and recovery. PERRP social mobilizers were expected to coordinate with them. The idea was to build relations and rapport before help might be needed and, especially from government officials, to take their direction and encourage them to visit the project and take part in any related activities. With so much reconstruction activity going on, it was often difficult to get government staff to play leading roles or even visit, but social team members regularly visited key stakeholders to keep them informed.

Throughout the project, the stakeholder list served as a reminder to all project staff about who was responsible for dealing with which stakeholders and, very basically, what was to be done. It helped maintain awareness, foresee stakeholder involvement, and coordinate the work of project staff. It provided the foundation for identifying specific stakeholders who should participate. Importantly, it meant that when something went wrong, PERRP already knew the right people to help solve the problem. Finally, all staff members shared in the responsibility of collaborating with the implementing agency, CDM Smith, including with the staff at its head office in the US and at project offices in Pakistan.

Exercise 2: Capacities/Vulnerabilities and Conflict Sensitivity Analysis

Purpose
As discussed above, projects are often planned without knowing the strengths or capacities of a community. This oversight results in missed opportunities both for the people and for the projects. With this in mind,

the basis of the PERRP social program was a capacities approach. Taking this kind of positive approach was the single most important decision in the social program, and it guided PERRP to set up the social process with each community. This approach proved to be highly motivating among project staff and communities. Recognizing existing community strengths and encouraging these to be brought into the project helped build community self-confidence, willingness to contribute, and a sense of empowerment. Looking for the positives in the midst of poverty, disaster, and trauma raised awareness of communities' strengths and put a much higher value on them than would be usual. This built social mobilizers' confidence and the expectations of the people. Talking with leaders about their communities' strengths, resources, ideas, and opinions helped mobilizers to encourage and mobilize people and build their self-confidence. In such a postdisaster situation, it is not necessarily easy to see the positives. In 2006, amid the almost overwhelming results of the earthquake, PERRP social team members needed to be encouraged to search out the strengths, attitudes, and resources that may have existed long before the disaster and that could still be present in each community. This is the main advantage of conducting such an analysis: it brings to light a new set of attitudes that teach others a new way to see.

These approaches particularly suited the PERRP project area, with its stratified, hierarchical social structure and ever-present risk of conflict. The project needed to be aware of what caused frictions, what the project needed to do to not cause conflict, what conflict prevention and management capacities existed in the community, and what the project could add to support those efforts.

Conducting This Exercise
This analysis began in a workshop setting as part of the social mobilizer training, but observation, discussion, and analysis continued throughout the project and guided the social mobilizers' work as situations changed in communities.

From living and working in such communities, social team members had experience observing, hearing, and seeing community realities. It was well known in the team that, although each community was very poor, little had ever happened in these remote communities unless the people themselves made it happen. Government and elected officials hardly ever helped, and outsider help either had never been provided or was scant.

The Capacities/Vulnerabilities and Conflict Sensitivity Analysis drew out observations from social team members who themselves were somewhat representative of project beneficiaries: they also were earthquake survivors from different social groups and from different villages within the project districts. As certain factors were identified, we engaged in a long discussion as to whether something was a strength or a weakness, how bias affected our judgements, and how other matters were simply facts, neither negative nor positive. Social mobilizers' own critical analysis capacities were developed through these discussions and continued to evolve throughout the project.

To analyze the postquake project communities in a workshop setting, social mobilizers were asked to consider capacities and vulnerabilities in four realms: physical/material, social/organizational, conflict/collaboration/security, and motivational/attitude. Table 4.4 summarizes results of the analysis, showing a balanced picture: while there were many challenges and risks, there were also strengths. The analysis highlighted that, since the quake, much had already been achieved by the communities with minimal outside assistance.

The Findings and How They Were Used

There are frequently weaknesses in the design of development and disaster recovery projects as the strengths of the communities they intend to help are overlooked. In PERRP's case, when there was deliberate effort to find the positives and capacities, it provided an unusual view of these communities. As intended, the exercise showed that, no matter the many problems, divisions, or vulnerabilities, there are also significant strengths, resources, capacities, and connectors that, if tapped effectively, can gain productive results.

Physical/Material Capacities and Vulnerabilities: Findings

Considered first were the physical or material realities, as these were the most visible and were where most outside assistance went, if any had come. On the vulnerabilities side, there had been much loss and trauma. Houses, schools, health facilities, and much of the infrastructure had been heavily damaged or destroyed. In these regions that were already the poorest in the country, poverty was prevalent, and families had few productive resources with small landholdings. Complex land issues were already a source of much conflict.

However, on the capacities side, there were many strengths. In only one year since the quake, most people had already rebuilt their houses, often using materials or cash assistance from government or aid agencies. Although schools and health facilities had been heavily damaged or destroyed, most families still sent their children to school and still sought medical attention, with these services being provided in the open air, in tents, or in temporary structures crudely put together by community members. Students attended class sometimes only sitting on the ground or on the

Table 4.4. Capacities/Vulnerabilities and Conflict Sensitivity Analysis: The Findings.

Vulnerabilities and Dividers	Capacities, Strengths, and Connectors
Physical/Material	
Houses destroyed. Public buildings, schools, health facilities, roads, bridges and other infrastructure were heavily damaged or destroyed.	By one year after the quake, most houses were rebuilt, children were going to school outdoors. Teachers and health workers were still doing their jobs.
Existing poverty, very small landholdings (average under two acres)	Despite poverty, community members had resources to contribute: influence, time, land, water, materials, etc.
Earthquake destruction, loss, and trauma	People had already taken reconstruction actions in the first year after quake and had a strong desire to do more.
Complex historical issues with land, a main source of conflict	With a fair and transparent process facilitated by PERRP, people were willing to settle land issues.
Social/Organizational	
Communities had many differences based on social stratifications by caste, sect, political affiliations, ethnicity, etc.	Each community had influential people or connectors able to bring or keep the peace.
Lack of unified, representative leadership	Individuals had a strong desire for community recovery and development.
Weak local organization for disaster recovery or development	Organizational skills had been developed in other activities (e.g., organizing political or religious events and family weddings, etc.).
Conflict/Collaboration/Security	
Disputes and conflicts were common, creating high risk to people and the progress of construction. General insecurity and tensions in the region	Each community had "connectors"—people and traditional conflict resolution practices that could be applied to construction.
Motivational/Attitudinal	
Loss of hope in the future, and low level of self-confidence	Getting organized to support construction helped restore confidence and hope. The construction site was seen as a symbol of recovery.
Mistrust. Earlier, other agencies had promised to help but had not. Surrounding reconstruction sites were often stalled or abandoned so people asked, 'Why should we trust PERRP?'	Trust grew as people saw PERRP do what the project said it would do: build. With trust, enthusiasm spread to help get the new facility built.

rubble, and lessons were written on broken pieces of chalkboard. Teachers and health workers were still doing their jobs, winter and summer.

In most villages, the mosques had also been rebuilt, a clear sign of motivation and the ability to find resources. Despite the poverty, influential community members often had connections or resources that they could access to contribute to the project in the form of loans of land and water. Complex historical land issues were a main challenge for any construction; however, as PERRP found, these issues could be settled through a fair, transparent process that was developed and used by the project.

Social/Organizational Capacities and Vulnerabilities: Findings

On the vulnerabilities side, the communities were heterogeneous, with many divisions and differences based on social stratifications by caste, sect, political affiliations, and ethnicity, and they were divided into separate power groups. Even before the quake, disputes and conflict were common, resulting in much tension and loss to local people; such conflicts had the same effects on reconstruction projects. There was a lack of unified local leadership and the organization for disaster recovery or development was weak.

While such differences are common in the project area, almost every community had the capacity to deal with disputes and conflict. There were numerous people with leadership skills and a generally strong desire to help with recovery and the rebuilding of schools and health facilities. These influential local people included elders, retired or active government employees (such as head teachers and military or forestry officers), businesspeople, social workers, and religious leaders. Such community members were often relied upon for solving community problems using negotiation, their social capital, alliances and connections to others, or pressure tactics. As demonstrated in PERRP, with appropriate facilitation, even communities in which major differences existed could be brought together to help the community and construction. It was also common for some community members to have organizational skills and connections developed through other activities (such as organizing family weddings and political or religious events), which they put to use in the committees.

Conflict/Collaboration/Security Capacities and Vulnerabilities: Findings

As stated above, common vulnerabilities included disputes and conflicts, resulting in much loss. Such risks of sectarian and communal frictions and violence, along with general insecurity and tensions in the country at the time of the project, were a high risk for construction. However, each community had capacities—most importantly, the capacities provided by influential connectors and traditional conflict resolution practices that could be applied to construction-related problems. Much of PERRP's approach to community participation was built around this capacity and conflict sensitivity.

Motivational/Attitudinal Capacities and Vulnerabilities: Findings
At the beginning of PERRP, a year after the earthquake, the region was still in the early recovery stage. There was a general and often-expressed loss of hope and lack of confidence in the future. There was also, at first, a general lack of trust in PERRP, which had developed because of other agencies' unfulfilled promises.

On the capacities side, as soon as people saw PERRP doing what it said it would do—building new facilities in a way that was culturally sensitive and respectful of the recipient communities—trust was established. Later, leaders often expressed how getting organized and participating in the project helped restore and build confidence. People saw construction as a symbol of hope for recovery and the future. By the time the project had wrapped up, the committees that had formed were strong, confident, prominent, and respected in the communities.

How These Findings Were Used
The strongest capacities were immediately drawn upon. The presence of influencers, connectors, and people with leadership skills—and the strong sense of self-help demonstrated by the reconstruction they had already achieved on their own—were strong indicators that these communities could achieve even more. This strength-focused approach served to be highly motivating for PERRP staff members, whose enthusiasm then encouraged community members, having a ripple effect. Many people now wanted to participate and contribute to an extent even they had not envisioned. Its empowering results were textbook—exactly what scholars and theorists like Anderson had predicted.

Exercise 3: "What Could Go Wrong?" Analysis

Purpose
A wide variety of things can go wrong in construction or reconstruction: matters to do with administration, management, finance, and scheduling; navigating regulations and obtaining permits; performance of designers, construction contractors, and workers; getting supplies and equipment; and challenging weather conditions. In a postdisaster situation, the challenges can be multiplied many times over, with the abnormally high demand for construction creating shortages and competition for resources. Instead of waiting to see what problems would arise in PERRP, the social team consulted early on to get a range of perspectives about the most likely problems.

This consultation covered several subjects, and each problem that was identified became the basis for the solutions-based, capacity-driven approaches and strategies that our team used in PERRP community participation.

Conducting This Exercise: Gathering Perspectives

This exercise was conducted by the social team, who limited their discussion to asking only about potential construction problems that involved local people. As opinions could vary greatly over what constituted a "wrong" or something "going wrong," different perspectives were sought from five main sources:

- The other donor and implementing agencies also doing reconstruction
- PERRP's own highly experienced construction engineers
- Social mobilizers who were from the same districts as the beneficiaries
- Community leaders who were watching the slow progress of reconstruction in other projects around them
- Contractors hired by PERRP to do the reconstruction work

Donor and Implementing Agency Perspectives

At coordination meetings with other donor and implementing agencies that had been active in the region following the quake, these agencies reported slow or stopped construction. The main challenges were consistent: land issues, blockages of access to the site, unreliable contractors, and conflict between the community members and contractors. Such challenges were repeated at every coordination meeting.

Construction Manager and Engineer Perspectives

Early in the project, we held a workshop with PERRP's social team and the construction manager and engineers, in which the technical team looked to the challenges ahead and all participants started deciding on the approaches that could be used to handle them. We consulted eleven engineers with a combined total of 240 years' experience working as construction managers for contractors in hundreds of other construction projects. We asked: In their experience, what was a typical construction site like? If there were any problems involving local people, what happened? Who handled the problems and how?

The PERRP engineers pieced together this typical scenario: the client—for instance, the government's Ministry of Education, Health, or Roads—selects a construction contractor and assigns them to go to a place and carry out construction. There usually is no local organization to work with the project, and often even the responsible government department is not effective in dealing with the local people. This situation means that the contractor is expected to do everything. They need to build the new building and fend off any problems that might arise from people near the construction site. When such problems arise, the engineers might try to deal with a few prominent people who actually help. Or somebody from the project might have to run after the responsible government department to get them to act, but the department will be slow and is often ineffective. There are rarely any grievance procedures at all. Occasionally, a book will be kept at the gate in which people can write their complaints, but such an approach depends on literacy and can easily be ignored. Typical projects do not have any staff who are specialists in working with communities. The community members are not involved in any planning; there are no formal agreements and very little information is shared. Communities and contractors can often get into conflict, sometimes prompting court stay orders that force projects to come to a halt.

Social Mobilizer Perspectives
Project social mobilizers, speaking from their experience as local citizens, pointed out that contractors frequently arrive with a dominating attitude, almost like an invasion. Since they have been assigned to work in a location, they act like their assignment gives them the authority to take over. They do not ask local people for permission to take or use things. Because there was a shortage of skilled laborers in the earthquake zone, contractors brought their own laborers from other parts of Pakistan, where the culture was different. These outside laborers did not know how to behave in these conservative villages, leading to a lot of trouble. In general, across Pakistan, contractors have a negative reputation and communities' mistrust of them is reciprocated. Because there is no community organization to work with construction, virtually all the problems come from individuals or small groups who take their complaints directly to the contractor. There is no transparency; deals are made privately and without written agreement, and when things go wrong, there is no recourse, which is a cause of much of the fighting. For example, a local man might agree to rent a house to the contractor and verbally agree to terms, but later the man might accuse the contractor of not paying as promised.

Community Leader Perspectives
In informal discussion in numerous communities, when asked about their experience with construction, community leaders were consistent, outspoken, and clear about the problems. From the earliest community meetings, complaints about other construction contractors were frequent. Construction contractors often were seen as corrupt, inept, and keen to use inexpensive low-quality materials and to take short cuts that reduced

the quality of construction. They were said to use and overuse local resources (land, water, and electricity) without permission, to disappear or stop working, and to refuse to listen to community members. We were told, "They make agreements with us, to pay us for something or rent something from us, but then they don't keep that promise. Their workers disrespect cultural norms and cause big problems among people in the community."

Construction Contractor Perspectives

As PERRP engaged contractors to carry out the project's construction, some of their company representatives and construction managers were consulted. We asked, in their many other projects around the country, had they experienced any problems that involved local people? Their list of complaints was as long as the others' lists. We were told that individuals or groups in the communities sometimes interfere or try to control what the contractor does, they use coercion to get undue benefits (materials, favors, or services), they exert pressure or make threats to get jobs, they steal or damage equipment, and they get into fights with each other and with the construction staff. A consistent remark was: "People are always coming to us with complaints and demands, telling us what to do and how to do construction. The 'big men' try to force us to give them things or do work for them that is not part of the project contract. People sometimes give wrong information and at times don't honor the agreements that were made."

The Findings

These frank analyses were compiled into a long list (table 4.5). Based on this list, PERRP chose project approaches based on what was needed to prevent or solve each problem with the support of local capacities.

"What Could Go Wrong?" Analysis: How the Findings Were Used

According to the "What Could Go Wrong?" Analysis and PERRP's consultations with different stakeholders, the potential for conflict was the number one issue. This was followed by concerns about construction contractors, especially the way contractors managed—or failed to manage—things on or around the construction site. Other main issues included the behavior of community members and laborers. Foreseeing these issues, the project developed several approaches geared toward prevention and problem-solving, including:

- conflict sensitivity
- committee formation and collaboration
- Communication protocol with grievance procedures
- Committee-Contractor Agreements

Table 4.5. "What Could Go Wrong?" Analysis: The Findings.

Most common problems in construction in Pakistan that involve local people:	Responsibilities and strategies in PERRP:
• Common local differences and conflict • Land issues: ownership, boundary issues, and encroachment • Access blockages across private or other land • Community member–construction worker conflict • Court stay orders to stop construction • Elite capture and "big people" demanding benefits • Uncertain water supply and access (critical for water-intensive concrete work) • Competition for an unreliable electricity supply • Damage or loss of community or contractor property • Placement and storage of construction vehicles, machinery, materials, and equipment • Traffic disruption and damage to roads and bridges • Dust, noise, and hours of work • Loss of privacy and use of visual barriers • Uncertainty of disposal site for rubble and construction debris • Discrimination against workers (by origin, ethnicity, language, caste, etc.) • Pressure and threats to hire local contractors and provide jobs • Mutual mistrust of local people and contractors • Building design features that ignore the culture • Cultural insensitivity of laborers from other parts and cultures of Pakistan • Disrespect for cultural norms, resulting in fights, losses, and risks • Issues at laborers' camps (noise, overuse of resources, firewood, water, etc.)	For each of the problems listed, the social team and committees, in cooperation with the site engineers, worked to prevent conflict and to make and enforce agreements. For the above purposes, several tools were introduced including the communication protocol, lines of communication, grievance procedures, formal Committee-Contractor Agreements, "Do-no-harm" guidelines, Workers' Code of Conduct. All are described in detail in this and other chapters. Architects were directed to follow community design requests where feasible.
• Pre-existing public reputation of contractors in general: blamed for being corrupt, using faulty materials, and taking dangerous shortcuts • Safety on and around the site • Contractors' quality of construction • Late or nonpayment of workers and suppliers	Strict enforcement of contractual requirements, multilayered monitoring, and PERRP control over quality, cost, and time Local committees also invited by project team to be involved in monitoring work.

Conflict Sensitivity

Of high priority was sensitivity to the frictions and conflicts that already existed and how reconstruction was exacerbating these. In the project areas, construction sometimes sparked specific problems: encroachment; undesired cultural change brought by outsiders; rejection of ideas by others due to old conflict or rivalries; real or perceived loss of land, water, or other precious and scarce assets; and previous negative experience with, and distrust of, contractors and construction. A vicious cycle can be created where one of the above problems adds to another.

For example, an accusation of encroachment might actually be retaliation against an old political rival, and this latest accusation just added to the enmity. A group from one caste might refuse to share water for construction, as the spring was on their land and they didn't want the other caste to benefit from it, renewing caste-based disputes. Locals beat up construction workers, risking full-blown conflict, because the workers who came with the contractor were from another ethnic group and were perceived to be taking jobs from locals. One community could not come to an agreement over land even though they were all from one caste and part of one large extended family; they were split by old political differences. Combining each community's capacities, especially for conflict resolution, with other features introduced in the project helped prevent and solve conflicts.

Committee Formation and Collaboration

A main source of conflict was the relations among different social groups, including those among castes, sects, ethnicities, or political groups, as discussed above and in chapter 2. In a public forum in each location, PERRP led community members in forming a committee that was representative of the geographic area and its social groups—a highly unusual collaboration. This committee then led the community in working with the project and being responsible for preventing and solving community conflict related to construction. This was a critical first step in participation and conflict prevention.

Communication Protocol with Grievance Procedures

What was clear from discussions with both community members and contractors was that the conflict between them was common and that it was caused by ineffective communications, lack of agreements, and lack of effective methods to handle complaints. The project introduced protocols that separated but coordinated communications between community members and contractors, serving as a way for anyone to make a complaint and get a response quickly. Tensions were reduced simply by knowing whom to talk to, and by having a place to make a complaint and get an answer. For more detail, see chapter 5.

Committee-Contractor Agreement

As conflict was often caused by contractors' and community members' mutual mistrust, poor treatment of each other, and lack of communication, the social team led the two parties to establish friendly relations and make agreements before construction started. Conflict was significantly reduced by the process, and the resulting written document was used as a reference throughout the project.

"Do No Harm" Guidelines for Contractors

Construction contractors are normally given no guidelines at all about how they should relate to local people, and the result is often conflict. To prevent conflict and loss in PERRP, contractors were given directives to do no harm to people, their property, their relations, or their culture. They were directed to not use land, water, or anything without permission; to not damage buildings, land, water sources, or other natural resources; and to not break cultural norms or create problems between local people. These guidelines became part of the Committee-Contractor Agreement. Having such standards was new to the contractors in PERRP, but the project's site engineers enforced these expectations, reducing reasons for public reaction against construction.

Construction Workers' Code of Conduct

Construction workers who were brought from other locations due to local labor shortages could often be a source of conflict. Having a written code of conduct reduced problems by helping construction workers to be clear about expectations for their behavior.

Part 3: How Communities Participated and Contributed—Monitoring

How did the communities in PERRP participate and contribute, and to what extent? How was all this monitored? To answer these questions, we first must ask: can participation be quantified? While some of the most important forms of participation cannot be counted, aspects of it—for instance, activities—can be quantified at least to a certain extent. As part of the project's overall performance monitoring plan, the social program developed a participation index, with detailed metrics to monitor our work, make certain points measurable, and establish a minimum threshold or goal of 50 percent. This was to be a participatory assessment, and the idea was that these new committees would be able to rate their participation above the minimum threshold.

Monitoring the Social Component

To establish formal monitoring and the participation index, members of both the social team and the committees set up two main methods: social step tracking and periodic performance assessment.

Social Step Tracking at Each Construction Site

As described in chapter 5, the community participation process—working alongside construction and its innumerable technical steps—was set out in twenty-four main social steps (see table 5.1). Since each committee had its own unique factors and each construction site was at different social and technical stages, and because each social mobilizer was looking after several sites, a way to record this detail was needed.

To help monitor progress, a chart was developed that listed each of the sites, as well as each of their social steps. Table 4.6 shows the twenty-four

Table 4.6. Monitoring—Social Steps Tracking Chart: Monthly Progress.

	Social Steps: Note: see table 5.1 for more details on each social step	GGHS Noman Pura	GGMS Kahna Mohri	Basic Health Unit Harighel	Basic Health Unit Khawja Ratnoi	GBPS Phel	GBMS Chaknari	GGHS Chowki	GGHS Dhal Qazian	GBHS Afzalabad	GBPS/HS Mohandri	GGHS Behali
	Stage 1: Before Construction											
1	Rapid social assessment	✓	✓	✓	✓	✓	✓	✓	✓	✓	✓	✓
2	Introductory meetings	✓	✓	✓	✓	✓	✓	✓	✓	✓	✓	✓
3	Public meetings, willingness resolution	✓	✓	✓	✓	✓	✓	✓	✓	✓	✓	✓
4	Committee formation	✓	✓	✓	✓	✓	✓	✓	✓	✓	✓	✓
5	Communication protocol with grievance procedures introduced	✓	✓	✓	✓	✓	✓	✓	✓			✓
6	Settle the land issues	✓	✓	✓	✓	✓	✓	✓	✓			✓
7	Arrange land for temporary tent setup	✓	✓	✓	✓	✓	✓	✓				✓
8	Committee input to design	✓	✓	✓	✓	✓	✓	✓				✓
9	Committee hosts prebid site visit	✓	✓	✓	✓	✓	✓	✓				✓

Social Steps: Note: see table 5.1 for more details on each social step	GGHS Noman Pura	GGMS Kahna Mohri	Basic Health Unit Harighel	Basic Health Unit Khawja Ratnoi	GBPS Phel	GBMS Chaknari	GGHS Chowki	GGHS Dhal Qazian	GBHS Afzalabad	GBPS/HS Mohandri	GGHS Behali
Stage 2: At Start of and during Construction											
10 Contractor briefing on social component	✔	✔	✔	✔	✔	✔	✔				✔
11 Committee-Contractor Agreement made	✔	✔	✔	✔	✔	✔	✔				✔
12 Committee organizes construction launch event	✔	✔	✔	✔	✔	✔	✔				✔
13 Relocate to temporary site	✔	✔	✔	✔	✔	✔	✔				✔
14 Construction worker code of conduct introduced	✔	✔	✔	✔		✔					✔
15 Make management and maintenance plan #1	✔	✔	✔	✔							✔
16 Committee capacity building	✔	✔	✔	✔							✔
17 Exit plan developed with committees	✔	✔	✔	✔							✔
18 Make management and maintenance plan #2	✔	✔	✔	✔							✔
19 Operation and maintenance training	✔		✔								
Stage 3: End of Construction											
20 Committee in final inspection	✔	✔	✔								
21 Committee organizes inauguration	✔	✔	✔								
22 Contractor cleanup, restorations	✔	✔	✔								
23 PERRP exits, committees continue	✔	✔	✔								
24 Committee and contractor defects liability period	✔	✔	✔								

Notes:
✔ = step achieved
G (Government), G (Girls'), B (Boys'), PS (Primary School), MS (Middle School), HS (High School)
This is a sample of one month's progress at eleven of the seventy-seven schools and health facilities constructed in PERRP.

steps and an example monthly reporting chart that details the progress made in of eleven of the seventy-seven construction sites at a certain point during the project. Social mobilizers updated the chart monthly, marking each step that was reached. The chart was kept in two forms: one on large paper for display in a prominent office location, and the other in a digital spreadsheet format to use in monthly reports. Both gave a bird's-eye view of the participation activities as they were reached and what step needed to be done next, helping to communicate progress to others.

Participation Index: Periodic Participatory Performance Assessment
For the participation index's minimum threshold or passing mark, the social team arbitrarily chose 50 percent and developed twenty questions to be answered periodically during the project period. The participation index allowed them to compare total scores at any given time, allowing them to see each community site's progress.

The first time the committees were assessed, only one quarter of them ranked above the minimum threshold of 50 percent—but three years later, all of the committees were above the minimum threshold. By the end of the project, all the committees scored 70–100 percent on the participation index. These scores indicated the high levels of local participation as well as the significant in-kind and monetary contributions. By then, the committees had become deft in project approaches and in dealing with their communities.

For general project purposes and this assessment, social mobilizers trained and monitored committee members in record keeping to collect data on topics such as contractor compliance with the Committee-Contractor Agreement, school maintenance, gifts in kind, attendance at events, and frequency of meetings. This training not only increased skills but also raised awareness and appreciation among committee members about the range of their own contributions and their value, creating a level of competition within and between communities. Recording and accounting for these contributions was another new experience for committee members.

Methodology
The social team developed a questionnaire with twenty questions on group representativeness, formal and informal skills, problem-solving, sharing of responsibility, and other factors. This assessment was conducted four times. Early in the project, the first assessment was conducted by social mobilizers alone, who assessed the committees as an office exercise, assigning scores and checking each other, as mobilizers were often familiar with one another's assigned schools. Friendly competition over who had

the highest-scoring schools helped keep unreasonably high scores in check. The second and third assessments were fully participatory, with social mobilizers facilitating school committees in scoring their own performance. After first scoffing at the idea of marking performance—it was "too much like school"—the social mobilizers and community members soon came to enjoy the chance to officially criticize or praise what they were witnessing.

By the fourth assessment, the same participatory scoring was done in workshop settings in each community, with committee and community members participating. This time, in several places, a community member led the process with mobilizers being only observers. Scores were decided by participants after much debate over what was deserved. Of course, self-scoring like this can be subjective—even highly subjective—but what was much more important was that local people were asked to give their opinions and to make such assessments. This kind of collaborative analytical process among people who often had many differences was likely more important than the score itself.

Participation Index Questions

Questions posed were the same each time: there were twenty questions that were scored from zero to five, with zero meaning "no, not at all," and five meaning "yes, excellent or outstanding." The questions assessed six main subject areas:

1) **Formal group skills**: Has the committee elected officers, held monthly meetings, kept quorum at each meeting, kept written records, and opened a bank account as required by the government?
2) **Nonformal group skills**: Has the committee shown an ability to obtain resources (e.g., land, water, time, money) and to keep or develop relations with the government, NGOs, and other stakeholders?
3) **Representativeness**: What percentage of members are from beneficiary hamlets and social groups? What percentage are women? How does the gender representativeness compare to that of other local events or organized efforts?
4) **Problem prevention, problem-solving, and responsibility sharing**: Has the committee prevented problems that could lead to loss or delays in construction? What number of days were lost due to conflict? What level of assistance was provided by the committee to help prevent construction delays? To what degree is the committee sharing responsibility for facility maintenance? Do they have a written maintenance plan? If yes, how well is it being implemented?
5) **Quality of education (for schools)**: Has the committee initiated school activities or helped the school improve education? What

is the level of communication between school staff and parents? What is the likelihood of the committee continuing after PERRP is completed?

6) **Miscellaneous impressions**: Overall, how do committee members rate their community's relationship with the contractor, social team, and engineers?

With scores for each answer tallied and expressed in percentages, each committee got an indication of their participation and progress over the duration of the project.

Main Forms of Participation and Contribution

In any project with community participation, consideration needs to be given to what is feasible, needed, and within local means, while also keeping in mind that communities, as well as outsiders, frequently underestimate existing local capacities. A capacities/vulnerability analysis is valuable because it can facilitate such understanding, and, in PERRP's case, it identified significant potential. However, it wasn't enough for PERRP's social team to understand the capabilities of local people: communities still needed to be convinced of their own potential to participate and contribute. Once motivated to try a participatory approach, they found they were often able to mobilize far more than they had previously believed was possible.

From the committees' feedback, we learned that people found it helpful that PERRP was specific about what the project would need, which motivated the committee to get other local people involved—and that started the ball rolling. For example, at the start of the process in each community, the committee was informed that the project would install a temporary tent school or health facility to use until construction of the new building was completed. To set up the tent facilities, flat land of sufficient size would be needed. In mountainous areas where flat land is scarce and the average land ownership size is under two acres, the committee went out, identified suitable land, and convinced the owners to lend it for the tent facilities—a major achievement in itself, as flat land is usually productive for food and resources. Then, at their own initiative, most committees also asked the landowner to donate its use at no cost. PERRP had not asked for free use of land; it was the committees' choice to have others contribute in this way. Committees' success in this request started the long sequence of many more contributions.

To facilitate voluntary contributions, committee members used friendly persuasion, calling on their family and fellow community members to contribute as part of a collective expression of gratitude for being promised a beautiful, safe facility. It undoubtedly made a difference that the committees and social mobilizers developed strong working relationships, with the mobilizers providing information, guidance, and encouragement throughout the project. Committee members and many other volunteers in each community contributed in different forms, including through time, decision-making, and problem-solving; gifts in kind and cash; event organizing; data collection; and performance assessment. For schools, the levels of participation and contribution in PERRP are all the more remarkable given that, in many parts of the country including the project area, School Management Committees existed in name only. As schools are government owned and operated, it is normal for communities to not be involved at all.

Representative Participation

Committee membership criteria included the need for members to come from and represent the places, ethnicities, castes, and sects in the school catchment area. Assessing this subject in an index question, we found the average score was 91 percent—a high level, and one verified by using membership lists with names and addresses (the names revealing ethnicity, sect, community, and gender) and by observation. Of the 606 committee members, women comprised about 22 percent, which may seem low by standards in other parts of the world, but locally this percentage was reasonably high. Considering that such committees did not exist at all before PERRP, this level of overall representativeness was exceptionally high.

Time and Decision-Making

The greatest contributions to the project were in time and decision-making. Our records show that, altogether, the committees had just over 600 members, who volunteered over 53,000 person-hours—roughly 18 years, collectively—and attended a total of 3,800 meetings! These included the committees' monthly meetings and occasional public meetings or events, but the majority of hours were for the work involved and the many ad hoc meetings held on the construction site, in which social mobilizers and site engineers solved community-related issues. This level of attention, with quick responses to situations as they arose, allowed construction to continue unhindered while also quickly alleviating problems for community members.

Problem-Solving and Conflict Prevention and Resolution

The other outstanding contributions to this project were the quantity and variety of problems solved and the conflicts that were prevented and solved by the committees. Many of the situations that arose could have easily led to conflict, work stoppages, or court cases, which might have resulted in long, costly delays or even the abandonment of the construction work. Although these contributions are unquantifiable, it is likely that they saved significant amounts of money for the project and prevented common or typical losses for local people.

Being responsible for preventing or resolving community-related conflict in the project, committee members used both their social capital and the community's conventional methods: pressure to conform to community or committee obligations or decisions; friendly persuasion; calling in influential people; use of reciprocity ("another community member has already done X, so you should too"); reminding others of religious obligations for education or health; appealing to those in dispute or conflict, to stop it in honor of those who died in the disaster; and reminding them to think of the future or to show respect for the outside help being received. If these methods of persuasion did not work, the last resort was to threaten shunning, a local practice; but in the end it did not have to be enacted in any of these communities. These traditional approaches, combined with those introduced by PERRP (the communication protocol with grievance procedures and other conflict-sensitive tools), resulted in far less conflict than is common in such projects.

Gifts in Kind and Cash

We also kept records for gifts in kind, especially those of land and water, which have the highest cash value. In almost all cases, contractors needed additional land outside the project site's boundaries—for instance, for a site office or a place to store materials or equipment. Also, in these water-scarce areas, getting the large quantities of water that were needed for concrete- mixing during construction was a major challenge. But as committees had started early, successfully obtaining free land for the temporary tent facilities, they took the same initiative with their next needs, again asking community members to lend free land or give free water for construction purposes. Each contribution was made completely at the initiative of the committee and was not a requirement of the project. Where land was lent without charge, PERRP's construction managers calculated the value of the donation based on current rental rates. Similarly, where communities allowed the contractors to take water, PERRP engineers calculated the value according to what it would have cost for the project to bring tanker truck loads of water. Along with donations of cash and materials for school events, the total market value of these contributions from poor communities was nearly a half a million US dollars.

The committees also decided that they needed to find and manage cash to carry out any special school events they chose, such as their first-ever parent days, exam results announcement days, construction launch celebrations, and inaugurations. To do this, members usually contributed some cash themselves, but more often, representatives went into the community, asking people in the better-off households, businesses, or the mosque for cash or for loans of goods. For example, committees were responsible for hosting all public events and would have to pay for them themselves—but they were urged to do so cheaply and within their own means. Committee members decided it was important to go all in and make these large events special, which would mean they needed chairs, portable stages, sound systems, and overhead sunshade or tent structures. So committee members tapped the many wedding equipment rental places in the area, asking them to lend these goods as each business's contribution.

For the communities where schools were built, the idea that they could raise funds for these buildings seemed highly unlikely, as communities rarely are involved in the government-run education system. However, not only did these committees choose to fundraise, but they figured out how to do so even in poor communities that were in the early disaster recovery phase. Considering that the daily income in the project area was under $2 and that a teacher's average monthly salary was about $110, it was remarkable that communities raised nearly $40,000 (not even counting the funds they raised for the Library Challenge, described in chapter 7).

Organizing of School Events and Public Attendance

Besides large special events such as the Library Challenge, construction launch celebrations, and building inaugurations, it was part of each committee's responsibility to help improve education. This meant getting involved in school business. They worked with teachers, parents, students, and local officials to organize and host school-based activities, such as public speaking, debates, poetry recitations, arts and crafts, essay writing, sports days, and performances. For schools that normally had few to no such activities, these new efforts and the resulting attendance were a welcome change for the school community. When the head teachers were surveyed to see what they recalled of any such events before PERRP, they reported remembering a total of only two hundred events in all their years of teaching. In contrast, since PERRP had started working in their communities, about one thousand events had been organized. PERRP kept attendance at such events, showing that about seventy thousand people had attended, many of whom had not been to the school before.

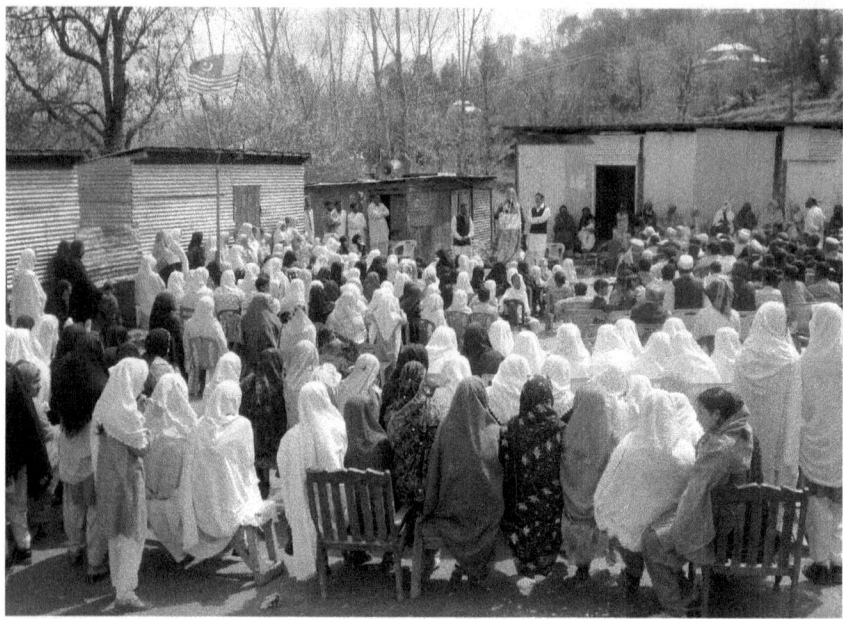

Figure 4.1. Committee-Organized School Activities. In addition to assisting construction, committees formed in PERRP helped with school activities such as this event, a public speaking contest at Government Girls' High School Juglari, 2010. © Asya Tabassum.

Benefits for Committee Members

There is a risk that the rich and powerful get more benefits out of a community project than the intended beneficiaries. Such outcomes can occur when a project has not found ways to prevent the well-off from capturing the benefits. In PERRP, committee members received no monetary or other material benefit for their involvement. As it had been made public information from the beginning of the project, committee members worked purely as volunteers, with no allowances or fees of any kind, even though it was common practice for NGOs to pay at least token fees for attendance or participation in certain efforts. From the day the committees were formed, it also had been a criterion of membership that anyone hoping to benefit financially from the construction—such as a supplier or subcontractor—did not qualify to be a member. Besides gaining new skills, committee members gained some amount of admiration and prestige in the community for having helped the new school be built in each place. In terms of material gain, however, committee members brought far more to the project than they individually got out of it.

What Happened to the Committees?

It is common in many countries that local organizational efforts, which are started by a temporarily present project or agency, fold once the project has been completed or its agency has left the scene. This also happened with the PERRP committees. Despite early exit planning and extensive ongoing discussion on this subject with the committees—and despite the skills they had built up, and the frequently expressed optimism and the preparation by members to continue and to even form their own umbrella group—all the committees stopped functioning once PERRP was completed and project operations closed down. The reasons for this are numerous and not unique to PERRP or Pakistan. The local history of organizing and the local social structure make such groups fragile, especially when they are without some neutral entity that provides an ongoing and long-term platform or acts as a catalyst. During the project, the power structures outside the groups still existed, and once the independent catalyst was removed, the old power arrangements and struggles took over again. People did not stay organized for many of the same reasons that they were not organized earlier. Without change in the surrounding social structure, and without lasting shifts in power, the sustainability of such groups is commonly at risk.

The longevity of such groups often depends on long-term, regular follow-up by some entity such as an NGO, a self-initiated entity, or a government agency, which would provide structure and maintain community motivation—but that did not happen in this case. Although the committees were legally mandated to exist at each school, the Department of Education had no central office or personnel that could specifically work with these committees. That responsibility was given to the district education officers, who were already overstretched.

Knowing there would not likely be another entity to provide long-term facilitation or a neutral platform after PERRP was completed, the committees had been encouraged to form their own umbrella group to work proactively for their own future, and to continue the highly popular Library Challenge. While this continuity was welcomed by many, when meetings to discuss the establishment of an umbrella group began, power struggles started. When other groups with commercial interests assumed they would take over (inevitably involving matters of caste, political and ethnic groups, and other alliances), the committees walked away.

While the project was present, the committees were strong local institutions. Had they continued, the schools could have benefitted from them significantly. Nevertheless, with the skills they developed and with higher expectations within communities about how they should be treated and how projects can be managed, committee members and others are undoubtedly putting this new experience to use in other endeavors, including building capacities in other institutions.

"Participate? Nobody Had Ever Asked Us to Do That Before"

One of the most common remarks made by community members to social mobilizers was: "When you first came here, we did not understand what you were talking about. You said you wanted us to participate, but nobody had ever asked us to do that before, so we didn't know what you meant. But now we know, and we like it a lot. We wish others would ask us to do it too."

See the Difference? Participation versus No Participation

With so much construction being planned or attempted by different donors and projects in so many places all at once, reconstruction, and peoples' varied experiences with it, was a common topic of discussion.

A committee chairperson asked, "Have you seen the school that was under construction down the road? Now there is no activity there, no equipment, no workers. It's all empty since the contractor left, and we don't know why he left. That construction got started in the usual way that government does it, even before the disaster. They hire a contractor who comes to the place and builds. He works alone without a local organization or committee in the community, except for maybe asking some local individuals if he needs help; he goes back to the government if there's a bigger problem to solve. But that is very slow, and all kinds of problems happen that don't get solved. People in the community don't know anything about that construction, even who the contractor is or what exactly they were going to build."

He continued, "But with the community participation in PERRP everything is different. From the beginning we knew lots of details. Things were explained to us: who is the contractor, where the funds come from to build our school, and what are the details of the construction schedule and the building design. The reason we know this is because the social mobilizers and engineers told us. And we are still surprised we were asked to give our opinions about the design! Our committee is in charge for the community to work with the contractor, and we made a written agreement with the contractor that we are both obliged to follow. If there are any problems or complaints, we have good ways to settle them. Before this project we never heard of community participation: nobody ever asked us to participate, but we like very much to do it! And we've never seen construction go on so steadily like this."

An Elite's Demands—Attempting to Capture Benefits

In projects, it can be common for powerful individuals to try to grab benefits for themselves. As found in PERRP, the most effective ways to deal with or prevent this was to first have a public agreement about it, and to have other local influential people taking responsibility to stop it.

Along the road to one of the PERRP construction sites lived a prominent political figure—an elite—who was used to getting personal favors from many sources. He started demanding that the construction team install drainage he needed on his property, which had nothing to do with the construction of a new building. The contractor took this demand to the PERRP site engineer, who, according to PERRP's communication protocol, then told the social mobilizer about it. As the man's demands escalated, the social mobilizer asked the committee to reason with this man and help him to understand that this project would not do unrelated work. They succeeded, and he stopped his demands.

Blocked Access to Construction Site

Regardless of all the effort put into the project preparation and agreements with communities, elites sometimes still rejected community requests or decisions.

Three separate times in one location, despite significant community intervention, the contractor's access to the construction site was blocked by a powerful landowner. In this community's Committee-Contractor Agreement, the owner of the land that provided the only access to the construction site committed to free access without charge. However, a few months later, after differences with the contractor, he changed his mind and blocked access, demanding a large sum of money. Pressure from the community forced the man to honor the agreement and it seemed to be solved—yet a couple of months later, the landowner made the same demands. In a committee meeting with the contractor, on a day when the man was out of the village, his elder brother took charge of honoring the promise on behalf of the family. However, when he returned, the owner rejected his older brother's promise and again demanded payment from the contractor to use the land. Rather than hold up construction any longer, the social mobilizer and resident engineer had the landowner and contractor negotiate a monthly charge for the use of this land, even though this broke the original agreement.

"My Parents Never Set Foot in My School"

A PERRP social mobilizer explained that, when he was younger, his parents had never met his teachers or saw inside his school. When first visiting schools early in the PERRP project, he remarked, "Nothing has changed in these government schools since I was a student in the primary levels over twenty-five years ago. Back then it was unimaginable for a parent to go to the school, and so my parents never set foot in my school. Just like everybody else, they thought the teacher was in charge, so education was the teacher's responsibility. We showed our respect to them but, frankly, my parents were a little afraid of the teacher. But since the school committees have become active in this project, change has started. They are bringing parents and other community members into the schools for the first time."

Parents Locked the School and Led a Protest against the Head Teacher

Change occurred at all the schools in this project. When PERRP first arrived in a community, parents had never been involved in their children's schools in any way. With time, however, the newly activated committees—for the first time ever—encouraged parents to get involved at the school and in education. One school went much further than the others.

At this school, with the completion of the building only one month away, parents—mainly mothers—led a protest against the school's head teacher when they heard of the poor board exam results of all the students. They put a lock on the school door, and when the head teacher failed to attend a meeting that they had requested, they went to the Department of Education and demanded the head teacher and staff be replaced, or else they would transfer their children to other schools. Project social mobilizers, all of whom were from nearby locations, observed that not only was this parental action unprecedented, the Department of Education's reaction was also unheard of. In only a few days, the District Education Officer attended a meeting at the school with the parents, school staff, and the committee, and, admitting the Department of Education had failed this school, took responsibility and agreed to replace the head teacher. They then appointed an acting head teacher, who was the chairman of the committee and was also the headmaster at a nearby school. The Department of Education had committed not only to finding a new head teacher, but had done so with the input of the committee!

This was almost a textbook case of people's empowerment. The parents involved had participated in the school's first-ever parent events, which were initiated by their first-ever functioning School Management Committee. These brief meetings appeared to have convinced parents that the education of their children was their responsibility and that they had the right to make demands of the education system. Now the committee could be of even more benefit by harnessing the energy and commitment of these parents.

Not participating in the protest, the committee members acted wisely, cautiously, and diplomatically, as they were reluctant to be perceived as campaigning against school staff or as revolutionaries in the education system—actions that could have put their committee in jeopardy.

Community Helping Construction Drew Attention to Girls' Education

All the activity around design and construction—the activation of prominent people in a school committee, the presence of a large number of workers, the frequent visitors from PERRP, and accessible information about the reconstruction project—served to draw attention to education in general, and in this case, to girls' education.

One girls' school was situated in the middle of densely packed houses and the mosque, with the river on one side. It lacked road access, and was accessible only by a steep, twisting footpath between buildings. Rebuilding this school at first seemed impossible, as there was barely enough space left for a new building and there would be no way to truck in supplies or equipment. In addition, this community was deeply divided—separated into two groups with a long history of conflict—and it was not noted for its efforts for girls' education.

Despite these challenges, the social team was able to work through the design and preconstruction phase. They helped the community to organize and make the Committee-Contractor Agreement, in which the seemingly impossible land and access issues were solved one by one. With the social mobilizers' encouragement, the committee members, surrounding landowners, and local notables provided solutions and made important contributions—including guaranteed access across other private land to move equipment and supplies, and a donation of the use of land for water storage, dumping of excavated material, site offices, and a laborers' camp. Despite the long-standing differences, this committee made it all happen.

Two years after the completion of the school, the head teacher was asked if she saw any differences in her community, besides having a new school. She replied proudly, "Yes, very many differences! Now the community has so many expectations of us! Before the earthquake and our new school, nobody in the community was interested in the school and they didn't care at all, but the work they did to help construction made them pay attention to the school for the first time ever. Our committee has drawn a lot of attention to the school and to girls' education. It's all very different now."

Within the first year of the school's completion, enrollment had tripled, and it was expected to grow even more in the next few years.

Brother Who Refused to Lend Land after His Family Agreed to It

In one community, a piece of property was subdivided many times among family members, but ownership had never been formally transferred, and now two brothers were fighting over it. A piece of land had been loaned by the family to serve as a place for the temporary tent school—but when one of the brothers returned home from his job in the Gulf States, he vehemently opposed the loan.

The brother's refusal occurred only a few days before the contractor had planned to set up the tent school. If that could not go ahead, all subsequent steps would be delayed. Knowing this family and community, the social team and committee identified the person most likely to have an influence on the brother—his uncle—and asked him to take charge. The uncle did so, reminding the dissenting brother that this loan had been agreed upon by the family, and that agreement had been written into the Committee-Contractor Agreement. He told his nephew that now the family would be dishonored if they withdrew the offer. After much arguing, he relented. No construction time was lost.

Meeting a Main Stakeholder on the Snow-Blocked Road

Although in the social team we thought we had done a thorough job of listing stakeholders (see Stakeholder Analysis, table 4.3), a few months into our work, we realized we had forgotten to include one quite important stakeholder: the executive engineer of the AJ&K government's road maintenance department. The reminder came in a practical way. One day, driving through a narrow mountain road to meet people in a far-off community, two social mobilizers and I found ourselves driving into deeper and deeper snow. Soon we were stalled in a long lineup of vehicles waiting for the snowplow to carve a corridor through the roof-deep snow ahead.

We decided to join many others who had left their vehicles, walking ahead and mingling with the crowd to see the heavy equipment at work. At the front of the lineup, the crowd stood back from a small group of men directing the work. As I was the only foreigner in an area where non-Kashmiris or non-Pakistanis were unusual, the man in charge noticed me and came forward to meet our team for the first time, shaking my hand in greeting. He was the district executive engineer in charge of roads, who happened to be traveling to the same town for his own meeting. He had seen PERRP construction underway and now wanted to hear about it.

As we stood and watched the action, he realized that PERRP would need him, and he told me that when we have issues with roads, the project should call on him and his department. Only a few weeks later we had to start taking him up on his offer, as road issues appeared around a few construction sites. He was good on his word, and readily solved a problem between two contractors. See, in chapter 6, the anecdote "Two Contractors in a Road Dispute."

Why We Want This School

A chairman explained why their committee put in so much effort to get a new school:

> "At any time, construction of anything in this area is very difficult. Our school is at 5,900 feet above sea level but, with no roads in most areas, we have students walking down mountain paths from 2,500 feet further above. Even with severe weather conditions they walk down here every day to attend classes in these rough sheds that the community put together when our school collapsed. The families want their children to get this education, so rather than having these students drop out due to distance or these tough conditions, or having them go away to attend other schools, our hope is to give them the opportunity to study closer to home. With the new building we will be able to do that."
>
> —SMC chairman, Government Girls' High School Kheral Abbasian

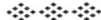

Bherkund Snake Infestation

In some cases, committees had to tackle unusual and difficult challenges. Around the town of Bherkund, one story that was told by the people for a long time was how snakes came out of the old school building when it was demolished. The contractor had first established the temporary tent school site on a separate area of the school ground and then shifted the students to the tents before proceeding to demolish the old building. Unbeknownst to all, snakes had made nests in a hidden part of the school and somehow survived both the demolition and being trucked in the rubble to the dumping site. When the snakes scurried out of the rocks in the dumping site and into surrounding fields and houses, the local people became so terrified—erroneously believing these were poisonous snakes—that they forbade any more dumping of excavated materials. Without a place to get rid of the materials, all preparations for construction would have to stop.

The committee was so anxious for construction work to continue that its members rapidly went around the community appealing to local people to allow the dumping of the materials on their land. Several hours later, at midnight, the committee convinced one man to let his land be used, and in the morning, dumping of the excavated material was moved to the new location. If this situation had happened in a typical construction project that had no community participation, the contractor would have been left to solve the problem alone, and so an alternate location might never have been found—meaning that construction could have been delayed indefinitely.

Ethnography—Government Girls' High School Long Valley*

Long Valley is a pseudonym. To maintain confidentiality, the names of schools and villages have been changed.

The people of Long Valley suffered a great tragedy in the quake: eighty-four students were killed when the local girls' high school collapsed. Because of this great loss, Pakistan's Earthquake Reconstruction and Rehabilitation Authority (ERRA) and USAID assigned PERRP to consider building a new school here. The original site was at a high altitude in AJ&K, and despite being in the roughest of conditions, classes were being run both in the open air and in a rough shed built by community members, even in freezing winter conditions.

From the technical assessment at the Long Valley school site, PERRP at first rejected this location due to its limited accessibility and the small amount of land available. The school land was located about eight hundred yards below the road on the steep mountainside. It was also blocked in: the site was surrounded by terraced agricultural land with no access to roads, only a footpath to the school. Therefore, it would be impossible to move even the smallest construction equipment here.

However, as it was the only girls' high school in such a large area, rather than give up on this site, social mobilizers appealed to the engineers to find solutions. Both teams discussed options together. It was clear that the technical challenges could only be overcome with special cooperation from the community—but the social assessment had revealed that community participation would also be a major challenge. In the social assessment, social mobilizers had already learned that this community was one extended family from a single caste, which had split into two factions due to old differences and opposing political party affiliations. For many years, disputes had consistently flared up, keeping the village in a state of tension. In that assessment, ownership of the land had also been identified as a potential problem. The terraced land between the road and school ground was made up of six small separate plots of land, each having at least two or three co-owners who were all brothers and cousins from the family's opposing factions.

The social team called the first public meeting, and an audience of about two hundred men and women from the community attended. The social mobilizers explained that ERRA and USAID had asked PERRP to consider building a school here, but the idea had already been rejected due to poor accessibility and the small land size. If the community knew ways to solve these issues, the project might once again consider building here.

Social mobilizers then left community members to discuss this situation among themselves for the next few weeks. People stayed in their political divisions, discouraging their own members from cooperating, but the social team pointed out that building a school would not be for anybody's political gain and appealed to people to stop politicizing the matter. At the most critical meeting, one of the most influential community members stepped up and asked everyone to remember that eighty-four lives had been lost in the old school, yet not a single political party was helping here. He asked everyone to put their differences aside and to join together to take this huge opportunity. Finally, enough people were convinced to try to figure out solutions.

The biggest technical challenge would be for a contractor to get equipment and materials to the site. A rough road or path was needed, but the only feasible route would be across the terraced land with multiple co-owners. The community asked its most influential people to talk to all the co-owners involved, and after much arguing and dissension, they obtained written agreement from the co-owners to proceed with their request. With this much agreement, the social team asked the project engineers and survey team to visit the site again. Working together with the community leaders and landowners, they first sketched out where a rough access track would need to go. Engineers assured the owners that this would be only a temporary track. After construction was completed, they could choose to leave the track there or, according to their wishes, the contractor could be directed to restore the land. With much negotiation, the track's alignment was moved this way or that way on each little piece of land, with co-owners eventually agreeing to a finalized route. This agreement made it possible for PERRP to proceed. The school was designed to fit the site and it went on to be a landmark that is visible all the way across the valley, with 350 girls attending classes.

This is another example of the benefits of having a dedicated social team. When the project's technical assessment had deemed construction on one location not feasible, the chances that this badly needed school would be rebuilt were very low. To make things more complicated, the local people were so divided that they might have never been able to solve this problem. However, the persistence of PERRP's social team paid off.

CHAPTER 5

Social and Technical Integration

Introduction

The Pakistan Earthquake Reconstruction and Recovery Project worked to integrate the sociocultural and technical matters, bringing together the main actors: the local people, social mobilizers, project engineers, and contractors. This was especially important to undertake, as differences and conflict frequently had major negative effects in this general disaster reconstruction scene. Figuring out how to get cooperation would reduce losses and allow PERRP's reconstruction to be completed in a timely manner so that the urgently needed educational and health facilities could operate again.

Efforts for integration of the technical and social disciplines not only helped in moving each building along on schedule—such efforts were also related to main principles of disaster risk reduction, which posit that disaster reconstruction needs to be about more than physical rebuilding: "Although short-term needs may be fulfilled by reconstruction projects sponsored by governments or by donor agencies, the real success of reconstruction is determined by the extent to which reconstruction considers and influences the contextual parameters that create vulnerability of the impacted communities in the long term" (Jigyasu 2013). PERRP's social program was designed around these kinds of contextual parameters, especially the area's highly stratified social structure comprising different social groups who normally did not work together and among whom the risk of conflict was high. PERRP worked to integrate the social and technical staff who worked for the project and the steps they took to get design and construction done. The processes chosen also helped integrate the people of the differing social groups, often for the first time, at least over the limited time span of the project.

This chapter examines how the integration was tackled, with content presented in four parts:

- **Part 1** introduces the coordinated technical and social steps selected to carry out all the work before, during, and after construction.

- **Part 2** provides specific details about the project's community participation and how it was decided by the social team, in consultation with project engineers.
- **Part 3** is about the procedural tools and training developed for the social and technical staff to understand each other's roles and coordinate their work.
- **Part 4** addresses relationship building: what it took for technical and social specialists to work together effectively so that community participation could be brought into such a project. It is a look at the rarely considered subject of the challenges and benefits of technical and social specialists working together, and at the factors that support this collaboration.

Part 1: Coordinated Social and Technical Steps

Given the scale of PERRP construction and the limited project time, coordination and integration of the elements was essential. The project involved thousands of people spread over several hundred square miles, at seventy-seven construction sites, all running simultaneously but at various stages over an average time of about three years at each site. With such a large audience in so many public locations it was important for all project staff to be consistent, to sing the same song, to be reading from the same page.

To start this coordination and integration the social team needed to understand more about what design and construction managers would do and how construction would be organized, and to then assess how the community could actually help. From meetings with the responsible project engineers a clear picture emerged of this design and construction's sequence of work and its critical path. From this discussion, we created a list of the main steps the project would need to take—before, during, and after construction. This list is available as table 5.1. The right-hand column shows the main steps that would be taken by the engineers to manage construction, starting with environmental and rapid technical assessments and ending with issuing completion certificates for the one-year defects liability period.

Table 5.1 shows the skeleton of activity throughout the project. It was used as a checklist by the social mobilizers and construction managers, as a reminder of what came next and, for monitoring the social program, of what progress had been made (see table 4.6, Monitoring—Social Steps Tracking Chart).

The left-hand column in table 5.1 lists the social or community participation steps taken. According to the main technical steps to be taken,

Table 5.1. PERRP's Step-by-Step Process.

Social Steps (Community Participation)	Technical Steps (Design and Construction)
Each of the below social steps are described in detail in the following pages. See also table 4.6 for how the social steps were monitored.	

Stage 1: Before Construction

1. Rapid social assessment 2. Introductory meetings 3. Public meetings, willingness resolution, and partnership formation 4. Committee formation 5. Communication protocol and grievance procedures 6. Settlement of land issues 7. Arrangement of land for temporary setup 8. Committee input on design 9. Committee hosts contractors' pre-bid visit	1. Environmental and technical assessment 2. Approval from USAID of design budget 3. Topographical survey and soil testing 4. Solicitation for design contractor 5. Approval of design contractor from USAID 6. Preparation and approval of design 7. Prequalification of construction contractors 8. Solicitation of construction contractors 9. USAID approval of construction budget 10. USAID approval of construction contractor

Stage 2: At the Start of and During Construction

10. Contractor briefing on social component 11. Contractor-committee agreement made 12. Construction launch event 13. Relocation to temporary site 14. Construction workers' code of conduct 15. First management and maintenance plan 16. Committee capacity building 17. Exit plan developed with committees. 18. Second management and maintenance plan 19. Basic operation and maintenance training	11. Award of construction contract 12. Contractor preconstruction meeting 13. Notice to proceed 14. Routine inspections and quality assurance 15. Health, safety, and environmental compliance 16. Scheduling and cost control 17. Contract administration 18. Progress review meetings 19. Prefinal inspection 20. Punch list items

Stage 3: End of Construction

20. Committee participation in final inspection 21. Public handover and inauguration 22. Contractor cleanup and restorations as agreed 23. Exit from community, continuation of committees 24. Committee monitors for liability defects	21. Final inspection 22. Substantial completion certificate 23. Operation and maintenance (O&M) training 24. Removal of temporary facilities 25. Handing over of building to owner 26. Contractor one-year defects liability period 27. Completion certificates issued

Note: In this table, as elsewhere in the book, "contractor" refers to the local companies hired to carry out design and construction with supervision by the implementing agency, CDM Smith.

the social steps were decided: what could be done by the social team and committees to support the technical steps in each stage of the project? The committee support was to be provided in several ways, from preventing and solving community-related conflict and other problems to helping develop member and organizational capacities. As shown, the social or participation process was set out in twenty-four main steps, starting with rapid social assessments in each location and ending with the committee having a role in the contractor's defects liability period. Following is a detailed explanation of each of the twenty-four social steps.

Part 2: Community Participation in PERRP— The Step-by-Step Process

Stage 1: Before Construction

1. Rapid Social Assessment
Along with a rapid technical assessment by project engineers, which was conducted to determine which schools or health units were technically feasible for this project to build, the social team carried out a rapid social assessment to determine if there were any strong social reasons for or against building there. Some of PERRP's social assessment criteria included: Had the school been fully functional before the disaster? Was it operating now? Were there any land issues? Did the school have a functioning community-based organization that could work with the project? Was there any conflict?

2. Introductory Meetings
Once a school location was deemed technically feasible for PERRP to construct, the social team began introductory meetings with the head teachers and respected, influential people, as detailed in the first part of chapter 4. After further discussion, the first public meetings were called, beginning the wider participation.

3. Public Meetings, Willingness Resolution, and Partnership Formation
At the first public meeting at each location, which was usually attended by a few hundred people, the social team informed the community about the potential project to rebuild their school or health facility. We explained that the government had requested this construction and that the donor was willing to pay for the design and construction, but that going ahead with the project would depend on community interest and their willingness to participate and contribute. In short, we explained that we would like to form a partnership, where both partners—the community

and PERRP—would have demanding responsibilities. In this partnership, PERRP would take responsibility to build the new building, but since there were no functioning community-based organizations, the community needed to form a committee to carry out a long list of duties—notably, to help the construction process, keep it on schedule, and prevent it from causing problems for the local people. The partnership was also offered on the condition that land issues, if any, were settled before PERRP would take any further steps for design or construction.

In regions where construction and contractors often have a negative reputation, and where construction is often associated with trouble, loss, and conflict, the first public meeting was also an opportunity to start talking about working together and preventing conflict (as related in the anecdote "Introducing Grievance Procedures," page 205). For many, it was possibly the first time that they heard, in public, that their complaints would be addressed, along with the planned process for doing so. They were introduced to the communication protocol with the grievance procedures, and they were informed that the use of these procedures could prevent conflict and should reduce the need for court cases.

After we answered audience questions, they voted with a show of hands. Did the audience members agree to take on such a partnership, form a committee, participate in the project, settle land issues expedi-

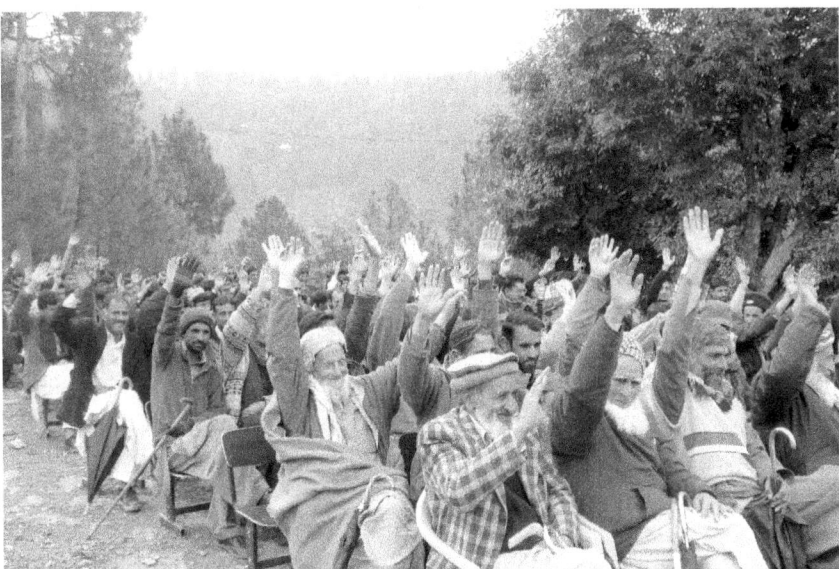

Figure 5.1. Voting on a Willingness Resolution. To form a partnership with the PERRP project, community members in each location voted, making a formal Willingness Resolution to form a committee and participate, 2008. © Zia Ahmed.

tiously, and carry out many other volunteer duties? In every case, the answer was an enthusiastic "yes."

At this point, community members were asked to write a simple willingness resolution that formally invited and requested PERRP to proceed, and to state their willingness to accept the duties that were assigned. With this agreement between the project and community, the partnership was formed. Such willingness resolutions have become customary among NGOs working in different fields in the region, as implementing agencies have learned to avoid assuming that help from outside—or help from particular sources—is welcomed by all. Some reconstruction projects have also learned to make sure that community representatives issue a formal invitation and request to work in the community to show the project is not being imposed. This written resolution was kept by the project and committee as part of meeting minutes and other documentation.

4. Committee Formation
At this first public meeting, those in attendance—who often numbered in the hundreds—were requested to ask people to form a committee that would work with PERRP, choosing only members that fit criteria established in earlier introductory meetings with key community members, as discussed on page 133. The process for committee formation applied in both AJ&K and KP province, with one exception. According to the government guidelines, girls' schools in KP province had women-only Parent Teacher Councils, in accordance with the customs of *purdah*. In those cases, a separate committee of men formed based on the same criteria to advise the Parent Teacher Councils and work directly with the project for construction.

5. Communication Protocol with Grievance Procedures
To coordinate the social and technical aspects of work and prevent conflict, the social team introduced the project's communication protocol, which applied to the committee, community members, contractors, and all project social and technical staff. This important management tool is discussed later in this chapter. One of the committee's key responsibilities was to help prevent and resolve construction-related conflict. As some of the committee members were elders or other prominent people whom the community relied on for dispute resolution, this responsibility was highlighted in the first public meeting. PERRP built on communities' dispute-solving traditions, adding new tools to prevent and deal with complaints and conflict, such as the communication protocol with its grievance procedures, written agreements, a code of conduct, and other measures discussed later in this chapter.

6. Settlement of Land Issues

Issues about land ownership can be a significant risk in construction at any time and, as discussed in chapter 2, they were one of the reasons for long delays in other projects in this disaster reconstruction. It is common that differences over land lead to conflict and violence, as well as to court cases that are pursued either for valid reasons or for retribution. These are some of the many ways that power is used or misused by individuals, families, or groups who oppose each other, creating situations that have lasted for years or even decades.

Foreseeing land issues as one of the main things that could go wrong in this project, PERRP made a condition with communities that they would settle any disputes over land before design or construction would proceed. Since committee members were respected, influential people with strong capacities for problem-solving, they were given this task as their first major challenge. PERRP offered a fair, transparent, participatory process to help settle the land issues, enabling the people themselves to settle them.

Despite the *patwari* culture and the reputation for corruption in the land revenue system, these locally based government offices and officials are the authorities, and settling land issues in PERRP could not be achieved without them. To establish the cooperation needed for a fair and transparent process, the social team worked first on getting the buy-in and support of the district's highest administrator, the Deputy Commissioner (DC) or District Coordination Officer (DCO). Meetings were held with the DC or DCO to introduce the project, and have them direct the Revenue Department to assist as needed on the ground. PERRP then had the Revenue Department agree that no fees would be paid by anyone for any reason for their service. Other preparations for the day of the *patwari* survey at each site included an open invitation for any community members interested to attend and witness the survey.

Since many years earlier the government had purchased the land on which PERRP would construct high schools and health facilities, the most common land issue was about exact property boundary lines. Each school or health facility needed to provide PERRP with copies of their ownership or mutation documents, as well as the original cadastral survey map showing the land boundaries, but almost none had these documents on-site and instead had to search for them in faraway government offices. Even if it was claimed that there were no land issues, the same process was conducted to verify this claim.

On the day of the *patwari* survey—which took place on the prospective construction site with a small crowd attending as observers and informal witnesses—PERRP's social team and committee members facilitated a discussion among adjoining landowners and government officials or their authorized representatives. Participants were informed that:

- discussions and agreements to solve the land issue must be public (with no separate or private negotiations), so that it would be public information with many witnesses
- as a result of the agreement made in public at this event, the Revenue Department and *patwari* would formalize the agreement and promptly issue the renewed or revised legal documents
- no money was to change hands for any reason
- whatever would be agreed on in the meeting would be binding, according to local custom
- negotiation was between the landowners, not between the landowners and the project, as this was their land and school or health facility at stake
- if any landowner would not cooperate or made unreasonable demands to settle a land issue that could affect the design or construction of a new facility (as assessed by project construction engineers also attending), it was up to community leaders and members to persuade settlement on the spot, without delay.

Using the original documents, local knowledge, and debate, participants compared the boundaries in the documents with what the boundaries were understood to be today. In most cases, the boundaries had never been demarcated on the ground and were only noted on the rough hand-drawn map made decades earlier, or remembered in relation to natural features, such as "from that big rock to that big rock" or "to that point of land." The *patwari* conducted a new cadastral survey on the spot, marking out the boundary lines according to the final agreement. As an innovation within this process, community members watched and helped the *patwari* install pegs in the ground to show the boundary line according to what had been agreed on, often for the first time. As they had participated in making the decisions about the boundary rather than having decisions imposed on them, as is normally the case, they protected the pegs until the end of construction. In contrast, when decisions are imposed, pegs are often removed in protest.

By the end of this one day, all paperwork was completed and signed on the spot, or taken back to the Revenue Department. As settling land issues in Pakistan can often take years, doing it in only one day created a celebratory mood and an excitement that design and construction would proceed. For the community members, forming a representative committee had been their first big achievement, but the transparent process offered by PERRP helped them quickly settle land issues, which proved to be highly motivating in taking the next steps.

Within a few days, the *patwari*'s office issued the new survey and other legal documents, and for the first time ever, copies of these documents were provided to the school or health facility to keep for their own reference. Some head teachers remarked that this alone was of value, as having documents on-site would help them argue against future cases of encroachment or other intrusions on school land. At times, even government officials expressed surprise with how well this process worked.

7. Arrangement of Land for Temporary Setup

In order for construction to start, the rubble of the destroyed building needed to be cleared away. Teachers and students were attending class either in remaining dangerous buildings or outdoors on the same land, sometimes sitting on the stones from the old building or on damaged furniture. Patients were visiting health clinics in the same condition as schools. For construction to be underway, the students, teachers, patients, and health staff had to be relocated. But to where?

For this purpose, the third challenge given to the committee was to arrange a loan of land for a temporary school or health unit site for up to two years. On this land, PERRP would install a temporary tent school or clinic for use during construction of the new building—and for such large tents, flat land was needed. This loan was often difficult for them to achieve, as such land was needed for crops and other productive purposes; in this mountainous region, flat land was scarce and precious. However, somewhat buoyed by the early success of settling land issues, local inhabitants also succeeded at this assignment. In every location, committee members convinced someone to forfeit their land and crop for a few growing seasons so that the tent facilities could be put there. Moreover, most of the owners donated the use of the land with no charges, prodded to do so by committee members. In a couple of cases where land was not available for free, committee members—at their own initiative—paid the rent out of their own pockets or secured other donations for it. These donations had not been suggested by the project, but instead were initiated by the committee members who chose to ask fellow community members to contribute. The courage it took to do this, and to succeed at it, formed the basis for future initiatives, especially the Library Challenge, during which the schools were led to put together their first-ever libraries (see chapter 7).

This process worked because the committee members took their responsibilities seriously and were anxious and enthusiastic to get a school built. Few other reconstruction projects were offering a temporary place to continue classes. As expressed at the time, land was lent as a gesture of gratitude for the new school.

8. Committee Input on Design
The design of the new buildings was driven by many factors, but part of the participatory process was to get community and end user input. This not only increased buy-in but also helped to prevent costly mistakes and save time. Details of this process are outlined in chapter 6.

9. Committee Hosting of Contractor's Prebid Visit
As normally there is no relationship between contractors and community members—or there is only an adversarial relationship—PERRP took early steps to prevent conflict by putting the committee into an unusual position of power: because they were prepared, they had more power. As part of PERRP's tendering process, a mandatory prebid site visit was held in each community and was attended by all representatives of the shortlisted construction companies. By this point, the local committee had been functioning for months and was well organized. To show contractors that this project and this community were going to be quite different from those at other places they had done construction—places where communities are not organized or involved at all—PERRP had each committee host the shortlisted contractors. This friendly visit showed that the committee was in charge for the community, and that its members would be of unusual help to the contractor. PERRP engineers and committee members walked company representatives around the site and surroundings, pointing out the technical considerations and giving general ideas about the availability of land, water, and electricity. Such preliminary steps helped establish friendly relations between the community and whoever won the contract.

Stage 2: At Start of and During Construction

By the time construction was ready to start, the social program was well established, and the communities were well informed and prepared. Social mobilizers and engineers had a clear picture of each other's roles and what they could depend on each other for. The technical component had prepared the design, obtained the needed approvals, conducted the tendering process, and selected the contractors.

10. Contractor Briefing on the Social Component
Since a structured social component in construction projects is uncommon, if not unprecedented, the companies who won the bids to be PERRP

construction contractors had no experience with such community participation. As part of their preparation to start work, the companies attended a contractor briefing on community participation, on the communication protocol with grievance procedures, and on the "do no harm" guidelines.

The medical imperative to do no harm has been adopted by many other fields, and while the concept applies well to construction, it is rarely used. In PERRP, it was an important tool in conflict prevention: the project asked the contractors to be careful and respectful of the committee and community members, and in turn, the committee would help them during the project. Contractors were asked to do no damage or harm to people, their property, their relations, or their culture; to not assume they could use people's land, water, or resources without their permission; to not do any damage to buildings, other land, trees, or natural resources; to not break cultural norms; and to not cause problems between local people. These and other requests were written into the Committee-Contractor Agreement.

11. Committee-Contractor Agreement
As obvious as it might seem, many problems could be prevented by making an agreement prior to construction, but this is rarely done. As discussed in detail in the second part of this chapter, "Integration Tools and Training," committees and contractors were led to make a point-by-point agreement in writing.

12. Committee Organization of Construction Launch Event
As soon as the contractor was ready to put shovels in the ground, the committees organized public events to launch the construction. Such events were large gatherings, and were attended by the teachers, students, parents, local officials, donor representatives, and hundreds of community members. After suffering the destruction of their old school or health facility, the loss of life, and doubts that these facilities might ever be rebuilt, the public launch was a big celebration. Speeches by local officials, students, school or health facility staff, and prominent people usually attested to the hope that the project gave them. To emphasize that the committees were in charge, the project did not organize this event or pay for any of it, as might otherwise be standard practice for a foreign-funded project. Committees were advised to stay within their means: they were advised to hold no-cost events, but it was up to them what to do.

13. Relocation to Temporary Site
Now that construction was ready to start and the committee had arranged land for the temporary tent school or health unit, the contractor was re-

sponsible for setting up that site's temporary tent classrooms, offices, water supply, toilets, wash basins, and other necessary facilities. Once set up, teachers and committee members helped move students and school operations from their old destroyed facility to the new site, freeing up the original land for construction to begin. In the same way, health unit staff and their committees moved their operation to the temporary tent clinic.

14. Construction Workers' Code of Conduct

Contractors from different parts of Pakistan brought their work crews to do the earthquake reconstruction. Following the first life-threatening incidents around construction sites in response to workers breaking local cultural norms, the social team developed a construction workers' code of conduct to try to prevent these kinds of problems. Workers from other regions and cultures of Pakistan needed to be briefed on the kinds of behavior expected in these conservative rural areas. Serious breaches of the norms could damage local people and cause retaliation against workers and construction. See anecdote "Serious Cultural Breach," page 68.

To develop the construction workers' code of conduct, social mobilizers worked with each committee to draw up a list of the most common cultural breaches, along with specific ways to prevent them. For example, in their off-hours, workers often wandered around the close-knit, conservative community, sometimes getting into private or sensitive locations where women might be gathered together—for instance, at water wells. The solution was for each community to identify the places the workers could not go. Another problem was that the laborers would sometimes act or speak disrespectfully to local people or get into heated political arguments. In the code of conduct, they were asked to avoid political discussion and to respect local people like they respect their own family members.

At each site, workers were briefed on the code, and contractors were obliged to have their workers honor it. At the briefings, elders welcomed the laborers to the community, thanked them for coming to this far off place, and appealed to the workers to respect the norms. Although there still were a few instances of significant breaches of cultural norms during PERRP's six years, some causing serious fights, the frequency was significantly reduced by the community, contractor, and construction workers' clear and firm expectations.

15. First Management and Maintenance Plan

Once the new buildings were constructed, the committees were to be responsible for sharing maintenance of the new buildings with the government. To raise awareness about these duties, they were started at the temporary tent sites. The social team led the committee in analyzing maintenance needs and determining what work would have to be done, by whom, and when, how, and with what resources. This first management and maintenance plan was made and then executed by the teachers, students, and paid cleaning staff (if any), with the committee acting as monitors. These duties were also part of the Committee-Contractor Agreement.

16. Committee Capacity Building
While even the poorest, most remote communities can have significant capacities, these strengths are often overlooked by external agencies. On the other hand, if agencies were to seek out these strengths, such as was done with PERRP's capacities and vulnerabilities analysis exercise (see chapter 4), they would find potential and opportunities in the local communities. For example, in the school and health committees, members' abilities and interest in helping construction were apparent early on, and the project introduced additional activities to enable the committee members to increase their knowledge about construction and, in the case of school committees, how to help improve education. Other activities included participatory performance assessment, the introduction of cocurricular activities, and fundraising for their schools' first-ever libraries.

As committees at health facilities were only for the purpose of facilitating construction and had no community participation in health activities—as per the directive of the Department of Health, and related in the anecdote on page 110, "No to Community Participation!"—committee member activity was limited to construction-related matters. But for the communities in which schools were being built, an important part of capacity building was regular attendance at joint workshops that, every few months, brought together the head teacher (as general secretary) and the chairperson (community representative) from all the PERRP school projects. The first school committee joint workshops included a visit to sites under construction, so that committee members could hear the latest plans from designers and engineers. These early workshops helped to build trust and confidence in the PERRP process. As projects developed, committee members began to develop their own agendas for the joint workshops. Members commented, "Now that we see our school's reconstruction actually is starting, we want to talk about our other problems too."

These joint workshops motivated committee members to share news and ideas from their own schools, and even to develop a healthy sense of competition as they told each other about what they had achieved: their first ever parent-teacher meetings, new and increased numbers of cocurricular events, and unprecedented attention and assistance from the community. The workshops were also used as a platform to carry out a participatory study on problems in education and to subsequently develop a plan of action. The unity and spirit developed through the committee joint workshops also grew into the remarkable Library Challenge, which is described in chapter 7. As with other community member participation, no fees or stipends were paid for any purpose on this project. Committee members attended all functions, including meetings and the workshops, at their own expense—a feat that is highly unusual in foreign aid projects in the region, which usually pay some level of fees or allowances. Even so, attendance at PERRP gatherings was almost always 100 percent.

As part of PERRP's internal monitoring to document and assess participation, the committees were led to collect, analyze, and report their own data on a yearly basis. This process was facilitated by a social mobilizer in a participatory performance assessment (see the participation index described in chapter 4). This was another new experience for committee members.

Before the earthquake, parents and teachers in this region normally had little or no contact with one another. Schools were considered the domain of head teachers and teachers. Parents were expected to leave their children's education up to the educators, and many did not feel welcome at the school. At the same time, there were normally no school activities other than classes. PERRP capacity-building led the committees to support teachers in different ways, including through the introduction of new activities. Committees did this by assisting with volunteer work and funds to run low-cost in-school activities such as contests, demonstrations of public speaking, drawing, spelling, essay writing, skits, poetry recitation, singing, sports days, plantation days, reunions, parents' days, and national holiday celebrations. Some committee members had related skills they could apply in such activities. Through these activities, committees brought together parents and teachers—in some places, for the first time ever.

17. Exit Plan Developed with Committees

To prepare committees for the time when construction would be finished and PERRP and the social mobilizers would leave the community, discussions about an exit plan began about midway through the project. What would the committees do when the project was finished? Would they continue to meet? For what purposes and activities? Plans were made for committees' continuation after the project.

18. Second Management and Maintenance Plan

After practicing maintenance of the temporary tent school or health facility for several months, and when construction of the new building was in its final state, the maintenance planning exercise was repeated, and a second management and maintenance plan was created for the new facility.

19. Basic Operation and Maintenance Training

Once teachers and students were moved into the new school, or staff into the new health facilities, PERRP provided basic operation and maintenance training to facility users and staff. This training covered what to do if the building had an emergency, including how to use a fire extinguisher and circuit breaker, shut off the water valves, and control the water pump.

Stage 3: At End of Construction

20. Committee Participation in Final Inspection

In Pakistan, when construction of a new public building is complete, it is normally handed over to the owner without any community involvement. In PERRP, since the committee had taken responsibility all along and deserved recognition for it, they were invited—along with government officials, the construction contractor, PERRP engineers, social mobilizers, and representatives from either the Department of Education or Department of Health—to walk through the building and to participate in the final inspection. As a final show of recognition of the committee's contribution to getting the school or health clinic built, PERRP placed a series of construction photographs in the entryway of each building, as well as a permanent plaque listing the committee members' names. For committee members, this was an unexpected honor and, for many, an emotional time.

21. Public Handover and Inauguration

With all construction and interiors completed and furniture moved into place, responsibility for the new building was handed over to either the Department of Education or Department of Health at a special public event organized by the committee. This was a special celebration, and the committee put their new organizational skills to use for this event. Such events were attended by hundreds or even thousands of people.

As with all such public events in this project, the committee was the organizer. Committee members once again called on their own skills and experience as organizers of large political, religious, or family events in planning these inauguration events. Members raised the funds and had businesses contribute by loaning the necessary resources, including stage and sound systems, chairs, overhead tent-like coverings, banners, and refreshments. Inaugurations were large events attended by representatives of USAID, the government of Pakistan, the government of AJ&K or KP province, and the media. Communities saw the completion and handover of the new building as a symbol of hope and a turning point in disaster recovery.

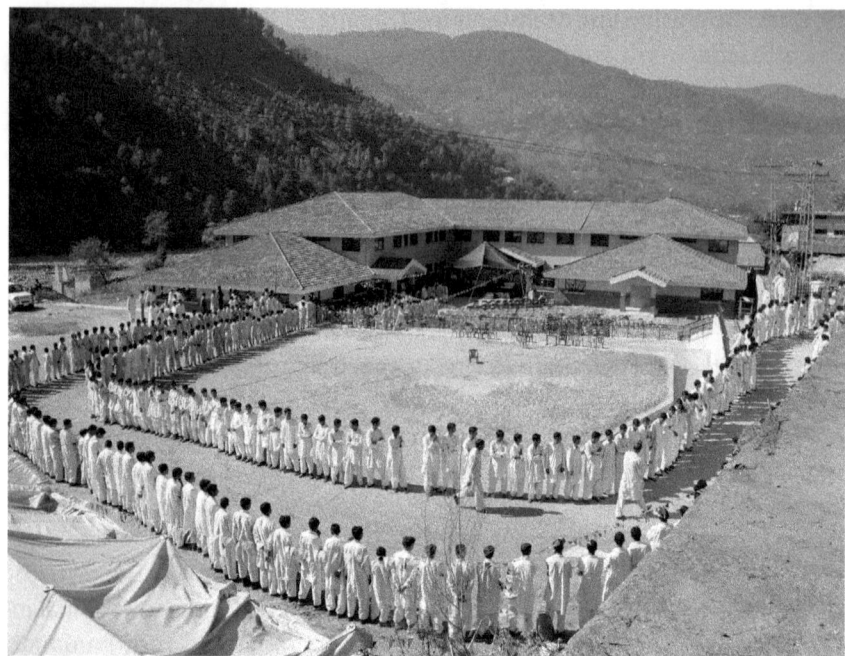

Figure 5.2. School Inauguration. Upon completion of construction of each facility, the committees organized inaugurations. Here in front of their new school, students formed an honor guard to welcome officials attending the celebration. Government Boys' Higher Secondary School Rerra, 2010. © Sardar Zaheer Mughal.

22. Contractor Cleanup and Restorations as Agreed

As per the Committee-Contractor Agreement, the contractor performed a cleanup and restoration before leaving the community, removing all materials and equipment and restoring all local land to its preconstruction state. For example, if a temporary track had been made to access the site by vehicle, and if the committee and involved landowners wanted it removed, it was removed.

23. PERRP Exit from Community and Continuation of Committees

When all work was completed, PERRP staff left the communities. Committees then were to continue and implement the plans they had made; however, this did not occur, as discussed in Chapter 4, Part 2.

24. Committee Monitoring during Contractor Liability Defects Period

For one year after the completion of construction, contractors were liable for any defects that might appear in their work. As PERRP was no longer present in the community, it was a duty of the committee to watch for any defects and report them to the PERRP office. PERRP would then have the contractor correct the defects.

Part 3: Integration Tools and Training

Three key tools developed in PERRP helped to create a friendly, responsible, and respectful atmosphere. These tools helped build the capacities of the technical and social staff, committee, and contractor; and they reduced conflict, preventing issues among the local people and saving a great deal of time that could have been lost in construction. These tools were designed to coordinate and integrate the social and technical components. At the end of the project, during "lessons learned" exercises with both social mobilizers and engineers, these tools were assessed as determining much of PERRP's success:

- the communication protocol with grievance procedures
- the Committee-Contractor Agreement
- the training together of the social and technical teams

Communication Protocol with Grievance Procedures

It was well known that disputes and conflict were common at other postquake reconstruction sites. We saw that these problems stemmed from a lack of organization and local leadership, from having no way to handle grievances, from a lack of coordination around the construction site, and from the resulting adversarial relationship between the contractor and local people. Having a committee for the purpose of facilitating construction allowed for a new organizational structure at the construction site. This put the committee in an unusual position of power, virtually equal to that of the contractor. Accordingly, PERRP encouraged and supported the development of friendly, mutually supportive committee-contractor relations.

To reflect this new arrangement of influence and power, and to coordinate and streamline information and activities, the social team introduced a communication protocol that included grievance procedures. The idea was that grievances would be handled the same way as other information. This completely changed the ineffective and risky ways in which community members and contractors usually would interact with each other. As much of the conflict around the construction site was a reaction from people having no way to have their complaints heard, the PERRP grievance procedures instructed project staff to listen to complaints and act on them immediately. This helped "people disengage and establish alternate systems for dealing with the problems that underlie the conflict" (Anderson 1999: 1).

The communication protocol with grievance procedures set out the lines of communication. As shown in figure 5.3, under this new structure all people involved would be treated according to the separate but coordinated social and technical sides of the project. The communication protocol with its grievance procedures included a set of rules about who would communicate with whom, and how grievances could be made and settled.

The protocol was simple. Social mobilizers worked exclusively with the committees, while the project's site engineers worked only with the contractor. For maximum transparency, community members and their com-

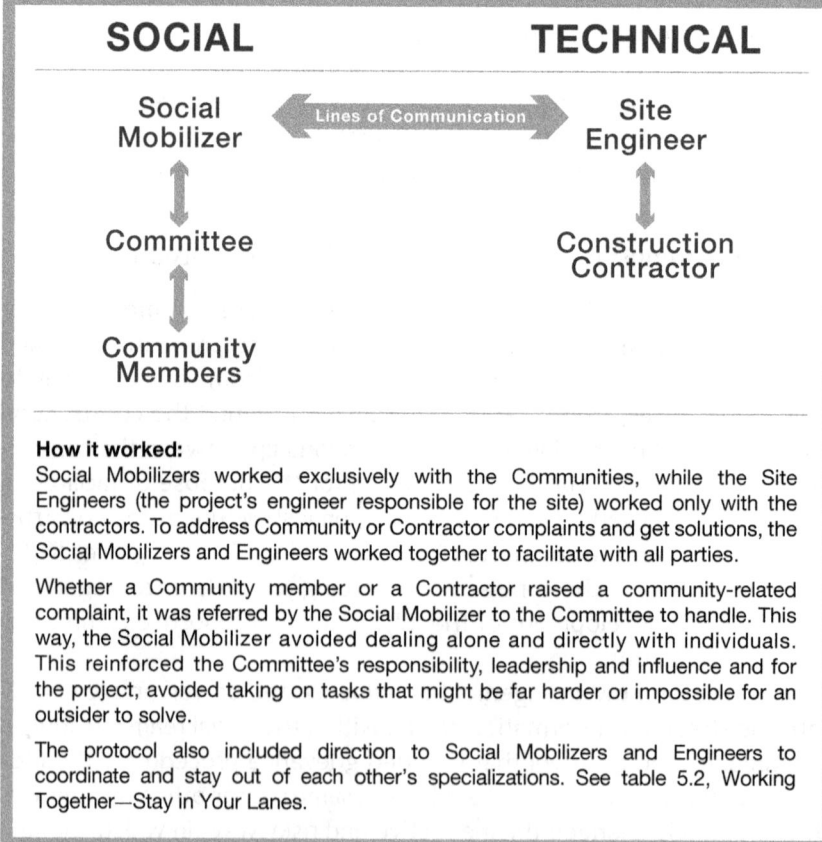

How it worked:
Social Mobilizers worked exclusively with the Communities, while the Site Engineers (the project's engineer responsible for the site) worked only with the contractors. To address Community or Contractor complaints and get solutions, the Social Mobilizers and Engineers worked together to facilitate with all parties.

Whether a Community member or a Contractor raised a community-related complaint, it was referred by the Social Mobilizer to the Committee to handle. This way, the Social Mobilizer avoided dealing alone and directly with individuals. This reinforced the Committee's responsibility, leadership and influence and for the project, avoided taking on tasks that might be far harder or impossible for an outsider to solve.

The protocol also included direction to Social Mobilizers and Engineers to coordinate and stay out of each other's specializations. See table 5.2, Working Together—Stay in Your Lanes.

Figure 5.3. Communication Protocol with Grievance Procedures. Also see table 5.2 for how the social mobilizers and site engineers were to work together by staying in their lanes.

mittees were discouraged from dealing directly with the contractor, and vice versa, unless it was an emergency. Whether a community member or a contractor raised a community-related complaint, it was referred by the social mobilizer to the committee to handle. This way, the social mobilizer avoided dealing alone and directly with individuals. Assigning local responsibility this way reinforced the committee's responsibility, leadership, and influence and avoided having the project take on tasks that might be far harder or impossible for outsiders to solve. All such complaints were to be dealt with right away, and were usually handled within minutes or hours, either face to face or by cell phone. The protocol also included direction to the social mobilizers and engineers to coordinate and stay out of each other's specializations (see table 5.2).

Committee-Contractor Agreements

In PERRP's "lessons learned" workshops, there was consensus that the innovation of a Committee-Contractor Agreement was one of the main reasons for cooperation between the community and the contractor. This agreement reduced local loss and conflict, which helped reduce the number of lost construction days. This relatively simple document, which had been made in mere hours, was probably responsible for saving months of lost construction time and also establishing the respectful working relationship.

When the construction contract was awarded, and even before the formal notice to proceed was issued to the contractor to start construction, each project site required a community-contractor agreement. While the community was informed well ahead of time of what the contractor would likely need, thus allowing committees to start working out solutions, the agreement would come together the day the contractor arrived at the site.

On the designated day, a meeting was held to create and sign the agreement. Held on-site, the meeting was attended by the full committee, the contractor, and the key technical people who would work on site. The meeting was facilitated by the social mobilizer and site engineer. In each case, the contractor was asked to list the things they would need—for example, a certain amount of water supply, electricity, access across other land, or a rental agreement. Then, point by point, the committee was asked for their suggestions. Could they help supply each need, whether paid or free of charge? Likewise, the committee was asked about what the community wanted to happen and what they wanted to avoid. For example, they were asked about traffic, dust, noise, a laborers' camp, the potential for loss of privacy, and the behavior of workers.

On each point, the consensus was put into writing as the Committee-Contractor Agreement. Over time and as needed, the Committee-Contractor Agreement was altered or added to, as long as both parties agreed. It was treated as a valuable document and used as a reference by all parties for the entirety of the project. It was also often used by community members among one another, as reminders of what they promised to do. The agreements included many different terms, with each one custom made in each location by the people involved.

While these agreements varied place to place, typical content included:

- **Land.** Outside the school land, what other land or space was needed, for what purposes (e.g., for a site office or residence, or to store equipment or materials), and for how long? Who owns the land, and what would be the terms of use?
- **Water.** How much water was needed for what purposes, when, for how long, and from what locations? What would be the terms of use?
- **Electricity.** What amount of electricity was needed, for what purposes, for how long, when, and from where? What would be the terms of use?
- **Site access across other land or sensitive areas.** To reach the construction site, would the contractor need access across other land where direct access might be blocked? What land would they need to cross, and who owns it? How could access be guaranteed? How long was it needed? What would be the terms of use?
- **Safety precautions.** What safety precautions would be needed? Who will take them and when? If blasting for excavation had to happen, would advance notice and protection be given to local people?
- **Laborer camp.** Would this community allow a laborer camp here? If yes, where, for how long, and under what terms? If no, where might be an alternate place?
- **Jobs.** Would the contractor hire any local workers?
- **Respecting cultural norms.** These communities are conservative with their own cultural norms. The contractor would need to protect the privacy of the surrounding buildings. How would the contractors' workers, who may be from other cultures, respect the norms and not cause disturbances?
- **Additional work outside construction.** What if someone were to make demands that work be done on their own property, which was not part of the construction contract? How would that be handled?
- **Days and hours of work.** Does the community agree with the proposed days and hours of work at the construction site? The commit-

tee usually asked the contractor to make sure there was at least one day per week that was free of noise or dust.

Training Together

Each site had a designated social mobilizer and site engineer who worked as counterparts. The social mobilizer worked with the committee, while the site engineer was on the site full-time to supervise the contractor. The social mobilizers and engineers were trained together and developed strong working relationships. The training exercise below—dubbed "Who is Going to Do What About This?"—shows how PERRP staff were trained to apply the communication protocol with grievance procedures. In this joint training exercise PERRP social mobilizers and site engineers were asked to sit together and analyze case studies from actual incidents, identifying the actions that should be taken—and who should take them—according to PERRP's communication protocol with grievance procedures or other agreed procedures.

Case 1: Petty Contractor Left the Job without Paying Local Suppliers
A petty contractor has left the job without paying local suppliers, who are threatening to block construction tomorrow and get a court stay order to stop construction. If the stay order is granted, it could disrupt or halt construction for months or even years. In the meantime, the local suppliers' businesses will suffer too. *Who is going to do what about this?*

Case 2: Elite Demands Unrelated Work
For their own benefit, powerful people sometimes try to get work done which has nothing to do with the planned construction. In one of the PERRP communities, the "big man" down the road is demanding that drainage pipes be installed on his land—drainage that has nothing to do with the construction project. He claims if he doesn't get this work done and soon, he will make trouble for the project. *Who is going to do what about this?*

Case 3: Stop the Water Supply until the Bridge Is Fixed
Although the community had agreed in the Committee-Contractor Agreement to let the contractor use their limited personal water supply in exchange for him making repairs to their nearby bridge, they have cut him off because he has failed to fix the bridge. Now there are two problems: the bridge is too weak to bring in heavy equipment, and there is no water for concrete work. Everything is stuck. *Who is going to do what about this?*

Case 4: Dispute within Family over Lending Land
Social mobilizers have worked for weeks to have the community identify a suitable site for a temporary tent school to be installed. In this mountainous area, the flat land needed for such a large arrangement of tents is scarce and always in use for crops. However, community members finally convince one family to let their land be used and make a loan agreement with the School Management Committee. However, when one of the landowning brothers returns from working abroad and hears about this agreement, he is furious and refuses to agree to the loan, making ominous threats. The contractor is arriving in the next couple of days to start installing the tents, and if this installation is delayed, it will postpone the construction of the new school. Community members, social mobilizers, the project's construction managers, and the contractor are all frantic. *Who is going to do what about this?*

Case 5: Threats for Jobs
Local men are making threats of violence against the construction contractor to hire them. They were making the threats even though it was part of the Committee-Contractor Agreement that the contractor would bring in skilled work crews and not hire from this location. *Who is going to do what about this?*

Case 6: Laborer Visiting Place Reserved for Women
A construction site laborer from another culture and part of Pakistan was caught by a local man hanging around the water spring where women were washing clothes—a location meant only for women. Taking this as an offense to local cultural norms, the local men beat up the laborer, and more community members rise up against the offender and his fellow laborers. Given that there are several dozen laborers on site, this situation could escalate into a community-wide fight, with potentially fatal injuries and stopped construction. *Who is going to do what about this?*

Case 7: Two Contractors Fighting over Road Construction
As PERRP construction of the new health unit was underway in a remote, mountainous area, the earthen road that passes by the construction site was being upgraded by another contractor for the government's Department of Roads. Each contractor is blaming the other for damage to the road near the entrance to the health unit. The anger is spreading and could easily turn into conflict between the two sets of laborers. *Who is going to do what about this?*

How Joint Training Worked

Occasional training and workshop-type discussions on the communication protocol, such as those in the above training exercises, served to refine and deepen understanding and usage of these protocols. Participating in these discussions were the social mobilizers, site engineers, and their supervisors; this was particularly important as this collaboration was a new experience for all. As construction projects rarely include social specialists, the engineers on previous projects had been left to deal with the people themselves, often unsuccessfully. In contrast, the social mobilizers had community expertise, but little or no experience with construction. The protocol helped delineate their roles while making them complementary, as discussed in "Relationship Building among PERRP Engineers and Social Mobilizers," next page.

The grievance procedures that were part of the communication protocol differed from normal practice in construction. Before, if construction projects had any grievance procedures at all, they were either informal and unknown to the people, or too weak to be effective. A PERRP engineer gave one example that he knew of from other construction sites: having a complaints book at the gate of the site. That process depended on complainants being literate, and on written complaints being attended to instead of ignored. In PERRP, the complaints process was part of day-to-day communications and action.

Normally, if contractors needed something locally, they would simply arrange it themselves in a private deal. If they needed a water supply, electricity, or a place to make a camp for their workers, they would find somebody willing to supply it, and make an informal verbal agreement with them. However, from the "What Could Go Wrong?" analysis, we knew these informal, private, verbal arrangements were the cause of many problems. In PERRP, the contractor was to make no private deals: all needs were to be funneled through the committee, and all such deals were made public, handled transparently, and put into written form in the Committee-Contractor Agreement. The site engineer and social mobilizer were responsible for ensuring that all business was handled this way.

There was only one exception to the communication protocol: in an emergency, or if any danger arose, it was not necessary to go through the prescribed channels. If a fire broke out, an injury occurred, or if members of the public came out on the construction site when banned from doing so for safety reasons, the normal protocol did not need to be followed. In such cases, the contractor, community members, or committee members were encouraged to take immediate action as needed.

Part 4: Relationship Building among PERRP Engineers and Social Mobilizers

Postdisaster reconstruction has drawn attention from a multidisciplinary community of specialists, which can be grouped into two broad categories: those dealing with the physical aspects of the built and natural environment such as architects, engineers, and planners, and those concerned about the social, cultural, political, and psychological aspects of reconstruction, led by anthropologists, sociologists, and other social scientists. "Unfortunately the disciplinary backgrounds that empower all these specialists with tools and methodological processes many times also act as blinkers restricting their vision from looking beyond their narrow disciplinary confines and seeing the complexity behind seemingly simple observations of reconstruction processes" (Jigyasu 2013: ix).

The above ideas raise the subject of technical and sociocultural specialists, and their ability and willingness to work together. Jigyasu posits that aspects of each discipline make it difficult for practitioners to understand other disciplines, while also making it easy to miss their complexities. But speaking as a sociocultural specialist with decades of experience working with specialists from many disciplines—including health, education, economics, law, agriculture, forestry, trade, microfinance, water management, and environment—no matter the specialty, there are often blinkers that hinder recognition of the complex cultural or social side of one's own field. For many, there simply is no awareness that there is a social side to their work. Either the education of such professionals offers no sensitization to the sociocultural dimension of their work, or that knowledge simply is not put into practice.

This also raises the subject of cultures and communities, specifically of engineers, sociocultural experts, and all their possible interrelations. If each of these two disciplines were analyzed individually, using the same vocabulary that is applied to the study of culture and communities, it could very well show that, even within the engineering community and the sociocultural specialist community, we can find heterogeneity, class-based hierarchies, arrangements of power, and many other similar divisions. How these disciplines view each other might not only be restricted by the blinkers described by Jigyasu but might also be a matter of culturally entrenched classes and hierarchies. This section, then, raises a rarely discussed question: how can technical and sociocultural specialists work together effectively? I do not attempt to answer this question broadly—this chapter will only recount how this work was undertaken in PERRP.

The Challenges

In PERRP, there were some initial challenges in having engineers and social mobilizers work together. Two sets of factors affected working relationships in the start-up period.

The first set of factors was the existing biases, prejudices, and stereotypes that the technical and sociocultural specialists each held regarding the other, along with the little knowledge they had of each other's expertise and usefulness. There was also the fact that engineers were used to working alone on any construction site. As projects do not normally have social expertise to resolve conflicts, engineers had been left to try to solve community-related problems. Not only had they been responsible for aspects of managing construction, but when something happened with local people, they or a delegate would have to try to address it. Depending on their style, they could ignore people, issue orders, take punitive steps, try to negotiate, or pass on the problem to authorities. Now that this project had a social team to look after all the social issues, there were mixed reactions: some were openly opposed, and others were just unsure what that would mean.

The second set of factors is common among any group of people, even those from the same discipline, who for the first time are coming together to work. These challenges, which are encountered by NGOs, corporations, and other institutions, fall into the realm of human resource development, group formation, or team building (Stein, n.d.). Stages in the framework used here are referred to as forming, storming, norming, performing, and adjourning. These are typical stages that groups of any kind go through. While at the beginning there can be uncertainty, misunderstanding, and friction, as members figure out how to work together, they can go on to perform effectively even in the most complex situations. These teams often form strong bonds and friendships, and they usually come to regret that the project and team must come to an end, which was the case in PERRP.

Team Building and Development

Year One: The Storming Stage

In PERRP, there were two distinct time periods in the development of working relations: the first year and the time that followed. Taking a frank look at those first few months, we can see that sociocultural and technical specialists sometimes perceived each other through stereotypes, throwing blunt accusations. To the social mobilizers, some of the engineers were heartless technocrats who were concerned only with the speed of work, their bricks and mortar, and their desire to get the job done. To engineers, the social mobilizers were overly protective of the local people's interests and inclined to raise unnecessary issues, inciting people who would make nuisance complaints, and interfering with the project's "real" work: building. One engineer often described what the social mobilizers were doing as only "drama." At first, the work of the social mobilizers was invisible to some engineers, who said that "the mobilizers are just out there sitting in the villages, drinking tea and chatting with the people." The engineers did not understand that such sincere and friendly discussion was building relationships that would lead to the problem-solving processes for construction. See anecdotes, pages 208–10.

Such stereotypes came from lack of experience in each other's disciplines. Only four of the twelve-member social team had any previous experience working with construction, but all had considerable experience organizing in their own or in other communities. In contrast, the dozens of engineers were highly experienced in construction, but none had experience working with social mobilizers in a structured community participation program. While community participation has been a well-developed subject in development projects in Pakistan, with projects in every sector at least claiming to include it, there was also the rhetoric of "community participation," which was often misused the in the reconstruction scene, as discussed in chapter 3.

While some engineers at first resisted the idea of community participation, some social mobilizers also questioned the way that construction would be carried out. Knowing little about the complexities of design and construction, some wondered: Why would the project contract out all the construction to commercial firms? Why not get the villagers (and train them if need be) to build the new facilities themselves? As engineers' ideas changed by witnessing the advantages of community participation, the social mobilizers' questions also vanished as they learned more about the level of skill and the number of skilled laborers needed for large-scale reinforced concrete work. Many skilled laborers from the project area were away working in the Gulf States, and with all the earthquake reconstruction occurring, the high demand for laborers meant they were scarce. It would not be practical to train others to the skill level needed in the finite time frame of the project, and contractors already had their own skilled work crews from other parts of Pakistan. While social mobilizers thought that local hiring might have been ideal to create jobs, it was a matter of not understanding the complexities of this reconstruction.

Building Understanding and Relationships
After the first few months, working relationships started to change, bridging the initial gaps in understanding. The change began as communications

improved: the counterparts developed an understanding of one another, their jobs and their joint process became clearer, and results were being seen. Both engineers and social mobilizers had to figure out what work needed to be done, which work needed to be done together, and how it would be done and when. Getting to this point came from a number of participatory critical analyses, including the "What Could Go Wrong?" analysis, the training they received together, and the creation of the joint step-by-step process.

Stay in Your Lanes

In the early months, one of the most commonly expressed concerns was that the social or technical teams would get into the other's business. In all their other construction projects, the engineers had been left with the responsibility of dealing with any community-related issues—however effectively or ineffectively they might have done so—and thus in PERRP, it was a challenge for them to drop that task and let the social mobilizers do it. Indeed, there were some examples in the early months where a few engineers bypassed social mobilizers to deal directly with the community about an issue. However, without understanding the complex social hierarchies in the communities, they inevitably complicated matters even further. At the same time, some engineers were sure that social mobilizers and community members would try to tell them and the contractors how to do construction. There was a strong, obvious need to delineate the

Table 5.2. Working Together—Stay in Your Lanes.

Social mobilizers, to stay in your lanes, you . . .		Site engineers, to stay in your lanes, you . . .	
SHOULD	SHOULD NOT	SHOULD	SHOULD NOT
• look after everything to do with the committee and community • refer any committee issues about the contractor or construction to the site engineer, who will deal with the contractor • ensure that site engineers are invited to community meetings	• try to solve any problem or talk directly to the contractor about anything to do with construction, except in an emergency, and ask the committee and community members to do the same	• look after everything to do with the contractors and construction • refer any issues involving community members to the social mobilizers, who will have the committee deal with them • attend meetings with social mobilizers and the community as much as possible	• try to solve issues directly with community members or ask them to do anything, even if it's the contractor making the complaint (unless it's an emergency) • ask the contractor to discuss any construction-related matters with community members

jobs while also building common understanding and being able to sing the same song in the midst of a very large audience.

While it was often not an easy subject to broach, social mobilizers and engineers were encouraged to have frank but friendly dialogue about how to keep out of each other's business. It was a matter of separating but coordinating the roles. Just as vehicles on the road need separate lanes to avoid crashing into each other, PERRP asked social mobilizers and engineers to learn about each other's roles, but to metaphorically stay in their own lanes. A social mobilizer should not try to direct, or give an opinion on, construction. The engineer should not direct, or give an opinion on, anything relating to the committee or community. They were encouraged to respect each other's professional expertise and take up the new skill of deferring to whoever has more expertise. Delineating the roles thusly was part of the communication protocol, which separated but coordinated the engineers' and social mobilizers' roles.

Year Two to Project Completion: From the Norming Stage to the Performing Stage

By the beginning of the second year, things were running far more smoothly. The social and technical teams, community members, and contractors had caught on to the new ways this construction project was being run. The step-by-step process was being followed, the communication protocol with grievance procedures was used daily, committees were fully functioning, and there was generally good cooperation between committees and contractors. PERRP had completed many of the designs for the first buildings and construction had already started.

There was a turning point in engineers' and social mobilizers' views of each other when both watched the other achieve what at first had seemed unimaginable. Engineers changed their views when they saw social mobilizers leading communities to organize, deal effectively with construction, and do what they had never seen before: quickly settle land issues, freely obtain loans of assets to help construction, and engage in community-wide problem-solving. For social mobilizers, respect for the engineers grew as new buildings started to appear even in the most challenging of construction locations, fulfilling the dreams of the villagers.

In this process, major lessons were learned about meeting each other's goals. While the engineers' goal was to finish high-quality construction as quickly as possible, the social mobilizers' goal was to have the people participate, to ensure their voices were heard in the project, and to build on their capacities. At first these seemed to be competing goals, but with time and effort, the technical and sociocultural sides realized that by helping to meet each other's goals, they were also meeting their own goals.

After months of working together, the counterparts were able to tackle the most ordinary and the most complex situations, as described in anecdotes and ethnographies throughout these chapters.

Factors Supporting Social and Technical Integration

While a disaster reconstruction project has a tangible end goal—which, in comparison to projects with less visible outcomes, may act as a focal point for the efforts of all those involved—a physical end product is no guarantee of a smooth process. Coordinating such a project requires certain management styles and features, such as the following.

Top-Down Management to Get Bottom-Up Participation

In the reconstruction research literature, there is some concurrence that "a very strong commitment and leadership from the top are needed to implement a bottom-up approach, because pressure is strong in an emergency to provide rapid top-down, autocratic solutions" (Jha et al. 2010: 183). People's participation in projects simply will not be thorough, or will not happen at all, unless it is initiated and reinforced from the top. In PERRP's case, the participation was initiated by USAID; this contractual obligation was taken on by the project's senior management team and then passed down to field staff, who implemented the work at the community level.

Making Sociocultural Expertise and Community Participation Part of Senior Management

USAID made the unusual move to specify that the head of the social component was to be part of the four-person senior management team. In projects in sectors such as agriculture, water, forestry, and health that involve community participation, it is more typical for a project to subcontract the community work (for example, to NGOs). However, community work is easily treated as extraneous to the project, and therefore as separate from the "real" work. Putting the social team leader into senior management emphasized the social component's importance and also made it partly responsible for the success of the whole project.

When asked about this decision after the project was completed, Robert MacLeod, former director of the USAID Pakistan Earthquake Reconstruction Office, said, "One of the most important decisions in designing the earthquake reconstruction program was to include an anthropologist familiar with rural Pakistan as one of the key personnel in the construction contract. Reconstruction is not just about bricks and mortar but rebuilding communities and the people who occupy them" (Hagan and Shuaib 2014: 2).

Consistent Message from Top Down

Within the senior management team, the chief of party—the head of the project, who was also the head engineer—and I invested time in developing a common vision, process, and communication procedure. Through an iterative process throughout the project, strong mutual support evolved. In the final workshops to evaluate the project experience, one of the points most commonly reported by engineers, social mobilizers, and others was the consistent message that field staff received from top management: "One of the main reasons the community participation program worked as well as it did was that we (social mobilizers, engineers, designers, and contractors in the field) heard a unified voice from the project's head office. Because the head of the social program and chief of party were consistent and backed each other up, we knew the project was serious about respecting the community and having the people involved."

Counterpart System

From the beginning, the project matched engineers and social mobilizers to work as counterparts: one pair per construction site. Each construction site had a PERRP site engineer, who remained there full-time to supervise the contractor, while the social mobilizer was responsible for the communities at four to five sites. Social team members and engineers were hired at the same time, shared side-by-side office spaces, and had orientation and training together, all of which helped integrate the social and technical work.

Communications and Reporting

While daily meetings and discussions were hosted at the two field offices in the Mansehra and Bagh districts, weekly conference call meetings at the main office in Islamabad were attended by the chief of party and key engineers and social team members, who reported on progress and raised issues to be addressed. Monthly written reports to USAID were compiled to document construction and participation progress. Addressing matters with both the technical and social sides present helped recognize and reinforce their interdependence.

Sample Willingness Resolution

In writing a willingness resolution, community members chose their own wording and wrote it themselves in Urdu. One community's translated willingness resolution read:

We, the people of Kafalgar and surrounding areas, testify that the social team of PERRP has briefed us about the project, its various components, and about the need for community participation. We have been informed about many responsibilities we will need to take on during the project, and we are willing to accept them and do so by consensus. We invite the project and request that construction proceed. We assure all our cooperation for whatever is needed and thank all those people who are making this new school possible.

Introducing Grievance Procedures

Even talking about conflict could be a delicate matter, but emphasis on prevention was welcomed. At the first large public meeting in each community, the social mobilizer assigned to that site gave a speech as part of the program. Speaking in the local languages and being from the same district and culture, the social mobilizer connected with the audience as an insider. They explained the unusual ways in which the project would work to prevent conflict, and that everyone's participation would be needed in this effort. This was going to be a new experience in these locations. The same message was repeated daily, and complaints were addressed by the committee and the project. The social mobilizer's introductory remarks included a variation on the following appeal:

> You know very well how easy it is for conflict to break out here. We have so many differences, and we know all too well what causes conflict: because people belonging to different political parties, different castes and sects, often don't get along very well. You know all too well how dangerous the conflict is, and how common it is for people to lose their lives and their property over such fighting. That's why PERRP is bringing a new idea here called "grievance procedures." What this means is that we have a way to handle everybody's complaints, so in this project, there will be no need to fight about anything. If you have any complaints, or if anything goes wrong, you should go right away to your committee. If they can't solve the problem, they will bring it to me as your social mobilizer. If the problem involves the contractor or construction, I will take the problem to the site engineer to get a solution."

"How Do You Do It? Be a Catalyst in Dispute Settlement"

A particularly active field officer in the Department of Education was keen to know how PERRP was settling land issues. Invited to attend community meetings to witness their process, he expressed surprise and wonder, saying, "In only a few hours, you were able to resolve this whole thing, but this would have taken us years in the court. Already we have over 150 court cases pending, mostly on land issues." On behalf of the Department of Education, he and others expressed the wish to replicate the PERRP process, but they also said that the changes that were needed to do it in the bureaucracy would be insurmountable. "In any case, independent projects from outside, like this, can be a catalyst, and can make change which may not be possible for a government because of our history together," he said.

Camel in a Tent School

Despite project supervision of contractors and the agreements made between contractors and committees, contractors still occasionally did not do as agreed.

For months, one local committee had been asking their construction contractor to put a fence around the temporary tent school site to keep out grazing animals and other unwanted visitors; however, the contractor did not do it. One weekend when the school was closed, a camel somehow got into one of the tents and could not get out again. Local people and the contractor tried to lead the camel back out of the tent, but it thrashed around, breaking the pipe to the main water tank. Finally, they were able to get the camel out. Soon after this, the contractor finally put in a fence.

A Deliberately Broken Water Pipe

The kinds of construction problems involving or affecting community members varied widely. Without a participatory process and agreements between the construction project and community, such problems could have had highly negative results for both. Sometimes the underlying cause of a technical problem was a long-standing social problem.

At a critical time when concrete was being mixed and poured for construction, the deliberate breaking of a water pipe that was supplying the construction site threatened the work. The damage to the pipe was done by a village man of one caste as revenge against a man from another caste for something unrelated. Without urgent cooperation, the concrete work would have had to stop, which would have ruined its quality and required a costly fix.

As soon as the site engineer discovered this sabotage, he informed the social mobilizer, who located committee members by cell phone and asked them to solve this immediately so that the concrete, which was already being poured, would not be damaged. With social mobilizers arriving at the site within the hour, the committee members had already identified the guilty man and called him, the man against whom he sought revenge, and elders of both castes together and condemned this behavior. The members reminded everyone that the community (in the Committee-Contractor Agreement) had agreed to provide water for construction, and that this kind of incident now was a shame on the community. Committee members asked the elders and the two men to settle their differences and the two men apologized. To be sure of no more water trouble, the committee had part of the water pipeline rerouted to land where it would get better protection. The problem was caught in time with no damage to the concrete, and construction was unaffected.

Construction Steel Stolen and Hidden in a Corn Field

Over the total of fifty thousand construction days in the project, only eight—an unusually small number—were lost because of conflict. Two of those eight lost days were over this incident: a misunderstanding about stolen property. A man had rented land to the contractor to dump excavated materials from the collapsed school, but he then withdrew his agreement and ordered the contractor to vacate the land in retaliation for the contractor having accused him of being a thief. Someone had stolen some steel reinforcing rods to be used in construction and hidden them in the man's field of fully grown corn stalks. Accusations and counteraccusations drew in the whole community, the contractor, and the construction workers.

In this uproar, the social mobilizer contacted the committee and the site engineer, and these two brought the man and the contractor together in one place. As the project assigned responsibility for conflict prevention and resolution to the committee, members heard both sides in the dispute. In the end, the two parties agreed that there had been a misunderstanding. They apologized to each other and made a new agreement about the land.

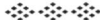

Fight Over the Road Being Blocked

Despite thorough preparation, agreements with communities, and public discussions on how to make and respond to complaints in order to prevent conflict and violence, it took about one year in each community for their agreed approaches to work. Conflict still sometimes happened, but the shared responsibility of PERRP and the committee served to resolve such problems.

As construction was about to start at one site, two local men had beat up the contractor's site inspector for unloading steel rods beside the road, partly blocking it. This was a situation that could have rapidly escalated into a wider fight between laborers and community members, which would have caused much loss, but it was resolved in only a few hours.

As soon as it happened, the contractor reported the incident to the police, but then, according to the communication protocol and the Committee-Contractor Agreement, he also contacted the PERRP engineer, who asked the social team to take action. As it was local men who had resorted to violence, and as the committee had promised to prevent or solve conflict, the social mobilizer went to the committee and asked the members to settle the dispute. They called an emergency meeting of the community, had the two local men apologize to the man they had assaulted, and issued a stern warning to the community: if anyone caused any more trouble, the committee would make them pay a huge fine of fifty thousand Pakistani rupees (roughly $550, about five times the monthly salary of a local teacher). Construction was not hindered.

"We Never Hear Complaints about this Project"

A government official, who was frequently in contact with the project, repeated this observation several times: "We are constantly contacted by community members about problems with construction on other projects, but we had never had a single complaint about the PERRP project." He wanted to know more about how PERRP worked with the communities. Committee members and social mobilizers explained to him how the project handled grievances inside the project:

> We try to make sure everybody in the community knows that, if they have any problems or any complaints at all regarding the construction, the contractor, or anything related to the site, they need to take that complaint right away to their committee—not the contractor. The committee, social mobilizer, and site engineer act quickly and reach a solution so people don't get upset and take action themselves. That's probably why you don't hear complaints. They are taken care of inside the project.

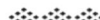

Two Views—Listening to the People

Looking back on the project's early months, a social mobilizer remembered:

> When we were first getting the project started, the engineers thought they knew everything needed and that they were superior. Some of

them looked down on us social mobilizers and on community involvement and even resented it. They didn't think that the local people were important at all. One of the engineers said to me, "We [engineers] already know how to do what's needed. We don't need a social program and we don't need the community. They will just waste our time and cause trouble." A few weeks later, when a big problem cropped up over a land issue at one of the schools, the same engineer phoned me to come urgently to the site and solve the problem. I reminded him, "But you said you know how to do everything"—he pleaded with me, however, so I went to the site, sat down with the community members, and in a couple of hours we solved the issue. After this kind of thing happened a few times, where the engineers heard the disputes, our negotiations, and the solutions we reached, it was a different tune. Their attitudes changed completely. They soon realized it was far more complicated in the communities than they had thought, and that it really does take special expertise to deal with it. They also got to see it was in their own benefit, too, to listen to the people.

Rough First Year

Near the end of the project, when looking back over their experience, a senior engineer said to a member of the social team, "Wow, things were pretty rough in the first year of the project. You social mobilizers were so stressed all the time trying to make things work." The social mobilizer replied, "That's because it took that much time for you [engineering] guys to listen to us!"

"Look Who Is in the Graveyard! Ha, Ha, Ha!"

Outside PERRP's compound walls in Bagh district, there was a local family's private graveyard, which had its tombstones clearly visible from the compound's entry gate. Sometimes an engineer, when bringing in visitors, would point to the graves and say, "See what we do with social mobilizers!" The joke reflected the rocky early relationship between project engineers and social mobilizers. If a social mobilizer was arriving with guests, they would also indicate the graves and say, "See what happens to engineers in this project?" While done in good fun, it should come as no surprise that the social and technical specialists at times had trouble getting along with one another, especially in the early months of the project. By the time they were able to joke about it like this, they had gained a deeper understanding of each other and their roles. It took time and effort for sociocultural and technical specialists to work together effectively, but after some time, they could draw on a shared sense of humor and joke about their differences.

Engineers Say, "Having a Social Team Saves a Lot of Time and Trouble"

Near the end of PERRP, windup exercises and discussions were held with engineers and social mobilizers to analyze their experience. Although highly experienced in other construction projects in the region, engineers reported that none of those projects had had a dedicated social team. When asked to compare and contrast community-related problem-solving in those other projects and in PERRP, there were a variety of answers, such as:

> In other projects I've worked in over the years, when there was a fight, we would just stop the work and go to the owner or client, but they often couldn't or wouldn't do anything about it, or it would take a long time. Sometimes the contractor would try to bargain with people, or pay them something to settle. When work got stopped, it meant a lot of time was lost and it multiplied the problems of the contractors too (site engineer, Mansehra).
>
> I watched PERRP social mobilizers working with the people and now I understand how complicated all that social stuff is. At first, I thought having a social team was not necessary, that it would just slow us down when all we wanted to do was get on with the job, but that turned out to not be true at all. Until I saw the social mobilizers doing what they do with communities, I had not realized how much skill that takes—and I don't have that skill. I changed my mind about how to deal with local people when I saw how they worked with the community and got the problems solved (site engineer, Bagh).
>
> When PERRP is finished and I will need to find a job on another construction project, I dread it, as other projects do not have social teams and that means somebody—probably me—will get stuck trying to solve these problems. I don't have the patience for it. And anyway, it means I have to run around doing that when I am supposed to be looking after all the details in the construction. Having a social team saves so much time and trouble (resident engineer, Bagh).

CHAPTER 6

PERRP Design and Construction

Introduction

With the destruction of buildings in a disaster and the need for reconstruction also comes the need for new buildings to be designed. This chapter discusses both design and construction in general terms, and then looks at how both were handled in PERRP.

The first part of this chapter brings in the subject of engineering and architectural design. It considers how the new design can be an opportunity to not only reconstruct using earthquake-resistant design criteria but also to construct new buildings that have improved function and relevance to community needs, including integrating features that are culturally appropriate. Content here draws on scholarly sources in architecture that argue that "design needs to respond to culture" (Rapoport 2005: 126). Accordingly, this section looks at how PERRP responded to cultural factors in its new building designs, and how by getting community input, designs were enhanced and some costly mistakes were avoided. Included are some examples of other factors that can affect design in a postdisaster scenario.

The second part of this chapter is about construction generally and then specifically in PERRP. Drawing on research literature referring to construction in many countries, I provide an overview of the challenges and hurdles faced by construction policy makers, planners, and managers even without a disaster. I discuss how reconstruction is likely to be affected by the state of the construction industry before a catastrophe occurs. I also raise the most relevant issues of stakeholder consultation and describe how, in the design and construction, the end users are often completely ignored.

This section also looks at how a disaster multiplies existing challenges in construction. I describe how construction was organized and managed in PERRP: its staffing, locations, site selection, subcontracting, scheduling, quality assurance, monitoring and supervision, and overall management. I include results from a focus group discussion with some of PERRP's most experienced field engineers, comparing "textbook construction project management" with what they had experienced as common in Pakistan and other countries.

Despite all the challenges, PERRP received international recognition from the Design-Build Institute of America for design-build excellence. For 2012, the institute conferred the "honor award for educational facilities" to CDM Smith based on the "design-build of four earthquake resistant schools in Pakistan" (PERRP 2013: 21).

Part 1: PERRP Design

When developing a building design, whether for construction in normal times or in disaster reconstruction, there are innumerable factors to consider. New construction in both situations provides opportunities to improve on earlier designs by taking in an even wider swath of considerations—seismic resistance, environmental aspects, sustainability, and suitability of design for the building's purpose—while still meeting the usual parameters for budget, timeline, design codes and standards, and client and funder requirements, among other factors. The purpose of these considerations is, of course, to create buildings that are long-lasting, safe, good-looking, comfortable, popular, culturally acceptable, and able to function according to needs. After a disaster, however, there are additional challenges for design: shortages of qualified building technologists, engineers, and architects; rapid changes in building codes, or standards that are poorly communicated in the chaos; client or funder constraints; long lag times for approvals; and abnormally strong time pressures to produce designs so reconstruction can get underway.

Additional issues are also considered in the design. First is the importance of community and end user input to the design of public buildings. While this is common practice and is even mandatory in many parts of the world, in other countries including Pakistan such stakeholder consultation is either unheard of or, if required by authorities, is often ignored by the companies involved. Next is the general subject of culturally sensitive building design, and how postdisaster times may provide opportunities that did not exist or were not pursued before the disaster. Taking advantage of such opportunities requires deliberate attention to, knowledge of, and respect for a culture—all of which are often missing according to the research literature. Also considered in this chapter are ideas about culture, design, and sustainability. Included too is a look at how cultural issues arose in PERRP concerning the design of the seventy-seven large facilities to be constructed, and a discussion of how they were addressed and what difference was made by doing so.

Culturally Sensitive Design

For public buildings, cultural sensitivity to design is critical but frequently overlooked. This is so in Pakistan and elsewhere, even as studies show that buildings that are designed for a culture help to improve their usage—for instance, school enrolments increase and health facility attendance goes up. Culturally specific design requires architects to be aware that building design is not only based on supposedly neutral science but is also culturally based, as much of modern design requirements, standards, and influences come from Western culture. This requires architects to be willing to take the time to consult with those who will be building users and to know and have respect for the local culture. In some cases, even the most basic cultural awareness is missing, and being of the same nationality is no guarantee the knowledge will be present, as with one architect who argued against culturally specific design. See anecdote, page 239.

When rebuilding after a disaster, aid workers, donors, government officials, architects, and other designers are often outsiders—whether "outside" means from a city in the same country or from the other side of the world. Even if of the same nationality, a designer may be of a different class or culture from the community where the building is to be constructed. Those who do the design are often from the educated urban elite, and they might never have visited the poor rural areas where destruction has occurred. They might have little understanding of that culture, or they could very well look down on it, as expressed in the anecdote below. There may be many others who are simply not aware that a particular design imposes cultural norms and values—especially Western ones.

Additionally, in postdisaster situations, there can be time pressures like at no other time. With much more design and construction work happening than normal, the pressure is on to get designs ready and approved for construction to start. To save time, decisions can get rushed and compressed into a one-design-fits-all template. This rush may also mean that designers are unable to visit the sites to be reconstructed, and so do not consult the end users. Instead, they may stay in the design office, urgently producing designs based only on the technical data received, building codes, budget, time allowed, and previous experience—the priority being to meet the deadlines and expectations of the client or donor. Bowing to such pressures can result in mistakes and loss and buildings that do not reflect user needs or priorities. See anecdotes, pages 240–44.

As demonstrated by the official who thought villagers know nothing about design, or the architects who were sure a modern building needed no considerations for culture, there can be lack of awareness—even outright rejection—of local, and especially rural and conservative, cultural features. Instead, some designers may seek to impose their choices, influenced at least partly by their design education. See anecdote, page 240.

This is not a new subject. For over fifty years, Amos Rapoport, an architect and pioneer of the intersection of culture and architecture, has been renowned for his work on the relations between culture, design, and the built environment. Rapoport wrote, "Design needs to respond to culture. There needs to be a change from designing for one's own culture to understanding and designing for the users' cultures" (2005: 126). He has argued that architects too often design for themselves, not the end user ("Interview" 1992). Similarly, according to Memmott and Keys, what is needed is a "conceptualization of architecture that is sensitive to cross-cultural contexts and values and not overly dominated by Western concepts of what architecture is" (2015: 1). The authors further contend:

> Without a more balanced definition of architecture, architects will be vulnerable to designing in an ethnocentric manner, possibly providing a good "fit" in the architecture for their own cultural group, but inadvertently creating a bad "fit" for other cultural groups ... Such a bad fit may result in users becoming stressed to varying degrees and/or being unable to cope with, or even un-wishing to enter the built environment with which they are presented. On the other hand, we would maintain a good "fit" between architecture and the user will result in a certain "well-being" experienced by the user and thereby contribute to a form of culturally sustainable architecture. (1)

While the above Memmot and Keys observations are general, they also apply to countries such as Pakistan where cultural oversights can cause people to be reluctant to enter or use a building out of protest or rejection of what they believe is wrong. When a school is rejected in this way it can cause a loss of face for school leaders or supporters who, among local people, might be seen as responsible for the design mistake. In a collectivist society where conformity to cultural norms is expected for all, using a building with features deemed inappropriate may bring stress and shame on the user. Fearful of being judged by others for using it, they avoid the building. Such design oversight can be a new problem or a repetition of design shortcomings from the past, such as toilets being put in the wrong places in some Nepali and Pakistani schools and visual barriers not included in some Pakistani schools. This reality already exists in many parts of Pakistan, and as evidenced by numerous studies, such design failures are part of the reason that significant numbers of children—especially girls—do not attend school.

Culture and Building Design in Pakistan

In Pakistan, attendance at school and usage of health facilities—and factors affecting attendance and usage—are common subjects of study by government and aid agencies. In schools, estimates on attendance rates and the number of out-of-school children vary widely. While there are many complex reasons for nonattendance, physical features of the building and lack of adherence to cultural preferences are at least partly responsible. Multiple studies have found what tends to be common knowledge among local inhabitants: that rural people are less likely to send their children, especially daughters, to school if the school is too far away to walk to, if the route is not safe, if the school does not provide the privacy or security of boundary walls, or if there are no toilet facilities (UNICEF 2014; World Bank 1996a; Alif Ailaan 2016). Although boundary walls, drinking water, electricity, and toilets are now considered basic essentials for enrollment in Pakistan's schools, only about 52 percent have such facilities (Alif Ailaan 2016).

From an outsider's perspective, having no toilets in schools may be unimaginable, but their presence or absence is a complex issue in itself, involving factors such as school planning and budget priorities, ideas of cleanliness, personal preferences, and the challenges to maintain them. In any case, change appears to be in the offing. In a part of the world where open defecation is still widely in practice, "studies suggest that access to useable toilets can increase school enrollment, attendance rates, and educational outcomes" (Hayat 2017: iii).

In Pakistan, schools are sometimes mixed-gender, but after puberty, students most commonly attend separate boys' and girls' schools, with teaching staff also separated by gender. Where the custom of *purdah* is in practice, there are additional design needs for modesty and privacy—especially different entry points and visual barriers using walls, window locations, or types. Lack of such privacy screening, and family and social pressure for modesty, can make it hard or even impossible for teenage girls and young women to go to school or on to higher education. Where such protection is not provided, it may be due to lack of budget, lack of awareness, rejection of or disbelief in the cultural needs, or simply a lack of care.

Culturally Sensitive Design in PERRP

One of the many roles taken on by the PERRP social team in the project's participatory process was to act as advocates for culturally appropriate building design, according to the wishes, preferences, and norms of the local people. We believed this would be best achieved through community input to design, and as result of this process there were in several cases some design modifications. The changes made not only helped shape design to fit cultural needs and values, but learning these preferences early also allowed for design changes to be made at the planning stage at no additional cost of money or time, whereas changes later would have been costly and might not have been possible. Schools built in PERRP included visual barriers such as boundary walls, window treatments, different drinking water sources, and culturally preferred placement of toilets. These were provided along with the new requirements for additional space per student and for rooms not previously common in most schools: science and computer labs, libraries, multipurpose halls, and office and staff space. Training in operation and maintenance of all these new facilities included how to maintain the toilets and, what was especially sensitive, how to use them.

In the first year of PERRP, when pressure was intense to produce designs for many new buildings at once, the subcontracted architectural firm insisted on working only from the survey and technical data they had been provided. Being located in a faraway city and under such pressure to produce designs meant they were at first reluctant to visit the building sites. However, the need for them to see the sites and speak directly with the people who would be using the buildings became all the more apparent and urgent as community input to design started, and as community-voiced design issues and requests arose. First needing to be heard were the teaching staff at schools and medical staff at health units: what were their needs and ideas for operating efficient schools or clinics? Next needing to be considered were the cultural preferences of local people, families of users, students, and patients. To avoid costly design mistakes and catch changes early, while the design was still only on paper, PERRP senior management directed the architects to start attending the community design input meetings. Their attendance had rapid benefits, as the designers then were able to make those changes that were feasible, as well as anticipate what would be needed in future designs.

In this disaster reconstruction, PERRP found several culture- and design-related issues, with a few examples shown in the following anecdotes.

End User and Community Input to Design: Process and Benefits

Rationale and Process
In normal times, schools would be designed in government offices or by a hired firm, with no local input. In PERRP, we invited communities to make input to the design of their new building early in the project, and consid-

ered this input to be a major step in the participatory process. In PERRP, we invited end users and community members to make input to the design of their new building early in the project. Teaching staff at schools and health personnel at the health facilities, committee members, and others attended design discussion sessions as an early and important step in the participation process. Their participation also raised interest and curiosity and, drawing on local knowledge, helped the project avoid culturally inappropriate design and costly mistakes and delays. With each partner community, the PERRP social team encouraged people in the communities to pay attention to the nature and quality of design and construction, as by then it was widely known that the high death rate associated with the earthquake was caused by shoddy construction.

Our review of related postquake reconstruction projects suggested that inviting such local input to the school and health facility design was probably unique among the hundreds of other schools being reconstructed at the time. But, as our work has shown, involving local people in this way avoided some of the problems foreseen through the social team's "What Could Go Wrong?" analysis, which identified main causes of delays in other school reconstructions, including disputes over culturally unacceptable actions and design features.

The design input was not a free-for-all; the community did not develop design from scratch. Realistically, the design was already dictated by many factors. Long before a preliminary design was shown to end users and community members for their input, the architects came up with draft designs using the parameters they were given: budget, timelines, sustainability, land available, donor and owner requirements, building standards, seismic requirements, and space allowances. At this point, the designs were taken to the community for review and input. Community input was only part of the design process. Design then passed through several layers of approval by USAID and ERRA, in conjunction with the national authority, the Government of Pakistan's National Engineering Services Pakistan (NESPAK).

Design input started in a short series of meetings. Local people had widely varied experience with such modern reinforced concrete building design. As this kind of formal design was new in these remote areas, to most people the technical drawings of floor and site plans were abstract, if not incomprehensible. A small number were familiar with design aspects—usually people who had returned home after having worked in construction elsewhere, especially the Gulf States. To begin basic familiarization before the visit of the architects, social team members brought their counterpart engineers together with community members to begin talking about the design and looking at the preliminary drawings printed out on large sheets of paper. This step enabled the community members to begin formulating their questions for the architects and envisioning what would be built.

In the second step, the project architects visited, walked around the site with community members and staff, then sat down with the people, reviewing the paper printouts and hearing what the people had to say. Designers asked the facility staff and people what they had liked about their old school. What did they think of the preliminary design? What should be included or avoided in the new school? In inviting such participation, some communities gave long wish lists to the architects. These wishes were accepted or rejected depending on feasibility, but such discussions also uncovered or highlighted some weaknesses or unpopular ideas in the preliminary design. Sometimes such discussion revealed that community members and architects had different priorities for use of the land, such as in the above anecdote where community members appealed to save their soccer field. In other projects and locations there were some newly reconstructed buildings that did not consider the culture at all. Through on-site discussion involving the architects, committee members, and clinic or school staff, what could have been a problem was avoided, as shown in above anecdotes.

As the third step in community input to design, and as a standard final step before construction started, the PERRP engineers, with the committee and contractor in attendance, had the design—according to the site and floor plans—marked on the bare ground with chalk powder for all to see. For the first time everyone got to see the exact planned location, actual size, placement, and orientation of the building. Sometimes this process revealed issues that no one had noticed before, again giving the designers time to make changes while the design was still on paper.

Benefits of Local Design Input
Being asked to make input had an empowering effect in the communities. This design input process gave people an unusual amount and type of information, and then encouraged them to analyze it and share their perspectives. This participation developed their sense of ownership, making people more interested in the design, which soon became a popular topic of conversation. In the process, the people built their capacity to analyze information in a new field and proactively share their point of view.

For PERRP, too, local design input had several benefits: it increased cultural appropriateness, enhanced the long-term functioning of the building, and helped avoid costly or impossible-to-correct design mistakes before construction started. Local people's input allowed for low-cost or no-cost changes to the still-on-paper preliminary designs. We never attempted to calculate how much construction time and money were saved by catching design problems early enough to change them—but those amounts, if they could be calculated, would be significant. Useful ideas, especially about visual barriers, came out of these early meetings, and PERRP began incorporating them as preferred design features in subsequent sites, instead of waiting for them to be requested. Recognizing the importance of these changes for design and construction is one thing, but they are, of course, even more valuable for people's comfort and use of the buildings in future.

Participants in the design input step varied from place to place. In some cases, the committees and school or health facility staff viewed the design plans as a small group. In other locations, committees chose to make the design input a public process, including other community members and large groups of the schools' own senior students. According to local practices of *purdah*, separate design meetings were held with men and women in some locations. Students also were asked for their design ideas in different forms. In a drawing exercise, students were asked to do two drawings, one to show what had happened to their school the day of the earthquake, the other to show what they would like in their new school. Students enthusiastically participated, submitting about four thousand drawings; one hundred fifty of them were selected for a special exhibition at the National Art Gallery in Islamabad, to commemorate the sixth anniversary of the quake.

Sustainability

At the design stage, the physical sustainability of new buildings was a major concern. The choices made at that time determined much about the building's physical future—not only how it would withstand future disasters but aspects of its daily operation and maintenance: how maintenance would be done, by whom, under what supervision, and with what skills and resources. The design determined what was needed to ensure the new building's maximum life and usefulness, as well as its affordability. In PERRP's case, there were a number of design considerations for sustainability of the new buildings. Earthquake resistance was of primary concern, following the ERRA and donor policies to "build back better." This was to not simply restore the level of development that had existed but to improve on it and reduce vulnerability in any future disasters.

Extreme weather conditions and low government budgets for operation and maintenance of these buildings were other major considerations. It was essential for the new buildings to be as easy and low cost to maintain as possible, as communities were to share responsibility for operation and maintenance with the government owners, and their budgets were minimal. Planning ahead for these realities involved several considerations:

- the building envelope and the kinds of floor materials and outer and inner wall treatments that would require the least attention and expense to maintain
- roof and drainage style, to help manage precipitation from monsoon rainwater and snow melt runoff while also preventing damage to the property
- placement of large windows to allow the maximum natural light, as electricity was scarce and expensive
- natural ventilation without electricity-dependent fans
- accessibility for those with physical disabilities

Due to the topography of the region and the subsequent variability of building sites, designs for each building were custom made individually, although PERRP buildings maintained a similar, recognizable style.

Location is another factor in sustainability. Some schools or other buildings had been destroyed in the earthquake or in earlier disasters because they were located in hazardous locations—particularly landslide- and flood-prone zones. In such cases, PERRP took measures to eliminate or reduce the risks, also acting upon local knowledge, such as that revealed when architects and local people took a walk together around the site where a destroyed BHU was to be rebuilt. See anecdote "Flash Floods," page 244.

Clearly, there is more to the sustainability of a new building than its technical features. One of the most important opportunities after a disaster is to design and construct buildings that are culturally sensitive and culturally sustainable, thereby making them more acceptable than the previous buildings to users. This requires knowledge of and respect for the culture, and willingness to design for what users consider culturally appropriate. As Skjerven writes, "the work of promoting sustainable development that explicitly concerns not only physical but also cultural matters is a relatively new occupation, thus there are many blank spots related to this endeavor on the map of knowledge and understanding" (2017: 19). PERRP tackled these challenges to construct buildings that would be both physically and culturally sustainable.

Part 2: PERRP Construction

Leading in to discussion of how PERRP's construction was organized and managed is some background on why the destruction rate was so high in the earthquake zone and how that damage was attributed to faults in earlier design and construction. Those observations are then set in the wider contexts of challenges to construction in Pakistan and other countries. This is especially important to consider, as much about any disaster reconstruction will be determined by the state of the construction industry before the catastrophe. While the research literature on the construction industry around the world finds many common issues and hurdles, one subject I found disturbingly common is failure to even mention the people who may be most affected by, and who may have the most effect on, the construction site: those living nearby who are expected to benefit from the construction. In this section, PERRP's main technical challenges are discussed, followed by details about the organization and management of the construction. This section ends with results of an engineer's focus group that compare this project's construction management with others. A detailed ethnography at the end of this chapter, "Boys' Primary and High School Glacier Way," illustrates how construction can have many unforeseen situations that require more than engineering or construction management expertise.

As stated elsewhere, almost all of PERRP's seventy-seven construction sites were completed on or ahead of schedule. Such an achievement not only benefitted the donor and the companies involved—it also helped build the capacities of local institutions and, for those who lost so much in the disaster, it meant people finally had facilities in which to study or get health services. When reviewing the range of challenges faced, PERRP's achievement is all the more remarkable.

First, Why the Destruction?

The 2005 quake killed over seventy thousand people and destroyed or damaged over half a million homes and almost all educational and health facilities. Why such devastating destruction? The most widely made observation about the cause of this destruction was the shoddy construction and unsuitable materials (Durrani et al. 2005). In Pakistan and around the world, hundreds of thousands of lives have been lost in recent decades due to poorly engineered and improperly constructed buildings in high seismic zones. What makes a building earthquake resistant? Some main features are "concrete (shear) walls, columns and beams that must have extra steel to withstand movement caused by the earthquake forces[,] and floors and roofs [that are] properly anchored to the beams and columns to reduce the probability of their collapse onto occupants" (PERRP 2011/2012:10).

In prequake Pakistan, building materials were often those available at hand—mainly stone, brick, or concrete, without the appropriate steel reinforcement needed to withstand seismic motion. One study by the Earthquake Engineering Research Institute (EERI), undertaken a month after the quake by a panel of seismic engineering experts from the USA and New Zealand, observed that "most of the buildings in the affected areas were of non-engineered reinforced masonry wall construction. Most of the structures consisted of one or two stories of unreinforced stone, solid brick or solid concrete block masonry bearing walls with reinforced floors" (EERI 2006: 7). Another study, this one by the Mid-America Earthquake (MAE) Center, came to similar conclusions: "The structural damage was expected owing to the poor quality of construction of traditional housing and modern reinforced concrete structures not designed to resist earthquake action" (Durrani et al. 2005: 6).

The MAE Center and EERI studies likewise determined that existing building codes in Pakistan were out of date and seldom enforced. The building codes referred to by these experts are those developed around the world from lessons learned from other seismic disasters. Comprehensive seismic building codes, guidelines, and standards, such as those in the 1997 Uniform Building Code (UBC) and subsequent updates, have been developed and used in many countries, including the USA, and in all the buildings constructed in PERRP.

Challenges in Construction in Pakistan and Other Countries

The fact is that Pakistan has a rich heritage of buildings that have lasted a very long time. The subcontinent, including Pakistan, is renowned for some of the world's oldest and most magnificent examples of design and construction. Pakistan has six UNESCO World Heritage sites, with eighteen other sites tentatively selected and untold others waiting. The six include the archaeological sites at Moenjodaro, dating from the 26th to 19th centuries BC; Taxila, from the 5th to 2nd centuries BC; the Buddhist monastery ruins at Takht-i-Bahi, from the 1st century BC; the Maki monuments at Thatta, Sindh province, from the 14th to 18th century; and the Lahore Fort and Shalimar Gardens from the Mughal era in the 17th century.

While such ancient structures are admired around the world, the challenges encountered when constructing them seem to be long forgotten. Not so with construction today. While construction is considered vital to development, it can also come with losses, complications, and controversies. The reputation of construction in Pakistan, even at the best of times before the earthquake, was frequently negative and assumed to be riddled with problems that all too frequently rendered construction projects stalled or even abandoned—whether the building was a mega project or one-room school.

The above realities indicate the challenges for construction even before the disaster and act as a reminder of how such realities will determine much about reconstruction. Such factors were what PERRP and other agencies involved in reconstruction were up against as each initiated and managed their own reconstruction projects.

Nowadays, there is a mushrooming literature on infrastructure construction challenges in Pakistan and around the world. Even without a disaster, comparative analyses indicate that Pakistan is not alone in facing barriers to getting safe, durable buildings completed. The problems they list could be categorized as managerial, technical, financial, policy related, procedural, and legal. The challenges listed barely hint at any social or "people" issues. A study by the Asian Institute of Technology on risk management in Pakistan's construction industry states its findings bluntly: construction there "is a high-risk business which haunts every participant in the business, the project owner, construction companies, consultants, bankers, financial institutions, vendors and suppliers, and even service providers, each has his own fears of facing risks in the conduct of business" (AIT 2010: 1). According to this study, the top ten problems as seen from the contractor's perspective are 1) delays in resolving contractual issues, 2) delayed payment on contracts, 3) political uncertainty, 4) financial failure, 5) scope of work definition, 6) war threats, 7) suppliers and subcontractors' poor performance, 8) change of work, 9) defective design and labor, and 10) equipment productivity.

Particularly revealing and relevant is a detailed series of studies by the World Bank to assess Pakistan's infrastructure implementation capacity. Based on literature reviews of construction challenges in several developing countries, a main conclusion in the World Bank series on Pakistan's construction industry is that "there is consensus on certain common issues that plague the construction industry in developing countries" (Mir, Tanvir, and Durrani 2007: 1)—implying that Pakistan is no exception. The same source adds that "the construction industry in Pakistan is well aware of the challenges it faces" (1). According to the World Bank series of studies, the problems in common include a lack of adequate education and training; a lack of government commitment; absence of long-term vision and planning for the industry; ineffective planning and budgetary procedures; fluctuations in work load; defective contract documents; corrupt contracting procedures; a lack of protection against adverse physical conditions; delays in payments to contractors; problems of bonding and insurance; absence of adequate credit; restrictions on imports; foreign exchange constraints; unfair competition from state-owned contractors and consultants and problems relating to availability of equipment and spare parts; and delays, cost overruns, and miscommunication of information (1).

A disaster of course multiplies existing challenges. A literature review (Hidayat and Egbu 2010) on the role of project management in postdisaster reconstruction drew comparisons from eleven disasters in different parts of the world, including the Mexico City earthquake (1985), the Kobe, Japan, earthquake (1995), the Turkey earthquake (1999), and the Indian Ocean tsunami (2004). Metrics included policies, funding, land ownership, construction material, contract abandonment, local capacities, political environment, and construction costs and quality. Not surprisingly, problems that were already common were intensified after the disaster, as costs escalated, supplies of materials and labor tightened, construction quality was compromised, and field staff struggled with insufficient relevant experience and training to manage such large and complex projects.

While construction problems are common knowledge in Pakistan, what is notable are the other factors that go unmentioned in these studies. In the studies consulted, nothing at all is mentioned about the social aspects or social context of reconstruction, or how these factors may play a large part in the success or failure of a project. The studies present a consistent, exclusive, top-down view, talking only about the concerns of the client, employer, contractor, engineer, or construction manager. Even the relatively exhaustive aforementioned World Bank series, in a 150-page analysis of "local stakeholders' perceptions" of the issues and hurdles in implementing large infrastructure projects in Pakistan, included as the only "key stakeholders" clients, consultants, and contractors (Gilani, Mir, and Malik 2007: viii). In none of the studies is anything at all mentioned about the local people: the stakeholders whom the project is intended to benefit, the people whose lives or property will be affected by the design and construction. There also is no mention of the key stakeholders' relations with the people. Unacknowledged in these one-sided studies is how the so-called key stakeholders' attitudes, actions, and behaviors can be the cause of many problems, resulting in threats, conflict, and court stay orders leading to a significant number of the work stoppages.

The above kinds of analysis miss the point that construction projects can be affected by sociocultural factors that appear to have little or nothing to do with construction, but which, if not acknowledged or if left unaddressed, can have serious impacts. Contractors in Pakistan and elsewhere frequently assume a stance similar to eminent domain—the government's right to take private land for public use—arriving invasion style, as if saying "we were sent here to build, so just get out of our way; you should be happy we are here." In many instances, there is little contractor acknowledgement of private property, and no thinking ahead as to the harms they can cause, including damage or destruction of private property; financial or material loss; local conflict and permanent damage to local relations;

and serious cultural offences, leading to loss of face or status or even loss of life. Without asking for permission, they may take over private land, cut trees, park their vehicles and unload their materials where they please, bring workers with them or hire people who may cause trouble or fail to pay what they owe locally, and so on. It is no surprise that adversarial relationships between community members and contractors are common.

There are a few reasons for the invisibility of local stakeholders. First, construction is inherently top-down and one of the last frontiers for more genuinely inclusive participation. Also, contractors tend to downplay or ignore the complaints of the poor and presumed-to-be-uneducated local people, whose concerns are often dismissed as mere irrational irritations that do not even rise to the level of legitimate problems.

There does, however, appear to be an incipient recognition—at least in the academic study of construction project management—that there is more to a construction site than steel and concrete. Construction management itself is, "in comparison with other areas, a relatively new field of academic inquiry," yet even within that field, the subject of culture—or "sociology of construction"—is underexplored (Harty 2008: 697). Harty suggests using sociological approaches to study construction management culture, as these approaches offer "a broad canvas of theories and approaches when we are thinking about the way people act when performing construction work" (706). Pink, Tutt, and Dainty have found that "[e]thnography is now emerging as part of the repertoire of approaches to understanding the construction industry" (2013: 1). As this latter work points out, for construction policy makers, planners, or managers, an ethnographic approach to construction means having direct contact with the end users "within the context of their daily lives (and cultures), watching what happens, listening to what is said, asking questions" (4)—in other words, using participant observer methods with the main stakeholders to develop an understanding of their needs and preferences, and then following up accordingly. Kivrak, Ross, and Arslan, too, have noticed that "[t]here is a growing interest in the studies on the culture of the construction industry, projects and the effects of culture and cultural differences on construction" (2008: 2).

As these scholars have noted, the need for awareness about sociocultural aspects of construction is being magnified by the enormous increase of construction firms working internationally in a highly competitive market. In this situation now, many sources are seeing cultural know-how as tied to the bottom line. "Understanding, respecting, accepting and managing cross-cultural differences effectively in construction projects can enhance the organization/project's effectiveness and provide competitive advantage, while ignoring or failing to manage cultural differences may lead to many problems in these projects, such as project delays and decreases in productivity" (Choi et al. 2015: 173-2). Occasionally, articles and papers on culture and construction appear in construction and engineering journals and at international conferences, such as the International Conference on Multi-National Construction Projects: Securing High Performance Through Cultural Awareness and Dispute Avoidance, which took place in Shanghai in 2008. Similarly, the subject of culture and construction was featured in the International Construction Specialty Conference of the Canadian Society for Civil Engineering in Vancouver in 2015.

The above does indicate growing awareness of the need for construction to include sociocultural programming. The challenge, however, is to avoid this being just more rhetoric. As discussed in chapter 3, there already is a large gap between theory and practice. To conceptualize, implement, and manage such work requires sociocultural experts specializing in people's participation—and for these specialists to be part of the project design from its early concept stages at senior levels, as was the case in PERRP. The most effective results will come when sociocultural experts, construction project managers, engineers, and other technicians work together.

Whether looking at postdisaster reconstruction or construction in normal times, whatever the country, questions need to be raised about these too often invisible or ignored stakeholders, especially because they—as users of the new facilities—may have the most at stake. As shown in PERRP, there are multiple benefits to bringing these stakeholders into the projects as partners. The question is, if construction problems are similar from country to country, could some of those challenges be reduced by structured community participation, such as occurred in PERRP?

PERRP's Main Technical Challenges

As described in detail in chapter 4, the scene was still quite chaotic when PERRP started about a year after the quake. Many dozens of international, national, and local agencies— NGOs, donors, the United Nations— had started their reconstruction projects months earlier but most of that construction was already in trouble, with many projects encountering a list of problems, including stalled work. Even so, the pressure was on to get construction started, get shovels in the ground, and get facilities completed so schools and health units could function again. Increasing this pressure were the technical challenges the project faced. The main challenges came from shortages of various kinds as well as the physical environment.

Shortage of Materials and High Prices

As the demand for construction materials was high, prices for these goods escalated dramatically. In this case, to save costs the project procured the materials in bulk—steel reinforcing rods, concrete, windows, doors, and tiles—and provided them to the contractors. This bulk buying helped to control costs, reduce speculative bidding, and maintain uniformity and quality of materials (PERRP 2013: 15).

Topography, Altitude, and Climate

The earthquake zone was spread out over an eighteen thousand square mile area on the southern edges of the Himalayas. The project's construction sites were in steep mountain locations, with few roads—and those that existed were narrow, sometimes single-lane dirt roads with many tight switchback corners that made it difficult for trucks and heavy equipment. In places, roads were not repaired after the quake or suffered other damage from landslides. All of the facilities built were at fairly high altitudes, an average of 5,500 ft. They ranged from schools at 7,900 ft at Naran, in the Kaghan Valley in KP, to schools and health units in Bagh, AJ&K, at 3,400 ft. Some of the sites were snowbound and inaccessible in the winter, while others were in monsoon areas in summer. Construction had to work around such weather conditions.

Shortages of Land, Water, Electricity, Reliable Construction Contractors, and Skilled Laborers

Land, of course, may be the number one need when it comes to construction. However, land issues throughout this project area—as discussed in chapter 2—were common and high risk, and these concerns were compounded by the disaster. The project's social team worked intensely with the communities to deal with land issues well before construction began, which helped prevent many of the problems suffered by other construction that made no such attempts.

The project was required to rebuild on the same amount of land already owned by the school or health facility, but given the new requirements, that land was often very small. The new building codes introduced or enforced following the earthquake required both more square footage per user and extra rooms not previously included in schools, such as laboratories, a library, and washrooms. As no additional land or new sites were possible, these codes were usually addressed by constructing a two-story building, whereas the destroyed building had been a single story. In one case, where a school was to be rebuilt in a risky location, the project workers and the community took extraordinary steps to reduce or eliminate the risk, as shown in the anecdote "Mohandri School, Mountainside Boulders." See anecdote, page 245.

Seismic construction involves mixing and pouring large amounts of concrete, which requires a high, consistent flow of water at crucial times. Electricity is also crucial at times, but in the project areas both were often scarce, even before the disaster—and the quake damaged electricity infrastructure as well. In many places, the earthquake had shifted the ground, causing some water sources to disappear, or appear in other places. The social team's work with communities helped deal with both these shortages.

How PERRP Organized and Managed Construction

At its peak, the project had 207 staff, including 93 engineers with various specializations and other technical staff to work at all the sites, 12 social team members, and 102 administration and support staff in finance, procurement, communications, logistics, security, transport, information technologies, and other areas. All but five of the positions were filled by Pakistanis. The majority of staff were located at the two field offices and on the construction sites. Senior management comprised four people: the project's manager or chief of party, who was also the chief engineer; the deputy chief of party, who was also the deputy chief engineer; the head of finance; and me, the head of the social component, also called the community liaison specialist. Our main office was in Islamabad, Pakistan's capital city, and we had two field offices: one in Mansehra city, KP province, and one in Bagh, AJ&K. Construction was carried out, monitored, and supervised from the Bagh field site.

The project's construction sites were spread out over Bagh district in AJ&K and the nearby Mansehra district of KP province, the sites being located from one hour's to five hours' drive from each of the two regional offices. The complete list of places built in PERRP is included in the appendix.

From the thousands of schools and health facilities destroyed, ERRA provided a list of 250 sites to USAID to consider reconstructing. These were then assigned to PERRP to conduct social, technical, and environmental assessments, and from the assessments, budget, time frame, and other factors, it was determined which places were most feasible for this project to build. To determine feasibility, small teams of PERRP engineers and technical surveyors conducted rapid assessments at each of the 250 sites. These rapid assessments sought to answer key questions: Was there access to roads, and if not, how far off the road was the site? Was there enough land to build on, given the building standards required? Did geotechnical tests indicate suitability? Were the needed water and electricity supplies available? What environmental impact could there be and what mitigation measures would be needed?

Using social criteria developed by the project, social mobilizers also visited each site for a quick assessment, talking with key informants such as teachers, medical staff, and others. This visit was to ascertain if there were any community factors that could negatively affect construction or the future operation of the school or health facility. As these communities were known to be heterogenous, the social mobilizer triangulated to identify local relations and conflict, if any, in the community. When conflict was found, we assessed its nature and risk level. We asked several key questions: Before the quake, how had the school or health facility actually been functioning? Were teachers and students, or health staff and potential patients, still present and needing these facilities? Would that need continue in the future? Who did the facility serve? Was the community involved in the school or health facility at all? Were there any sensitive areas, such as graves or monuments, that needed to be protected? Who owned the land where the facility was to be built, and the land adjacent to the building site? Did they have legal documentation of ownership—a mutation document, deed, or title? Was there the potential for conflict related to the land? If there was conflict, how feasible would it be for the social team to handle it in the time given?

In the first list of 250 schools—mostly one-room primary schools—many already had serious land ownership issues. When they were originally built, local people had donated the land, but the ownership was never officially transferred to the government and there were now many disputes over it. Settling such issues would take years—time that the project could not afford—so these sites were eliminated from the PERRP list and assigned by ERRA to local and international NGOs that would be present for the long term. ERRA and USAID redirected PERRP to construct only the larger facilities, mainly high schools where government had purchased the land so its ownership was settled.

Once the engineering, environmental, and social assessment questions were answered, a semifinal list was sent back to USAID, and—with ERRA's approval—the selection of sites was finalized.

Final Selection of Sites

From the original list of sites, the number was reduced to seventy-seven—sixty-one schools and sixteen health facilities. Places not chosen were rejected for a combination of reasons, such as intractable land issues, the size of the plot being incompatible with the new building standards, and the site being too far away from any roads. Only one site, a health unit, had to be eliminated due to a social conflict (see the anecdote "Who Should Attend the Meeting?"). In that case, the community was divided into two groups based on political affiliations with a long history of opposing each other on many subjects. Despite project efforts, they could not come to agreement, and the project declined to build there at all; instead, PERRP was assigned by the Department of Health to build a different health facility in another community. The seventy-seven selected PERRP sites were on government-owned land, with the mutation documents to prove it. While most of the communities where PERRP built still had land issues, those were due to a lack of agreement about exact boundary lines.

All of the sites in the final selection played significant roles in their regions. Most of the schools were high schools, where enrollment usually included children from preschool to grade ten, and higher secondary schools for students in grades eleven and twelve. While government primary schools are dotted throughout mountain villages, these higher-level schools are far less common, requiring students to walk far distances out of the mountains daily to attend high school. While schools for primary students were being built by other agencies, the multilevel high schools constructed by PERRP would give many more students from a wide area the opportunity to continue to a higher level of education. Of the total of sixty-one schools built, about half the students were girls, half boys. All of these schools were government owned and attended by children of the poorest families.

Subcontracts for Design and Construction

All the design and construction was carried out by Pakistani contractors who PERRP prequalified based on their technical and financial capabilities and their reputation for timely performance. From a pool of prequalified companies, the project selected construction contractors for each small group of two to seven buildings and awarded contracts based on competitive bidding. In total, twelve Pakistani construction firms, with a workforce of 5,800 workers, and over 250 local suppliers were contracted. In most cases, the construction contractors brought their own construction crews from other parts of Pakistan, as they were the skilled laborers needed, and skilled labor was scarce in the project area. Some unskilled laborers were hired locally. To design the buildings, four domestic architectural and engineering design firms were contracted.

Scheduling

Time was treated strictly. As a whole project, PERRP itself had strict beginning and ending dates by which all the work was to be completed. This required emphasizing to the contractors that they had to carry out all their work in a tightly controlled amount of time. If they got behind schedule, they were required to submit a "time-recovery schedule," a plan for making up for the lost time.

Each contract stipulated a specific maximum number of days by which all work had to be carried out for each building. The number of days was earlier estimated by PERRP design engineers according to size of the building, complexity, and other factors. For example, the 19,083-square-foot Government Girls' High School Chatter #2 was contracted to be completed in a maximum of 453 days—a goal that was achieved several weeks ahead of time. The largest in the project was the 84,031-square-foot Government Boys' Higher Secondary School Mansehra #1, which was built in 558 days. From the day USAID issued their formal notice to proceed with construction to the day the building was declared "substantially completed," each contractor's time was strictly counted. In each case, a plan was made that divided the total construction job into many stages, with dates agreed for completing each stage. At each site, the committees were also informed of the number of days the contractor was given to complete the construction, making that number of days common knowledge in the community. A countdown of days was started, adding to the committee's incentive to help prevent any interruptions. All the work was then monitored and supervised by the site and resident engineers for quality assurance. Time was also saved by having the community well prepared for the arrival of the construction contractor. As described in chapter 4, a main part of the community's responsibility was to help keep construction on schedule by preventing community-related problems, by making a formal agreement with the contractor, and by assisting whenever possible. Once the project got up and running, the average time for preparations—from first visit, to design and tendering, to the arrival of the construction contractor—was about five months. The period for construction then was on average eighteen months.

For the construction contractor, there were strong incentives to complete the contract as early as possible. As mentioned later in this chapter, contracts were awarded on a firm-fixed-price basis, meaning that the amount of money they would be paid was firmly fixed and agreed at the beginning in the contracting stage and would not be increased. To the contractor, this was the main incentive: the sooner completed, the lower the costs, and the greater the profit.

Monitoring, Quality Control, Quality Assurance, and Supervision

A common observation about construction in Pakistan and other countries is that it too often lacks supervision and quality control. However, PERRP's construction had four layers of management and monitoring to keep things on track. Full-time at each construction site was a site engineer to supervise the contractor to ensure they were building in compliance with the design provided to them, using the agreed materials, following safety regulations, and working within the agreed amount of time. At least weekly, the resident engineer visited to see the work of the site engineer, assess progress, and assist and guide as needed. At the higher level, a field-based overall construction manager monitored the sites and engineers and reported to the project's chief of party and deputy chief of party, who oversaw issues, compliance, and the progress of all of the sites.

With daily supervision on-site by site engineers and frequent visits by their superiors, weekly progress was quantified and reported. If the agreed progress had been made, the contractor continued on to the next stage. If the agreed progress had not been made, a time recovery plan was made and agreed upon. On a daily basis at each construction site, a social mobilizer and the site engineer worked closely together as counterparts—the engineer to deal with the contractor, the social mobilizer to work with the committee. Together, they were the frontline workers to keep things going. Such coordination was a key to successfully running construction in so many tough locations almost simultaneously.

During the early years of the project, the local contractors were sometimes found to lack the level of technical and managerial expertise needed, so they were mentored and trained by PERRP engineers on the building codes, scheduling, cost control, quality, health and safety, and contracting mechanisms. Project engineers themselves also upgraded their skills through both on-the-job training and online education from the implementing agency's subsidiary training organization, CDM Smith University online.

Corruption Prevention

Corruption in construction is a worldwide problem, and even in disaster reconstruction it is a reality requiring close scrutiny and control by donor and implementing agencies. Corruption is another complex subject and can happen in different forms, such as demands for cash, goods, services or favors, or illicit and often unsafe cost-cutting measures. In PERRP's construction management, this factor required multilevel involvement and stringent quality control procedures combining cost control and corruption prevention.

The project established for work on the ground a thorough selection process to vet potential contractors for their reputation for quality work, reliability, and being well-financed. Thorough costing was conducted ahead of time to know if contractor's bids and later claimed expenditures were legitimate. Bidders then were chosen based on realistic costs presented, not always on lowest bid terms (which tends to invite increased "costs" later). Contracts were detailed, specific, regularly scrutinized, and enforced to prevent loopholes and "extras," and each contract came with a firm fixed price or budget with no increases allowed. Each contractor was issued detailed scopes of work and procedures for change orders, which also helped prevent unauthorized work and payments.

In disaster reconstruction there can be additional possibilities for corruption when there is an extraordinarily high demand for and shortage of materials, and thus prices are far higher than normal. In such cases, to cut costs contractors may substitute cheaper, low-quality products and then try to cover them up by bribing inspectors, but when such costs did increase dramatically following the Pakistan quake, PERRP thwarted the problem by supplying the project's contractors with the main materials: cement and reinforcing steel.

Whereas delays in payments to contractors are a common problem, regular approvals and payments by USAID to CDM Smith allowed for the contractors to be paid regularly, keeping the needed cash flow. PERRP also kept close contact with high-ranking government officials to seek help in case of attempts at kickbacks. One situation where this did occur was when a lower-level official refused to acknowledge the government of Pakistan–approved import tax exemption for construction materials—a refusal that frequently signals a bribe demand. Reporting this to the higher officials resolved the issue with no illicit or illegal action in under twenty-four hours.

The key to corruption prevention was probably the selection, vetting, compensation, training, and monitoring of project staff. Recruiting qualified staff, with a pay scale that did not let staff fall prey to temptation, was essential. Also important was mandatory anticorruption training, with warnings of termination and potential criminal investigation if illicit activity was found. As described later in this chapter, unusually heavy monitoring was a deterrent. Besides daily, full-time monitoring on-site and from the regional office, weekly visits were made from the project head office.

Involved in the monitoring were engineering supervisors, social mobilizers, and committees. As part of the community participation, committees were asked to watch at construction sites and report any instances where they thought contractors were using substandard materials, resulting in a few such reports, which were checked and resolved. In the end, not a single issue of corruption was reported or detected.

Operation and Maintenance (O&M)
In PERRP, the committees agreed to share with the government the ongoing responsibility for the operation and maintenance of the new buildings.

This work was a completely new undertaking for such communities, because there was an expectation among the people that the government—which owns the buildings—would be responsible for looking after them.

To do their share, the social team had the committees draw up plans for what, when, and how maintenance needed to be done, as well as who would do the work and who would monitor it. The work was divided among cleaning staff (present in only a small minority of the schools), teachers, and students, with duties and a schedule posted for all to see. The committee visited regularly to see if the plan was being followed and to take action as needed. From the level of middle school upward, students, teachers, and any other staff were trained in "urgent operations," such as using a fire extinguisher, shutting off a water pump, or flipping a switch in the circuit breaker box. Nothing like this had been expected of the schools before, but most did it while the PERRP project was underway. Construction projects are often required to provide training or produce a detailed O&M manual for buildings, but the manuals are infamous for being dust collectors. Even though PERRP also produced the manuals, it encouraged teachers to post their own simple instructions and schedule where students could see it and check it off as duties were completed. Such hands-on experience raised some awareness of the need to keep up with O&M duties.

While the committees did an admirable job while PERRP was present, once PERRP was completed, the level of O&M dropped significantly in many cases, along with the committees ceasing to function as they had throughout the project. Government budgets and practices still allowed for only the minimum of O&M support, and people reverted to treating it as a government responsibility. However, general cleanliness was maintained at the female-led girls' schools by teachers and students themselves.

Reconstruction Site in Community Landscape

Most of the places built were in remote, rural areas throughout the mountains. Each construction site had high visibility in these quiet rural areas, and as such, it was the center of attention. Almost every day, visitors came from the community or other villages to watch the construction from a distance outside the marked safety boundary. Frequently, the site engineer, who was the project's full-time supervisor at the site, chatted with visiting committee members, groups of neighbors, elders, students, and families with out-of-town guests. From discussion about the earthquake features in the buildings under construction, a new seismic vocabulary of "shear walls," "columns," and "beams" was worked into the local languages.

Comparative Analysis of Construction Management

In the Public View

There may be a range of indicators of the quality of overall construction management, but in PERRP, the strongest evidence may have been the visible, concrete results seen daily by the public. Over the few years following the earthquake, reconstruction was to occur across the eighteen thousand square mile area of the destruction, at several thousand sites. In many places, these sites were visible along roads or in towns, making it easy to watch and compare construction progress—or lack of it—while traveling by. In this project's communities, construction status and comparisons were a daily topic of conversation among local people, PERRP engineers, social team members, and local officials. These ongoing observations were usually about PERRP construction as compared to the other construction happening nearby. Community people, often proud of their own involvement to help make it happen, frequently pointed out that the PERRP construction was continuing more consistently, without starts and stops, and was being completed more quickly than work in the other projects. In casual conversations and in meetings, local people talked about other nearby construction and recounted or speculated on the conflict over it, the court cases, the disappeared contractor, the funding problems, the reasons for it being slow or stopped, or other details.

As these local people were from the communities that had formed committees to work with PERRP, they often expressed pride in their roles in the project. The trouble experienced in other places was not happening in PERRP communities, partly because they had organized and were participating as partners with PERRP.

Engineers' Focus Group Analysis

As PERRP was ending, several internal assessment workshops were held. One such session was held especially for social team members, most of whom had little or no previous experience with construction, to ask project engineers about the construction management they had seen going on successfully in the previous six years. While the social team had introduced several innovations—the Committee-Contractor Agreements, the communication protocol with its grievance procedures, and so on—they wanted to understand from the engineers what construction was usually like in other projects and what these engineers did to keep PERRP moving forward.

These internal assessment workshops consisted of a focus group in which the engineers were asked to do an analysis based on their work experience inside and outside of Pakistan. This focus group was composed of eleven highly experienced Pakistani construction engineers with a combined total of 241 years of work in construction projects in Pakistan and other countries in the region. They were asked the following: Was construction in PERRP managed in any special or unique ways? How did it compare with their other construction experience? How were you, in PERRP, able to bring so much construction, in such tough conditions, in on schedule? They responded that nothing they were doing was unique. As one stated, "We did not invent any of what we do; we only applied textbook construction project management." They had learned these textbook practices in their own careers, from management training at university, from other companies, or from the implementing agency, CDM Smith. The focus group gave examples of what they meant by the "textbook construction management" strategies used in this project.

Selection of Contractors

Many of the most common problems in construction projects, according to the focus group, start with an improper process for choosing contractors. When construction is for government, the departments have a pool of enlisted contractors in different financial categories, with bid documents provided only to a select few. Only handpicked contractors are shortlisted, and these contractors can manipulate the rates or terms of payment, or deliberately underbid to try to get the job, and then demand more money later. In highly charged political environments, contracts are sometimes awarded under the table and paperwork is completed later.

However, in PERRP, potential design and construction contractors were chosen using a thorough, transparent five-step process to assess and prequalify them. First, invitations for applications were issued through the national media. A PERRP project committee of engineers then conducted a desk review of the submitted documents and made a preliminary short list of firms. Verification visits were made to those companies to see their organizational setup, including their completed and ongoing projects. From the visits, a final short list was made, prequalifying those companies to bid on "task orders"—small groups of schools or health facilities to be built. Contracts for that work were awarded based on a best-value basis. The focus group of engineers pointed out that, in Pakistan and other countries, such a thorough check is not the norm.

Contracts and Scope of Work

The focus group pointed out that contractors often are not given a detailed scope of work or assignment. There are unclear contract requirements, limited contract administration, and frequent requests for additions of unforeseen work. However, in PERRP, there were detailed contracts with each contractor, followed by close contract administration. Compliance to contractual obligations was strictly monitored and enforced.

Planning

According to the focus group, construction project planning in Pakistan and elsewhere is often not systematic or clear. Plans made at the head office do not get communicated down the line, and so are not implemented. But in PERRP, there were clear and detailed plans for each place to be constructed, and each plan was shared in detail at the different levels, managed, and monitored from beginning to end. There were clear organizational charts showing the chain of command and how all positions fit, as well as clear lines of communication and detailed job descriptions.

Timing and Schedule

Focus group members opined that it is common that the approved construction schedule is not followed in detail. Among staff there is limited sharing of the schedule and little understanding of time recovery scheduling, but in PERRP each site was on a strict construction schedule, developed along with time recovery plans as needed. Progress on the schedule was assessed weekly, with plans made to make up for lost time, if any, and with penalties for noncompliance.

Quality Control, Quality Assurance, and Monitoring

Frequently, there is little or no quality control or quality assurance and often even little conception of these, according to the focus group. They reported that, while the Pakistan Engineering Council decrees that a project is to be supervised by an engineer graduate, this requirement is seldom enforced. However, in PERRP there were four levels of monitoring and supervision for quality assurance (the responsibility of the implementing agency), in addition to the quality control (the responsibility of the contractor). Focus group members also observed that, normally, there is far less supervision and monitoring than occurred in PERRP.

Health and Safety

Members of the focus group pointed out that frequently there is little awareness of occupational health and safety requirements, including for gear like hard hats and protective clothing. Serious injuries are common but often not reported; in PERRP, however, there were strict health and safety requirements at all sites, and penalties for noncompliance. Regular incentives, briefings, and training were provided. PERRP received an award from the US National Safety Council for the project's safety record.

Payments
Reflecting on their other construction experience, focus group members pointed out how cash flow to contractors—and from contractors to workers, suppliers, and others—is commonly a major problem. Backlogs of payment result in hardship for workers and work stoppages, but as focus group members pointed out, in PERRP prompt monthly payments were made to contractors.

Cost Control
The focus group pointed out that in construction in Pakistan and elsewhere, strict project costs frequently are not given or are not firmly fixed, leading to cost overruns along with projects that take more and more time. It is a common industry practice to just keep extending the deadlines for completion and increasing the budgets allowed. However, in PERRP, careful cost estimating was carried out before contracts were let, and the contracts were awarded on a firm-fixed-price basis—meaning that the budget was agreed in the contract and cost increases or overruns of any amount were not allowed. Close financial monitoring helped keep costs as planned. The only exception to this was when the cost of certain building materials, such as steel and concrete, skyrocketed due to shortages; in those instances, PERRP purchased the materials in bulk and provided them to contractors, deducting those amounts from the contract's budget.

Leadership and Communications
According to the focus group, on other construction projects there often is not clear or consistent leadership, and information is not shared, so plans are not clear. However, as one focus group member stated, "On PERRP there was strong, consistent leadership from the top, which made the project work all the way down the ranks and into the field. This was true about the community participation too. If head office had not been definite and demanding about that, we [engineers] would have had a harder time, at least at first, to accept it."

Community Participation
As the focus group pointed out, community participation as practiced in PERRP is definitely not part of "textbook construction project management," but as it helped the construction go much more smoothly than normal, "it should be textbook." None of these engineers had any previous experience with community participation—at least, not in any deliberate, structured way, like it was in PERRP. Normally in construction in Pakistan and elsewhere, there is no organized community participation

and few ways are set up to prevent problems. Unlike in PERRP, there are normally no dedicated social teams to work with construction and the people, no agreements between the contractor and local people or committees (if any exist), no plans or protocols for communications or clear grievance procedures, and few attempts are made to guide construction worker behavior in communities. Focus group members opined that, of all aspects of community participation, what helped the construction management the most was the Committee-Contractor Agreements and the communication protocol with grievance procedures.

As the PERRP project was being completed soon after these windup workshops, many of the engineers expressed concern about going back to work in normal projects where there is no community participation as there was in PERRP, because it had helped construction and made their work go much smoother.

Architect—"There's Nothing about Culture in a Modern Building"

Visiting Nepal for a reconstruction conference following the 2015 earthquake there, I was introduced by a Nepali anthropologist to a small group of prominent local architects who had an established reputation for designing schools. Not so well informed on Nepali culture, I naively asked the architects what kinds of cultural considerations they had when designing schools. Much to our surprise, the main speaker of the group answered, "In a modern building, there doesn't need to be anything about culture. There's no need for cultural considerations." I listened intently while the local anthropologist and local architects went head to head. "How can you say there's nothing needed about culture in a modern building?" the anthropologist demanded. The architects seemed to not understand his concern.

Then the anthropologist, knowing where the cultural sensitivities lay, asked: "For example, in the schools you've designed, where did you place the washrooms or toilets?" The group was still somewhat dumbfounded and couldn't answer. The anthropologist listed off possibilities: Did the washrooms face inside the building with their doorways open into the hallways? Or did they face outdoors with their doors opening to the outside? Or were they put in another building outside the main building? Were male and female washrooms in sight of each other? Put on the spot like this, none of the architects could answer. Although these architects and the anthropologist were all the same nationality—Nepalis—the anthropologist explained to the architects the Nepali taboo against people of the opposite sex being seen going into or out of a washroom. Had they really designed so many schools in the past but never thought of such things? Apparently yes, and after the schools they had designed were constructed, they had not checked to see if there were any problems either.

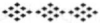

Official—"Village People Don't Know Anything about Design"

Even in the twenty-first century—after decades of social justice movements, sensitization, and lessons supposedly learned about "helping the poor" and the benefits of bottom-up development—some educated, urban officials still look down on rural people, being unable to imagine they could offer valuable input to such things as building design.

In one Asian country, I delivered a presentation on PERRP to a high-level international-aid decision maker. He was an engineer from a country in the region, and he listened intently until I described the Pakistani communities providing input to the design of the new schools and health facilities. At this point, he stopped the presentation, indignantly stating, "But village people don't know anything about design!" It took giving him several examples of how in PERRP community input had resulted in many good ideas and helped avoid costly mistakes before he decided to stop his protest against community input to design.

Toilet Orientation

As in many other cultures, certain aspects about toilets are delicate issues in Pakistan. In one of PERRP's preliminary school designs, washrooms had accidently been planned so that the toilet commodes faced southwest, toward Mecca, a taboo for toilets in Muslim culture. This mistake—noticed by community members in a design input session—was corrected while still on paper, a no-cost solution. Had these mistakes not been caught and corrected ahead of time, chances are high that the toilets would have been locked up, never used, a source of shame and embarrassment for the committee and school.

Boundary Walls

In areas of the subcontinent and other parts of the world, solid, high boundary walls are common around residential and other spaces. In Pakistan, such walls are used in both rural and urban spaces, especially at schools, for security purposes, for protection against unwanted visitors, and, in rural areas, also for protection from wild animals and grazing livestock. The walls demarcate the site, protecting the land from encroachment and providing the visual barriers preferred in the local culture.

For one of the large girls' colleges rebuilt in PERRP, designers had simply copied a design they had developed for a similar boys' high school. They had not planned to include a boundary wall. This cookie-cutter approach would not work in this case. When designers finally visited the girls' college and got local input, they had to make some fairly major changes to the preliminary design—major, at least, in the eyes of local people. When seeing the design on paper, the girls' college School Management Committee had noticed there were no plans for a boundary wall. This being a college for young women, they asked for a boundary wall as a priority. They also requested to have the main entry relocated from the front to the side of the building and the sports ground moved from the front to behind the school, both spots being out of sight of the busy road passing in front. As this was still early in the design phase, these requests were met at no cost to the project while making the college culturally suitable—and hence more comfortable and popular to attend. The building now has the reputation of being culturally appropriate, satisfying families who wish to send their daughters there for higher education.

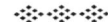

Unwanted Visibility

In another reconstruction project carried out by another donor and implementing agency, the school staff and community members raised several serious issues after the completion of the building, which by then were too expensive to correct. Had community members been consulted at this large girls' high school, a better, more culturally acceptable design may have been developed and at little or no extra cost.

The problem was that the new school was built on top of a mound, which meant that all sides of the two-story building were in plain view to everyone in the vicinity—in effect, putting the girls and young women on display, a cultural taboo. To provide a visual barrier would have required building a ten-foot-high boundary wall and gate, but this was considered an unreasonable expense, so it was not included.

Also, stairs to the upper floor were built on the outside of the building, further exposing the movement of the women. Had there been input from students, school staff, or the community, stairs could have been placed internally. To deal with this, the school administration covered the stairs with old banners and pieces of cloth, which gave the women some relief, but the fabrics were unsightly for the new building. Unfortunately, this school is now stuck forever with poorly thought-out design features that may be disappointing and stressful.

Glass Blocks in Windows

At a large boys' school already in an advanced stage of construction in PERRP, neighbors who had fully participated in the earlier design discussion meetings with project architects suddenly realized that the large windows of the new two-story school would overlook the private compounds of nearby houses, another cultural taboo. At the same time, although the architects were of the same nationality, they were not aware that this would be such a serious issue. An uproar ensued, and a neighbor threatened to go to court for a stay order to stop construction.

The social team intervened to try to find ways to deal with this, asking the project architects to visit and help find a solution. In a meeting on-site, some community members demanded that the whole window space, where wall-sized glass panes would be placed, instead be filled with bricks. Although this would mean almost total darkness in the classroom, the people considered the privacy invasion and potential for cultural offence as far more important to avoid. However, a solution was found by installing in the window spaces translucent glass blocks, which would block the view but still let in the light—building materials until then unknown in these areas.

With this solution, all the needs were met. The boys could not look into the neighboring family compounds, no one could see inside the classroom, the maximum light level was kept, there was no court case or stay order, and construction could proceed without any time lost.

After that incident, as a precaution and without being asked by anyone, the project as standard practice installed translucent glass blocks in window spaces at all other PERRP buildings constructed wherever windows might look into sensitive places.

Don't Waste the Land

At one of the schools, the community had valued their soccer field for decades, but the architects had other priorities. Without making a single visit to this site to be reconstructed, the architects—using only the technical survey data—decided to design the new school building to sit on the far end of the unusually large school ground leaving the old destroyed building as is, without demolition and removal. When community members were consulted about this, they protested loudly: That's wasting the land! We need our soccer field! They requested that the old building be removed and the new one built using the old footprint, as was the case with all the other schools constructed in this project. This way, the large plot of land would be saved to serve as the soccer ground and for other major community events as well. Since doing so would ensure better use of all the land, PERRP senior management directed the contracted architectural firm to follow the community input.

Respect for Graves

After discussing one school design with community representatives and implementing changes based on their input, as a final design step and standard practice project engineers visited the school site to lay out the design on location using chalk powder lines. It wasn't until community members saw the chalk lines on the ground that they realized there would be a problem with the planned location for the school's toilets. Located at one end of the new building, the toilet block's outer wall would be adjacent to the school's boundary wall, which separated the school from the graveyard. As it was considered insulting to the graves to have toilets so close, designers reconfigured the design, which was still on paper, putting toilets in another part of the building. Had this not been caught in time, it could have been a permanent problem.

"My School Is My Life"

Sometimes students were also included in the design process in order to make them feel part of this new thing happening in their community and to raise awareness about design. Some of the schools had older students study the floor plans and sit in at design meetings with the architects, so they were unusually aware of what was going to be built.

At some schools, the youngest students were also involved by being given fun drawing exercises. They were asked to draw what they thought their new school would look like and what they hoped for. As art is rarely taught here, and even the most basic materials are scarce, social mobilizers took sheets of simple computer printer paper and pencils to schools to get the kids to draw. At one location on a steep mountain slope, where the old school had collapsed but all its rubble had been removed, children continued to attend class in the open air, using the only furniture that remained—a few wooden benches. One of the seven-year-old girls took her piece of paper and pencil, and squatting on the ground using the bench as a table surface, drew her highest hope: to have another school. Penciling in Urdu, she drew a picture of a school and printed "my school is my life." Probably no one had thought of a school building as being so important to a child.

Flash Floods and Local Knowledge

A building's sustainability depends on many factors, not the least of which is its location and orientation. At one of the BHUs to be built, project surveyors had carried out all the geotechnical testing and measuring and reported it to the designers, but it was found out later that they had missed crucial information. As part of the community's design input process, community members accompanied the architects when they visited the site to discuss the preliminary design with the committee. On this walkabout, elder members pointed out the risk of flash floods in this location and informed them that, decades ago, one had destroyed the building then on the site. Although there were no longer any visible indications of flooding, the architects were able to take this local knowledge and make changes accordingly by raising the foundation and slightly reorienting the building while it was still only on paper. Without this input, the design could have added to the risks.

Honor the Committee-Contractor Agreement

A risky situation arose that needed quick resolution. In one location's Committee-Contractor Agreement, the contractor agreed with a landowner to rent his land for the storage of materials, a launching area, and a site office. The contractor was using the land for these purposes but not paying the rent. Making matters worse, the contractor refused to acknowledge the above agreement despite his having made and signed it in the presence of several community members at the time. An uproar was starting.

As per the communication protocol and the signed-in-public Committee-Contractor Agreement, the social mobilizer asked the site engineer to have the contractor attend a meeting with the committee. At the meeting, the engineer reminded the contractor that his contract with PERRP required him to pay his bills and do it on time, otherwise PERRP would deduct the amount owed to the landowner, plus penalty, from the contractor's own fee. A few days later, the contractor complied. There was no interruption of construction.

"Construction Here Is an Uphill Battle"

"The construction here at different mountainous sites is an uphill battle in its truest sense. The Government Girls' Middle School at Besuti was successfully constructed at an altitude of 6,875 ft, and the Basic Health Unit at Bani Minhasan at 6,586 ft. In such places with heavy snow, and other places that get the monsoon effect, work had to be planned around the seasons and weather. Single-lane dirt roads with many switchback corners made it hard to bring supplies and equipment. Still, the local people are amazed to see how we were able to bring workers and heavy construction material to our sites here in the mountains. In many places there were no roads, only footpaths to the school or health unit so we had to build a kind of rough track to some of the sites."

—PERRP Construction Manager

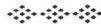

Mohandri School, Mountainside Boulders

In one case, where no other land was available, there was no choice but to build the new school in the same risky location as the school that had been destroyed, but the project and community took extraordinary steps to reduce or eliminate the risk.

Most of the destruction in the 2005 quake came from lateral movement, but other damage was caused when the quake set off landslides or rockfalls. At one project location assigned to PERRP, at Mohandri village in KP province, the quake had dislodged boulders from the nearby steep mountainside. They bounced down the steep slope, smashing through the roof into the school, killing four students and seriously injuring nine more. When no other land was available to rebuild this school in a safe place, steps were taken to remove the risks.

At first, only an extra solid wall was planned on the slope side of the school, to deflect stones should they fall again, but no one was comfortable with this choice alone. Imagine attending a new school in that location for decades to come, always fearful of more boulders rolling down—the root cause had to be addressed. Project engineers, the social team, committee members, and other local people began a rock-by-rock survey across the whole mountain slope. Aided by a teenage boy who hunted birds on the slope and who knew all its nooks and crannies, they identified all the loose rocks and boulders. At first the thought was to explode them to break them up, but that was too dangerous for the buildings and people down below. Instead, the engineers had the rocks and boulders broken into small pieces using a nonexplosive chemical, removing the threat. The new Government Boys' Primary and High School at Mohandri is now attended by more than five hundred students and their teachers, who are now free from the worry of falling boulders.

Hostel for Students from Farthest Valleys

In the mountainous areas, primary schools in villages are dotted throughout the mountains and valleys, but opportunities for continuing into higher levels of education are few and far between. Making it into PERRP's final selection of schools to reconstruct was the town of Jared's boys' higher secondary school, the only school of its kind in an enormous catchment area encompassing valleys and mountain ranges. After primary school, this was local boy's only chance for higher secondary education in a government school in their own vicinity. This school's committee made an appeal to the project to include a small hostel space in their new building, so that boys from faraway villages could attend school and have a place to stay, as needed, instead of walking back and forth the long distances every day.

Assisting the head teacher in putting together information to make their case to project management, a social team member asked about the boys who would need the hostel. "From how far away would those students come? From two mountain valleys away?" The head teacher replied, "Oh no, it's easy for those boys to get back and forth to home every day. I'm talking about the students who come from the fourth and fifth valleys away. A few of those kids come here every day already, walking up then back down or around the mountain sides, taking two to three hours every day one way. Sometimes the weather is just too bad for them to walk. If we had a hostel more of them would attend." Fortunately, the designers were able to include a hostel space. Soon after the new school building was completed the enrollment more than doubled.

Trouble over the Word "Local"

Even the most careful contractor selection and vetting process can hit snags. In this disaster reconstruction scenario, a different project advertised across Pakistan to locate qualified construction firms to rebuild schools. The advertisements in daily English newspapers specified the qualifications needed and encouraged "local contractors" to apply. Many applications were received and reviewed, a few companies were selected and contracted, and then they were sent to start work, causing an uproar at one site. There, from the same big town, was a contractor who had applied but been not accepted, since his company did not have the qualifications specified. But, as he pointed out, the company that won this contract was not "local" as the advertisement had stated. As he pointed out, the selected contractor was from another part of Pakistan, while his business was from here—local. Immediately, the man threatened court action to stop the start of construction, based on the "false advertising," and he also blamed the donor agency. This was an embarrassing situation for the project management who had placed the advertisements, as they had not foreseen how "local" is a relative thing. By "local" they had meant Pakistani, as opposed to non-Pakistani, while the nearby company interpreted "local" to mean from the same vicinity. Fortunately, influential people in the area convinced the local man to stop his actions, so that construction of the urgently needed school could get underway, and he did not follow through on his threats.

Pouring Concrete Roof, Community Members Stood By Overnight

The mood at this construction site was described by engineers as "euphoric," as the concrete roof of the Basic Health Unit was poured and completed all in one go, a sixteen-hour period. The resident engineer reported that local people came by the construction site, sitting on the ground outside the safety perimeter to watch for hours and repeatedly offering any assistance needed. They said they had never seen such modern (concrete and steel) construction before and they were especially delighted that it had gone so fast. Keeping with local custom for when the construction of a house is completed, community members brought food that night for the workers and recited prayers for the long life of the health unit, and for no rain to interrupt the concrete pouring. The main way they assisted, besides boosting the morale of the laborers and engineers, was making sure the crucial water supply needed was provided uninterrupted.

Locals Threaten to Be Given Jobs

There had been early and repeated announcements and agreement that contractors were not obliged to hire anyone local, as they usually would bring their skilled laborer crews with them. By the time the contractors arrived, this was widely understood and accepted; however, in a few instances, the agreement was ignored.

At one of the villages, a local man threatened the contractor and demanded he and his friends be hired. Instead of responding to the threat, the contractor followed the project communication protocol and its grievance procedures and reported the incident to the site engineer, who went to the social mobilizer, who then asked the committee to step in. Committee members said this threat was a power play by the local man against other locals who did get work. Since violence was threatened, an emergency meeting was called. Committee members asked the elder brothers of this man to attend, knowing they would be the most likely influence on him. At the meeting, the PERRP resident engineer reminded the elder brothers of the PERRP policy, while meeting participants confirmed this had been established as a rule from the beginning: that contractors could bring their own work crews and were not obliged to hire anybody local. The brothers went home and ordered the younger brother to stop making trouble and to find work someplace else. That was the end of the problem.

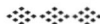

Two Contractors in a Road Dispute

Disputes and conflict among community members and contractors were expected, but less common were contractors in conflict with each other. As construction of one of the new clinics was underway by a PERRP contractor in a remote area, the dirt road that passed by was being upgraded by an unrelated contractor. Day by day, differences arose between the contractors over who had authorization to use the road. The matter came to a head one day when the PERRP contractor arrived with his heavy equipment and was hotly accused by the other contractor of damaging the newly repaired road.

As the argument between the two contractor's managers escalated—and with over a hundred laborers divided into two sides watching on—the social mobilizers followed up by phone with a contact made several months before. As part of the preparation for construction, they had met and had discussions with the main government stakeholder agencies to inform them about the project and solicit their participation and help when needed. As part of this, they had unexpectedly met with the district public works executive engineer responsible for roads while on a snowbound road a few months earlier. See anecdote "Meeting a Main Stakeholder on the Snow-Blocked Road," page 170. At that time, he had promised any help needed, and now they asked for it. As the road contractor was under the executive engineer's supervision, he directed the road contractor to allow the PERRP contractor to do whatever they needed. This intervention closed the case, and construction was not interrupted.

Ethnography: Boys' Primary and High School Glacier Way*

Glacier Way is a pseudonym. To maintain confidentiality, the names have been changed.

Construction or reconstruction can be affected by many seen and unforeseen situations. Here was another example of the importance of the social side of construction working in tandem with the technical side. At one PERRP site, a tragic accident occurred that could have had dire consequences for a far greater number of local people and brought construction of the new schools to a standstill.

While divisions by caste, sect, class, wealth, power, and politics are common in Pakistan and there are people and many kinds of incidents that serve to ignite the differences, the opposite can also be true. In such places, there are respected people who can bring situations back under control, who can restore calm and keep the peace. It all depends on the nature of the incident, how and when the situations are handled, and by whom.

Glacier Way is a major tourist destination in the north of the PERRP project area, a scenic mountainous area. In summer it is packed by people from the south of the country getting away from the oppressive heat. In the winter the whole population migrates out of this area to avoid being trapped in the valley by several feet of deep snow and the glacier that crosses the road in several places. The town has many hotels and other tourist services, but in the 2005 earthquake most of the facilities were damaged or destroyed, including the two government boys' schools, one primary and one secondary. ERRA had USAID assign PERRP to rebuild these schools.

As per the usual PERRP community participation process, the social team had the two schools form a committee from different interest groups in town: the hotel association, other businesses, retired people, parents, and the range of sects, castes, and political affiliations. As this construction was to happen in the center of town, in the midst of tightly packed houses, shops, hotels, and restaurants, it would take extra careful attention by all to avoid the most common construction problems. The committee was led through all the steps by the social team to prepare before construction started.

One day, tragically, as one of the contractor's trucks was returning to the construction site from dumping excavated materials and was passing through the narrow street, a small boy was hit and killed by the truck. He was the only son of one of the hotel owners.

When something like this happens in Pakistan it is not uncommon for people to take the law into their own hands and unite against the perpetrator, capturing, beating, or even killing him and destroying the vehicle and anything connected with the guilty party. In this case, however, some of the people who witnessed the accident grabbed the fleeing driver, took his truck away, and took him to the police, where the family had him charged with murder. As is the case in many parts of the country, such incidents can grow beyond the actual people involved and multiply the causes for fighting. A response was needed immediately to keep the situation under control.

Hearing this tragic news within minutes of it happening, social mobilizers in the PERRP office two hours away started contacting by cell phone the committee leaders and one of the town's most prominent members, the president of the Glacier Way Hotel Association, to organize a response in order to keep the incident from turning into a full-blown conflict between community members and the contractor and his laborers working on the construction site.

When social mobilizers arrived, the atmosphere was tense but it was not yet clear what retaliation, if any, would happen. Consulting with the hotel association president, committee members, religious leaders, and teachers (including the deceased boy's uncle, a teacher in the school under construction), they worked out a strategy for resolving the situation. Jointly it was decided a delegation should go to the family and give their condolences.

A group of forty to fifty prominent community members, project social mobilizers and engineers, and the contractor and his site engineers went to the home of the family. With the president of the hotel association acting as spokesman, he condemned the incident, expressed the sorrow of everyone, and apologized to the family for such great loss. The delegation appealed to the family to help keep the peace for the sake of continuing construction of the new school. They explained that the guilty man had been jailed and his truck had been taken but also that he was a poor man—an Afghan refugee. "If he's punished what good would that do?" reasoned the spokesman.

The *Kateeb*—a religious leader from the mosque—also appealed to the family, telling them that in Islam forgiving someone brings high rewards from Allah. As this was the holy month of Ramadan, he appealed to the family to be even more forgiving at this time. He requested that they forgive the driver as this had been an accident and not something done intentionally. He said the contractor was there for the benefit of future generations and that construction should continue. He asked them to withdraw the charges of murder.

In response, the family agreed, forgave the driver, and wrote a statement to say that they had nothing against him and that the conflict was resolved. Right away, the driver was released from jail and given back his truck. Still fearing for this life, he disappeared from town. The family refused compensation offered by the contractor.

Had this not been resolved so quickly and effectively, it could have led, like so many other cases in Pakistan, to further conflict and losses and to stalled construction that would never start again. It also could have become a much bigger incident. Since all the hotels and other local businesses have close relations with the country's top politicians, who also visit as tourists, such high-level connections could have been involved to punish the contractor. Journalists in town were already writing up the story for national news media coverage, which could have dragged in the donor and been made this into an international incident. They decided to stop for the good of the community.

Fortunately, this was another case in which, while there can be deep divisions among local people, respected people have strong abilities to keep problems from spiraling out of control.

Follow-Up
Some months after this incident, when all of the Glacier Way population had migrated out of the valley before deep snow would block all routes, the contractor won special favor in local hearts. As the last residents fled town for the winter, construction of the two new school buildings was still going full tilt—day and night—to complete as much construction as possible before they also would have to flee and close down construction for the winter. Even years later people still talked about seeing the contractor and laborers working late at night with snow swirling around in their flood lights. They said they had never seen a contractor working in such a dedicated way.

CHAPTER 7

The Library Challenge

Introduction

In project planning for community participation, the extent to which participation is likely or possible is always in question. What is reasonable to expect? To what extent and in what forms might people be interested to contribute, whether in tangible or intangible ways? Answers to those questions emerge over time and depend on many factors, the strongest of which may be trust, inspiration, motivation, and leadership. At first in PERRP, local people were reluctant to be involved, but in a short time that changed dramatically through local leadership and different sources of motivation. Sometimes each community contributed far in excess of what was imagined, as was the case with the Library Challenge.

The Library Challenge

Something remarkable happened about midway through PERRP: there was an event and process that brought all aspects of the project together. It was called the Library Challenge. Of all that occurred in the project, this challenge was probably a favorite memory for many people and was a textbook case of empowerment.

In the first two or three years of the project, the social team began to discuss the prospect of libraries for the new schools. Before the quake, none of the government schools had libraries or books because, in Pakistan, these are considered luxuries when education budgets are limited. But now, with the new building standards, all PERRP school designs included a dedicated library room that would be fully furnished. Without books, would these new facilities remain empty and unused? And wouldn't that be a pity? The debate about books carried on for months among social team members. Some of the mobilizers thought it would be a big waste of time and money to get books. They came from the same area where the schools were being built and said there was no culture of reading in the region. They were concerned that books would not be appreciated or looked after, or that the teachers would lock any library books in the cupboards. Others felt that stocking the library might be worthwhile.

All members of the social team had gone through the same government school system; knowing it all too well, they were divided in their opinions. In AJ&K, the literacy rate is 76 percent, as compared to 60 percent for other parts of Pakistan (Government of AJ&K 2018). Even with the highest literacy rate in Pakistan, there still was doubt about local interest in school libraries. The debate continued inside the social team: What do we mean by reading culture? Why don't schools have libraries already? Since there's practically no TV or Internet in these far-flung areas, what do kids do in their spare time? Do adults read? The *aha!* moment came one day when someone asked, "So why do you think people don't read here?" The answer decided the whole argument: "Because there's practically nothing to read! People are poor, they don't have books or anything else to read at home." If there is nothing to read, how can there be a reading culture? As one committee chairman later put it,

> I like reading, but before this, nobody was aware of the importance of school libraries. With the books our community has donated now, along with those from the Library Challenge project, we will have a great collection even in this remote village.

By three years into the project, about half the construction was completed or underway. All the committees had been active for much of that time. With facilitation by the social team, the committees had already made significant achievements and were busy fulfilling their duties with the project. By this time the project's protocols, routines, and committees were working relatively smoothly, to the point that the committees seemed to be ready for more.

Discussion had continued all along inside the social team and senior management about getting books. We would need an enormous number of books for the project's seventeen thousand students. How would we do it? What were the options? There was some thought about getting the CDM Smith head office in the USA involved to donate books, but that idea was nixed when it was realized that shipping costs would be exorbitant; that those books would all be only in English, and thus not very useful in these areas; and that it would be inconsistent with the participatory direction that had been used all along. We determined that the project should not be the gift-giver either of the books or the cash to buy them. Far more would be gained by once again sharing responsibility. If the community would get involved and take on the challenge to raise its own money to buy its own books, then it would feel a much stronger sense of ownership of them, be in a better position to sustain the libraries by making connections with publishers and booksellers, and at the same time generate wider interest in books and reading. In discussion first with PERRP's senior management, it was agreed that if the local committees decided they wanted to go ahead with this idea, then PERRP senior management would get CDM Smith—employees as well as the firm—involved to contribute books on a matching basis and have all the books purchased in Pakistan. The social team decided to present this "library challenge" to the committees.

Presenting the Challenge

By this point in time, PERRP was holding regular workshops attended by two representatives of each committee: the head teacher (the committee's general secretary) and the community representative (the committee's chairperson). During one of these workshops, I proposed the idea of the Library Challenge to these representatives. Reviewing architects' floor plans of a few of the schools, members of the social team pointed out the library rooms and said to each audience, "When we did the survey with you a few months ago, you told us you have no library books. What do you think of the idea of having no books in these wonderful new libraries?" The answer was unanimous: "We would love to have books, but the government has none to give to us, and no budget for us to buy them."

Speaking for the social team, I responded, "But why wait for government to do this? You have shown the project that you have very strong skills and resources in your communities. The way you have helped construction, it seems you can make anything happen! Now here is something else you can do: put together your own library!"

I told the assembled representatives that this was only an idea, and that it was completely up to them to try to get books or not. Their responses were mostly skeptical. Some were afraid to try to raise funds; some were a bit indignant, surprised, or in disbelief at having been asked. "But we are very poor!" they said. "Even before the quake, we were poor, but now we have lost everything. How can we possibly ask poor people to donate? Nobody has ever donated to a government school, so why would they start now? Money for schools is the government's responsibility!"

Members of the social team encouraged committee members to consider all the difficult things they had already achieved. They had arranged the loan of land for a temporary tent school while construction was underway, settled disputes over land ownership and other conflicts, got access to land, persuaded people and offices far outside the project to help with different hurdles, and made sure construction contractors got what they needed. It was their hard work that helped construction go ahead on schedule—a highly unusual achievement.

Most had made up their minds that they could not go out and ask for donations for books. The social team then introduced the idea of a Library Challenge: if the committees promised to donate at least one book per student in their own school, then CDM Smith had agreed to do the same. They also explained that since the PERRP budget was for construction only, CDM Smith volunteers would also have to raise funds for their contribution of books.

With this news, the hesitancy changed rapidly, with murmurs around the room expressing surprise. "What does this mean? An engineering and construction firm is willing to donate books to us?" One of the most gregarious head teachers spoke up: "This is a wonderful offer, and we will never get this chance again to start a library. We can do this!" He spoke enthusiastically, starting to generate ideas for how they could raise funds. By the end of the day-long workshop, participants had added many ideas, building each other's confidence. Within a few days they had taken on the challenge so seriously that they were in friendly competition with each other to see who could raise the most money and buy the most books. Their reactions went from reluctance to excitement to try, and they immediately went out to see about raising funds.

Finding the Books: Organizing AJ&K's First Bookfairs

Still, in the social team, we were not sure what possibilities there were for books for the libraries. Libraries simply did not exist anywhere else in government schools, and we were uncertain as to where we could source books. Having books shipped from the USA or elsewhere was discounted, as shipping would be far too expensive—plus, all those books would be in English, while abilities in the language were low in these schools. Project administrative staff in the central office in Islamabad took on the task of identifying Pakistani publishers by scouring bookstores for books in Urdu for children, bringing 150 samples back to the office. From these, we compiled a list of publishers, which helped us to identify hundreds of more book titles.

Given that even the Pakistani office staff—who had been educated in the city mainly in English—expressed surprise at finding children's books in Urdu, we wondered if the committee members and teachers would know about these. The project schools were in such remote areas, several hours from the nearest cities. When people visited the city, they tended to do so only for medical, business, or family reasons—not to go to book stores. At the next committee workshop, we laid out the 150 book samples, and even the highly experienced head teachers were astonished. In this display laid out for them, they walked around the tables, impressed and delighted—but also dismayed that they had not previously known such books existed. Anticipating their needs, we had compiled a set of fifty sample books for each school to take back to their communities to show around, so others could see the potential too and to help with their fundraising.

Six weeks later, at the next workshop, the committee members stated that, much to their surprise, raising money was not as hard as they had thought it would be. But now the big question was "Where do we buy the books?" With no local bookstores, and booksellers so far away, the social team suggested that booksellers be invited to Bagh city to hold a bookfair. Again, there was much doubt. Many wondered, "Why would book sellers come so far, over such small roads that are in such poor condition?" But soon this second hurdle of doubt was also overcome. To drum up interest in a bookfair in the communities, senior committee members joined other local people and officials to create a sixty-person organizing committee. The project became a PERRP-wide effort, with social mobilizers, engineers, office staff, and drivers all volunteering their support.

When we invited Urdu-language publishers to the bookfair, over a dozen companies responded. These publishers were aware of the higher literacy rate and potential audience in the communities, and the first-ever AJ&K bookfair was held in Bagh city in 2009, only five months after the idea of a library challenge was first discussed with the committees. Attended by eight thousand people, including busloads of children and teachers from the PERRP project, other schools, and the public, the bookfair was a wild success: the publishers sold out of books in two days. The local print media generated stories leading up to the fair, and the FM radio station, Voice of Azad Kashmir, broadcasted live from the event. The media attention drew in attendance from places far from Bagh city. To run the event—to administer first aid services, clean up, control traffic, and handle security, advertising, and logistics—we had contributions from local government, district administration, NGOs, and private-sector sponsors.

For the KP province schools, a separate bookfair was planned but had to be canceled due to security concerns. Instead, committee members went to the Lahore International Bookfair and Lahore's historic Urdu Bazaar, where they spent all the money they had raised. This included the Library Challenge's overall champion fundraising school: 120,000 rupees (roughly $1,300) raised by the Government Boys' Higher Secondary School Jared, in the remote Kaghan Valley.

By 2011, there was such a high demand for another bookfair in AJ&K that a second one was held. Because of the reputation of the first bookfair, many more publishers applied to participate in this second event but had to be turned away due to space limitations. Over twenty-five thousand people attended the fair, and the fifteen publishers almost sold out. For four days, a ten-thousand-square-foot college gymnasium site was jammed with parents, teachers, the public, and students of all ages. Whole families, dressed in their finest clothes, attended with their children. Local officials who inaugurated and closed the event observed that this was the largest event ever held in AJ&K Bagh district, outside a religious or political rally. Local news correspondents got the bookfair into international news, and soon committee members were getting phone calls from family in the UK and Gulf States saying they had seen it covered on TV.

In preparation for this second bookfair, the reach of community organizing in Bagh had grown even wider. Motivated by results they had already seen, twenty-seven AJ&K project committees gave themselves another challenge. Instead of focusing only on getting more books for their own schools, the committees decided to try to influence other schools in the region and to each show at least two more schools how to start their own libraries. Senior committee representatives then went to other schools and did the same, showing those communities how to raise money and come to the second bookfair to buy their books. This way, libraries were started in sixty-three schools outside those built by PERRP, even without the advantage of matched book donations from CDM Smith. Again, the city of Bagh provided all the services needed, and officials attended with their families. Along with PERRP's KP province schools, a total of 116 new libraries were established—the only libraries for children in the region.

Libraries Established

In the end, the number of books purchased for libraries in PERRP-built schools was more than double the Library Challenge goal. The fifty-three project schools raised 2.3 million rupees (almost $26,000), an enormous amount in local terms—the equivalent to 236 months (nineteen years!) of a typical teacher's salary. Maybe even more significant is that one book cost, on average, over half a day's income for a poor family. With these realities, for the 17,000 students altogether, the committees bought and donated 24,000 books, while CDM Smith and friends donated another 40,000 books. These were the first libraries in local government schools, and some opened their use to the community.

Following the bookfair, the agenda of the next committee workshop was an unusual and satisfying exercise: to analyze why the Library Challenge had been so successful. Participants concluded it depended on many factors. The first was the motivation received from the social team.

It helped that committee members were already known and respected, so they were able to go out into the community and ask for donations—and, in the process, spread wide awareness about the Library Challenge. People were also more interested to donate for a cause that was concrete and finite—to purchase one book for each student—and the books would be visible to everyone in the new school. In many cases, a further benefit had come when, upon request by the committees, imams made announcements at the mosques to encourage donations, adding to the awareness raising and providing an endorsement. For many, this was a legitimization, recalling the Quran and how it repeatedly urges Muslims to learn, get an education, and *ikra* (read)!

Following best practices for development proposed by scholars like Anderson and Woodrow (1989), PERRP focused almost exclusively on the strengths of the communities, encouraging the people to recognize their own capacities and to put them to work. These communities, like others, have certain strengths—pride in their kin, faith, and culture—even where there are many differences among their people. While the community members may know their own problems better than anyone else, it sometimes takes a catalyst for people to recognize their strengths, resources, and other capacities. However, sometimes it takes outsiders to recognize and encourage those capacities; encouraging poor communities can make their desires a reality.

The Library Challenge may have been a textbook example of community empowerment, but it was also just another step in a series of achievements that many people had doubted would be possible. First challenged with helping construction, each committee achieved one difficult task after another, each time building confidence. Such empowerment is the most important result of an effective mobilization process.

At community-wide celebrations to inaugurate each new school, which were attended by hundreds or even thousands of people, representatives spoke about how their participation had helped take them out of the despair and hopelessness they had felt following the earthquake. Frequently heard in speeches and conversations with committee members was the notion that "[PERRP] and the Library Challenge has got us organized, given us new hope and skills and made us now think of the future. Now we can do anything!"

However, as discussed, not long after the PERRP project was completed, the committees ceased to function as they had during the project. Although intentions had been expressed and some preparations made to continue the committees as well as the bookfairs, old competition and the power structures took over again. In any case, at least until PERRP was

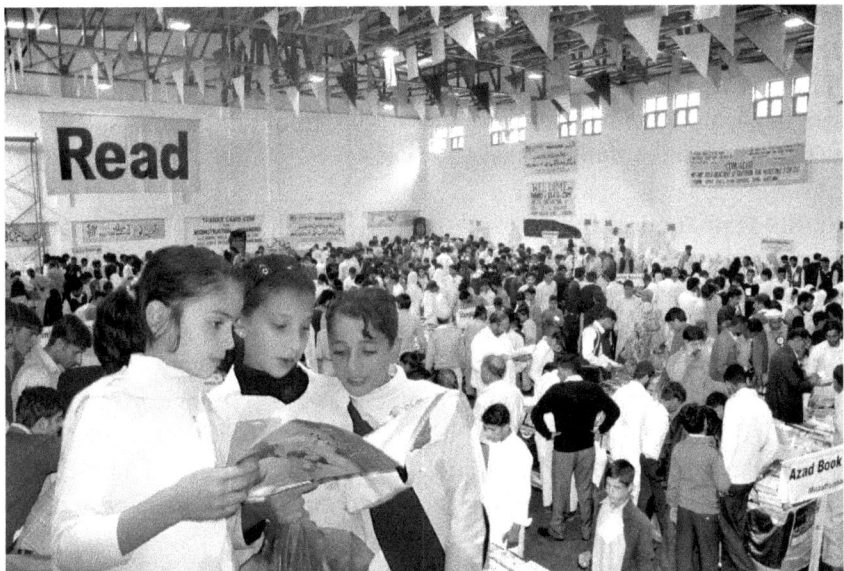

Figure 7.1. The Book Fairs. As part of the Library Challenge, PERRP and the committees organized two major book fairs, the first such events in AJ&K. Here at one of the book fairs in Bagh, students, teachers, families, and the general public attended to see, buy, and donate books to their schools, 2011. © Nadeem Anjum Kiani.

completed, the libraries were still intact and used. Capacities built could be used in other development and people's expectations were no doubt raised of what can be achieved by working together.

Library Challenge Notes

Each committee made its own fundraising plan. As prominent community members, they called on the wealthy, petitioned the shop owners in the bazaar, contacted alumni, had announcements made at Friday prayers asking for donations, sold odds and ends around the school, and had teachers, parents, and students contribute. Each school got hundreds of donations, even from the poorest parents, who gave perhaps one to five rupees. Some children even gave their pocket money.

All the books were new and most were published in Pakistan. About 80 percent were in Urdu, and 20 percent in English. Schools bought the subjects of their choice. The books donated by CDM Smith were chosen by social team members. Titles were not selected based on the curriculum; instead, subjects were chosen for the fun and enjoyment of reading. The books provided included general knowledge books, reference books (dictionaries, atlases, etc.), and books about the world, people, technology, households, science, health, the earth and earthquakes, art and design, nature, the environment, Islamic history, Pakistani history, sports, and language, along with jokebooks, storybooks, books of poems, and books with primary-level alphabets and numbers.

PERRP Staff Fundraising

Engineers in PERRP approached the Pakistani companies contracted to construct the schools and suggested they could give back by making cash donations to sponsor libraries in the schools they were building. Books for nineteen of the libraries were funded this way. From events at different embassies in Islamabad, from CDM offices in the USA, and from friends and relatives in many countries, PERRP staff raised funds from individuals by having them sponsor sets of books to be donated. Several project suppliers—including concrete, travel, and stationary—also made cash donations to buy and donate books.

Library Management Training

As government schools in Pakistan usually have no libraries, the project schools had no experience with library management. To address this in the most realistic way, guidelines on library management and monitoring were drawn up from participatory exercises. First, teachers and committee members were asked about having a library: What might the problems be? What would they worry about? How could they prevent or solve those problems? What would they need to do so? Who would monitor the library? When and how could they monitor it? Their answers were turned into guidelines made by the committees and schools themselves. Over the remaining time of PERRP, these self-made guidelines were used to set up and manage the libraries, and to do periodic self-assessments.

Each school set up its own borrowing and lending system, and its volunteer librarian was trained by the Punjab Library Resource Center. For schools still operating in tents before the new school was completed, their books were kept in metal storage boxes that were carried to a central point for the students to borrow books.

Library Days

Important to ongoing management and sustainability of the libraries was community knowledge of what books they could expect to see in the library. Committees acted as hosts at the schools' Library Days for community members whose donations had stocked the shelves. Library Day visitors were invited to look through the collection and come back again to read books themselves.

Related Activities

The Library Challenge introduced many different kinds of reading and related activities in the schools, such as students making, writing, and illustrating their own little books. An art project was introduced where students were asked to draw either their new school or what they saw at their old school on the day of the earthquake. In 2012, for the seventh anniversary of the quake, a selection of the two thousand entries received was exhibited at the National Art Gallery in Islamabad.

Impact

The Library Challenge made no attempt to measure the impact it had on reading, but even on unannounced visits to schools, PERRP staff could see students reading. We could hear the buzz in the libraries and classrooms as students carried out a wide range of reading activities: weekly or daily reading periods; displays of books that showed what was available; library art with drawings and slogans about reading; and students' own self-authored, self-made books of nonfiction, stories, and poems. Sometimes community members visited the school to read to classes. At other times, students read aloud to their peers and to younger children. Most such activities were new in these underfunded government schools.

Comments about the Library Challenge

School Management Committee Chairman: I like reading, but before this, nobody was aware of the importance of school libraries. With the books our community has donated now, along with those from the Library Challenge project, we will have a great collection even in this remote village.

Student in a Boys' High School: We have over 3,000 books in this library, and I'm going to read them all.

Teachers at the Government Boys' Primary School Mohandri, Khaghan Valley: We have never seen the students so excited. The only books they had seen before were their textbooks. Now they look at these new books full of color and pictures and they are surprised that they are able to read books they had not seen before!

Psychologist Working in Postdisaster Trauma Counseling, Bagh, AJ&K: The bookfair was likely the most fun many people have had since the earthquake. Such fun and recalling it for weeks and months to come will help heal the trauma that many people are still suffering.

First Student Donation to the Library Challenge

At Besuti, a girls' middle school at high altitude in a snowbound area, students attended school for the first year after the quake in a large tent, which was supplied by PERRP while construction was being prepared. One day, the school's SMC was using a corner of the tent classroom for a meeting space and was talking about the Library Challenge. A few of the students nearby overheard the talk about books and wanted to know more, so committee members explained that they were going to try to get money to start a library at their new school. These little girls were so excited by the idea of having books that, on the spot, they took out all their pocket money and handed it over to the members. The twenty-five girls, aged five to twelve, donated the first 250 Pakistani rupees (roughly $1.25) for this school's new library. Of all the schools, it was the first student donation in the whole Library Challenge.

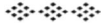

"Look! I Can Read This!"

Working in education-related fields, it is common to hear about poorly trained teachers and the resulting poor performance of their students. It is also a common complaint that students know only rote learning: memorizing without understanding. But the Library Challenge proved that wasn't entirely true. One of my fondest memories of this was at one of the most remote schools.

In my work as head of PERRP's social component, and as the founder of the Library Challenge, I frequently traveled from construction site to construction site to meet with social mobilizers, committees, and engineers, to discuss the progress of any community-related issues. I also visited the schools wherever they were operating, in their tent school or in their newly completed building.

In the earliest days, when the committees were only starting to establish their libraries, I often carried a box of brightly colored Urdu primary books that students had never seen before. This experience happened first in the third-grade class at Mohandri school in KP province, but it was repeated in many others. As I sat with the students on the floor, the books were distributed to each student, and we asked them to quickly look through them and tell us what they saw. All children eagerly did as asked, then one boy jumped to his feet and blurted out, "Look! I can read this!" He then proceeded excitedly and proudly to read aloud each page. Many other students followed with the same eagerness. Until then, the only books they'd seen in their lives were their textbooks, which they may very well have memorized. But being able to read new, unfamiliar material was a revelation to them. This was the first time they may have understood that reading was a skill that could be transferred to something outside the textbook. It was likely the first time many understood the actual reason for learning how to read.

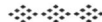

First Books Ever Owned

Sometimes we'd sit outside [of the bookfair] watching the masses of people eager to get inside or leave. One image sticks in my mind: a father and three children under about six years of age exited the large hall where the fair was held, each one carrying their own little plastic bag with a few books in it to take home. All were dressed in their old, worn-out, but finest clothes, and were clearly excited and proud. This would have been the first time any of them would have owned their own books, and somehow the poor father had found a few rupees to buy his children these gifts.

—PERRP social mobilizer

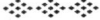

Roadside Chat about Books

The spring after all the books were delivered to the schools, I made a trip with the social team up the Kaghan Valley to visit several schools and talk with committee members, teachers, students, engineers, and local people about how everything was going. Had the new libraries got up and running? What did everybody have to say about the books? About reading? There were rave reviews, but I was concerned that much of that could have been people saying what they thought should be said.

On our way back down out of the valley on the narrow dirt road, which was barely wide enough for two cars to pass, we suddenly were stopped by the spring migration of *ghujars* (pastoralists) bringing their enormous flocks of sheep up the road and into the mountains to graze for the summer. We were stuck in sheep gridlock, when teenage boys in school uniforms began arriving on foot, struggling uphill and squeezing in with the slow-moving densely packed flock. The boys were on their daily trek home from the school, which was about three miles downhill.

As soon as the students recognized my car, which they'd seen a number of times at their school, a group of five boys fought their way through the mass of sheep to come and greet me at my car window. Taking this opportunity, with them being away from their teachers and so able speak frankly, I asked them about their library and books. What did they think of them? Always polite, they said all the right complimentary things—so, to test them further I asked, "Okay, which books have each of you looked at and like?"

A shouting match ensued over the sheep and the dust they were raising, as the boys proved they really did know what was in their libraries. "I like the books on astronomy." "Pakistan heroes and the ones about raising chickens!" "I've read all the novels already, the Urdu ones and the English ones." "I borrowed the one called *Where There is No Doctor* and took it home and read parts of it to my mother because she can't read." "I want more books on Islamic history. Can you get us more of those?" "I've read only the joke books, and now I'm writing down other jokes people tell me and I'll make a book of those too."

They all aced my test. Like all the other schools, these students had seen only textbooks before and had no idea other kinds of books existed, let alone ones they liked so much.

"But My Sons Won't Even Read Their Syllabus Books!"

When you first introduced the idea of the Library Challenge, I had my doubts as to whether anybody would get interested in reading. I told you that my teenage sons are lazy students and won't even read their syllabus books, so how could they ever get interested in library books? You told me, maybe they won't read because their textbooks are boring to them, and for the library, we have to find books that will interest them a lot.

Well, let me tell you this, now they pester me all the time to buy them books! They have read everything you put in the library on technical subjects which are not taught in the schools, like motorcycle and cell phone repair, welding, carpentry, growing trees, keeping bees, and even cooking—and now they want more of these books!

—Committee chairman

CHAPTER 8

The Social Anthropology of Reconstruction

Introduction

Considering and addressing the sociocultural side of construction by using anthropological and participatory approaches is—as the case of PERRP shows—a way to bring about two aims simultaneously: being responsible from a culturally appropriate, social justice–oriented, capacity-building, humanitarian perspective, and doing so while also increasing project efficiency and effectiveness. It is important to note that such approaches may be used by specialists who may or may not be anthropologists. There are many professionals, NGO staff, and staff at other organizations that have these kinds of skills and perspectives as practitioners, even though the work they do may not be labeled "anthropology." For this reason, I use the expressions "anthropologist," "sociocultural expert," and "specialist" interchangeably. At the same time, not all anthropologists would be suited to disaster reconstruction work.

This chapter takes a brief look at the background of anthropology and how it is now being applied far more widely than ever before, especially for its practical uses in addressing social problems. We look again at the disaster reconstruction site and its context, people, and power following a disaster, the impact of experience on perceptions of construction or reconstruction, and the effects that construction and local people can have on each other. This chapter closes with a look at the distinguishing features of social anthropology and how these were applied in PERRP, along with examples of problems this approach solved.

Reconstruction Sites Cannot Be Divorced from Their Surroundings

A reconstruction site cannot be divorced from its social context. In construction and reconstruction projects, managers often focus inward, looking only at the site itself—the contractors, labor, equipment, steel, and concrete. While this focus is necessary to produce high-quality work on schedule, it risks losing sight of other factors that will determine that success. Construction projects often assumed to be—even try to be—separate from the surrounding social environment, but such a disconnect is unlikely or impossible, and it can even be self-defeating. A construction site cannot be divorced from its surroundings. The social context of a construction project will, to varying degrees, have an impact on the construction, just as construction impacts the surrounding social context. And what may manifest as a problem for construction may have underlying sociocultural causes that need specialized attention to prevent or resolve.

In other words, construction is not just about bricks and mortar. As much as architects, engineers, and construction managers need to know in minute detail the composition and characteristics of concrete, steel, soil, and footing—and other factors that determine the new building's structural integrity—so too should the social specialists on a project get to know details of the cultural and social situation. From this knowledge, social specialists can predict local behavior that might affect construction and plan for it, helping to facilitate design and construction and so enable the project to proceed effectively. The activities of social specialists also free the project's technical experts to concentrate on what they need to do to manage construction, to reduce losses for both the project and the people, and to produce more positive long-term benefits for the building, its users, and the community.

People and Change in the Postdisaster Scenario

The challenges that existed before a disaster may be greatly magnified after it. Sometimes, new challenges arise that did not exist before. For reconstruction management efforts, there may be competition for and shortages of essential goods and service providers, including contractors, workers, spaces, equipment, and materials. There may also be changing policies, regulations, and standards that are not always well communicated, and lack of coordination and competition among aid agencies.

At the community level, the sudden arrival of projects and agencies—while necessary to save lives and be a bridge to the recovery process—can create competition or new rivalries. These sudden injections of relief goods, money, jobs, and people of other cultures have the potential to increase disputes and conflicts that already exist. A hand-out style of help can create disincentives: people sometimes begin to rely on the helping agencies to do what they used to do themselves. It is a delicate time, with the losses, trauma, change, movement of people, and fractured social supports. With such complexities, reconstruction projects benefit from sociocultural experts who know the local culture in its predisaster state, and so are best equipped to assess changes that have occurred and to draw people into the process of problem-solving while also building their capacities.

Perceptions of Construction and Reconstruction

While "construction" literally means the action or process of constructing roads, bridges, dams, shelter, housing, buildings, and other physical infrastructure, it will still have different connotations for different groups of people. To a donor or institution financing disaster reconstruction, their involvement could mean simply carrying out policy, budget, or financing arrangements. To a construction planner or manager, "reconstruction" may mean an exciting challenge to oversee and create a structure that will be of benefit to many for a long period of time. For-profit commercial organizations such as architectural, engineering, and construction firms—those most likely to be involved in infrastructure reconstruction—will see it as a business opportunity. To others, especially those who inhabit nearby areas, their view may be very different and not uniform. People's opinions will be affected by the reputation of construction before the disaster, by what they observe about other reconstruction sites, and by what they have heard—or have not heard—about the planned construction.

Part of an anthropological approach would be to find out these views from the people and, as needed, plan the preventative measures that the project would need to take. The kinds of questions to be addressed would include: Before and since the disaster, what is the people's experience with other construction and with construction contractors? Were they treated fairly? Has any harm occurred? Have they experienced or witnessed loss, damage, or destruction of property or other assets by construction contractors? Were they paid compensation if any was due? Do they suspect wrongdoing, cheating, corruption, wastage, or broken promises? Has previous construction caused problems among the local people? Does that experience make them anticipate it will happen again? Have they been consulted on the current reconstruction planned? Will they be involved? The answers to these questions will reveal the local people's impressions, which in turn will have a strong effect on how they interact with future construction or reconstruction.

Around the world there are countless examples of construction projects that have failed because they ignored the needs and ideas of local people. In chapter 3, in the anecdote about a flood control embankment construction project in Bangladesh, I described how the people violently opposed a construction project, but by managers and engineers listening to their concerns and finding feasible technical and administrative options, the project went ahead and, in the end, satisfied all stakeholders. As that project was being prepared, not only had the people not been consulted about the alignment of the planned embankment but the alignment chosen would have destroyed precious crop land; from past experience, the people were certain they would be cheated out of compensation and be forced off their land. By hearing their concerns, the project was able to proceed peacefully with the alignment changed; the government paid the compensation owed, and the new ownership documents were completed before construction started, with no resettlement needed. Using anthropological approaches that were culturally appropriate, conflict sensitive, and participatory resulted in another engineering and construction project that was able to get a technically sound embankment.

As table 8.1 shows, construction and local people can have positive or negative impacts on one another; their interactions can affect both the people and the implementing or contracting agencies.

Anthropology and Reconstruction: Foundations of Anthropology

So where does anthropology come into this picture? Cultural anthropology emerged first as a field of academic study in the UK in the late nineteenth century as the British Empire grew. The most prominent figures of this period included Edward B. Tylor and Lewis Henry Morgan. As the field grew in the twentieth century, a long list of other eminent scholars emerged in the US, UK, and Europe, including Bronislaw Malinowski, Radcliffe Brown, Claude Lévi-Strauss, James George Frazer, Raymond Firth, Edward Evans-Pritchard, Franz Boas, Alfred Kroeber, Ruth Benedict, and Margaret Mead. Subspecialties also emerged such as archaeology and linguistic, physical, biological (also called forensic), and social or applied anthropology.

While anthropology in its infancy had focused exclusively on culture, social anthropology grew to focus more on social structures and the relationships of groups. The fields of anthropology and sociology now share a fluid boundary. There is no universally agreed definition, but at its most basic, anthropology is the study of humanity, and social anthropology is the study of society, social structures, or groups of any kind. It could also be said that all anthropology can be applied. Anthropological approaches share common research methods—interviews, discussions, and surveys, for instance—but applying these approaches depends on the situation

Table 8.1. Negative or Positive Effects for Construction and the Local People.

	Negatively	Positively
How local people can affect construction:	• New differences among people may be created or existing differences exacerbated. • If not suitably treated or not participating in any way, the local people may be indifferent or even in opposition to the project. • They may file court stay orders or undertake other actions to stop construction.	• If effectively engaged to participate, local people can help to make things happen, donating their time, experience, resources, and influence. • They can prevent problems and serve as the main problem solvers of community concerns related to construction.
How construction can affect local people:	• Construction can damage property or other assets, and can overuse local resources. • Project leaders can overpromise and underdeliver, misleading people, creating mistrust or conflict. • The work may exemplify bad management, lacking transparency or accountability. • The local community may perceive the construction as a loss or something to resist.	• The construction can provide a new facility that will bring new benefits. • If the people participate effectively, they will increase skills and build their own institutions. • The work can exemplify promises kept, trustworthiness, transparency, and accountability. • The local community may perceive the construction as a gain and something to support. But for this to be the case, the local people must be treated fairly.
How results can affect the contracting or implementing agency and others:	• If a project fails, has long costly delays, or is abandoned for any reason—including opposition of the people—the reputation of the contractor or implementing agency may be damaged, affecting future contracts and their bottom line.	• If a favorable, respectful, and cooperative atmosphere is created, not only does it get better results for all on the ground, but it also adds to the positive reputation of the company involved and, possibly, to their future work.

and involves a range of other possible skills including action research, advocacy, and community mobilization and participation.

There are two main distinguishing features of anthropology: it is holistic and it involves extensive fieldwork as a participant observer, living and working among the people. Through this close contact, anthropologists may develop deep knowledge of situations, especially from the perspectives of the people being studied and/or assisted. In projects such as disaster reconstruction, social anthropology involves not just conducting research but also simultaneously putting that knowledge into practice and doing so in a scheduled amount of time.

Anthropology as Problem-Solving

To some, anthropology has an antiquated, esoteric ring to it. Anthropology has the reputation of being limited to academia, yet change has been occurring in recent decades, and anthropology is now being applied in practical ways across a vast array of subjects in dynamic, diverse situations around the world. Now it can be said that, wherever there are people, there is a case for anthropology, and whatever people do, there could be an anthropology of it.

Anthropology may be best described in the websites of universities promoting such studies, as well as in publications and by professional associations. The University of Manchester Department of Anthropology explains that social anthropologists "are concerned with such questions as: how societies are organized; the relationship between values and behavior; [and] why people do what they do" ("What is Social Anthropology," n.d.). The American Anthropological Association, the world's largest association of professional anthropologists, describes anthropology as working "to solve real world problems using anthropological methods and ideas" ("What is Anthropology," n.d.). In its website heading, the American Anthropological Association uses the slogan, "Advancing Knowledge, Solving Human Problems." The National Association for the Practice of Anthropology (NAPA), a US professional association, explains that anthropologists have three skills that make them "great cross-functional team players": the ability to "engage the underrepresented," to "observe and listen," and to "facilitate and translate" (NAPA, n.d.).

NAPA also lists a range of specializations among members, indicating the types of subjects and problems they tackle: business anthropology, medical anthropology, the anthropology of the workplace, public health, marketing, the arts, information technology systems, housing, social justice, mass media and communications, agriculture, computer science, military, artificial intelligence, international development, the design of facilities for e-sports, and so on. A glance through professional journals, conference topics, and new books adds to the range of subjects in which anthropology is being applied: disasters, aid, law, precious minerals, human rights, peace and conflict, the environment and climate change, gender and reproduction, health disparities in jails, and patient experience in the design of new hospitals. Additionally, the subjects are often location specific, such as refugee resettlement in Italy, artificial intelligence and virtual reality in China, the spread of malaria in central Africa, transboundary water issues in the Himalayas, microcredit in Bolivia, and Wall Street behavior. Also emerging is activist or advocacy anthropology "in the service of marginalized groups" (Schuller et al 2020: 6).

Because social anthropology helps identify, analyze, prevent, and solve real-world problems involving people, it can be applied to any subject—including construction and disaster reconstruction, as shown in this book.

Realities for the Sociocultural Expert in Reconstruction

With anthropology being applied to so many different subjects, it seems important to delineate the particular set of skills, attributes, or knowledge needed to do specific kinds of sociocultural work effectively—for example, to be a medical anthropologist in North America or to work on transboundary water issues in high mountains or in refugee resettlement in Europe. Certainly, not all sociocultural experts would be interested in or suited to all these roles. The same is true of the anthropology of disaster reconstruction.

While being well versed in the methods of anthropology discussed above, a sociocultural expert in a reconstruction project also needs to work within these realities:

- If it is a well-managed project, all design and construction work will be on a tight timeframe, around which the social program will need to be designed and carried out to help synchronize the technical and social steps.
- As infrastructure reconstruction is normally carried out by for-profit firms, this context will have considerations new to some anthropologists and other social experts.
- As construction can take years, projects need to include plans for how the sociocultural expertise can be kept in the field at or near the sites for the duration of the project.
- Construction engineers, planners, and managers can be thought of as from one culture, and sociocultural experts as from another. Besides bridging project understanding with the communities, it may be up to the sociocultural expert to initiate bridging the cross-cultural gaps between disciplines.
- While the sociocultural expert undertakes the work with communities and the technical expert launches all actions for design and construction, the two need to set up strong communications with one another to meet both the technical and sociocultural needs and goals.

Other essential skills include community analysis, participation, conflict prevention and resolution, and team leadership and management skills.

Social Anthropological Approaches as Applied in PERRP

In PERRP, our holistic approach involved first taking the widest possible view of the project's contexts, as described in chapter 2. At the construction site, this meant keeping the most immediate stakeholders in view: the design and construction teams. We strove to determine what they needed that the social team could provide from the community. This also required figuring out the community social structure, its blocs of power, and the steps required to have power shifted and shared so that the local people could work effectively with construction.

The fieldwork or participant observer component was built into the project. In academic terms, being a participant observer means living and working in a society, organization, institution, group, or community for extended periods of time, frequently counted in months. In PERRP's case, we worked six years full-time as participant observers.

Social anthropology now tends to be more participatory. In the past, it was typical for an outsider to go and study a group in top-down, extractive ways—collecting data, taking it away to be analyzed for assessment studies or academic papers, and never returning. While that approach unfortunately still happens, many contemporary anthropological approaches are collaborative, working with the people using participatory methods to jointly analyze data, identify needs, develop strategies, and monitor work—a kind of participatory anthropology. In disaster situations, in which speedy action is required, research methods such as rapid assessments and action research can be used, with the participant observation occurring simultaneously during these processes.

Advocacy is another important role for social expertise. While encouraging the community people themselves to speak up, using their own voices to get what they want, PERRP's social team members often played people's advocate with officials, architects, and construction managers, urging them to listen to the people.

Examples of Real-World Problems Solved

Almost all of the seventy-seven construction sites in this project had several problems involving local people. Some of the problems were caused by the construction teams, and some by a few local people. However, even the most complex situations were handled using culturally sensitive anthropological approaches with additional skills such as community mobilization, mediation, and conflict resolution. Being able to handle such challenges was—along with strong construction management—one of the reasons almost all of PERRP's construction was completed on or ahead of schedule. Examples of incidents and problems are given throughout this book, and below. In each case, the problem was solved by the social team, which had first concentrated its efforts in each community, working to understand the culture, the power arrangements, and the approaches necessary to facilitate formal agreements, allowing construction to proceed.

- In one remote conservative community, a serious cultural breach occurred involving one of the construction contractor's laborers. He was caught and severely beaten by villagers, but the incident so offended members of the local community—and generated so much fear about repetition of this behavior by the other laborers—that they demanded that the contractor be fired. They would have preferred to have no school built rather than suffer such humiliation again. A solution was agreed to when the contractor offered to replace all the laborers on the site, exchanging them with workers from another construction job, who would have their training in the code of conduct repeated.
- One girls' high school had already been deemed infeasible for this project to build, as engineers doing the assessment observed that the site for the school was not accessible from the road, being located in a precarious position on a terrace below the mountain road. Additionally, the surrounding six small plots of land had a total of about eighteen co-owners, all from the same extended family, who had a long history of conflict. Constructing the school depended on getting the access needed, and getting that access depended on people with serious differences coming to an agreement. While at first these landowners refused to cooperate with one another, peacemakers within the community, with the social team facilitating, convinced the landowners to resolve the matter. Had the agreement not been reached, the school could not have been built; with the land issues solved, work began immediately.
- At the critical time when volumes of concrete were about to start being mixed and poured, the water supply suddenly stopped. As the construction engineers urgently traced the cause, they found that someone had deliberately cut the water pipe bringing the water from the supply source. It was an act of revenge over an unrelated matter against the man who owned the land with the water pipe. The project's social process quickly and amicably solved the problem, allowing the concrete pouring to continue without hindrance.

- Located below is an ethnography that indicates how highly complex social problems can become manifest at a construction site. In this situation, there was a seven-way dispute involving two families, a renegade member of one of the families, a low-caste group, two government departments opposing each other's decisions, and an unscrupulous contractor who was attempting to have his own work stopped by court order. The final dispute was over the placement of a gate and walking path, a situation that again threatened to stop the nearly completed construction.

Ethnography—Government Boys' High School in Flat Land*

"Flat Land" is a pseudonym. To maintain confidentiality, the name of the school, village, and castes are changed.

This example illustrates how the problems that arise in construction or reconstruction can have underlying social causes that need to be sensitively addressed. The disputes in this location were power struggles between castes, classes, vested interests, and political connections, in the midst of rapid cultural change. This example shows the complexity of social structures in communities and how complicated it can be to prevent or solve community-related problems that could affect construction.

At one large school being constructed in PERRP, there were three particular incidents, each one threatening to interfere with construction and to cause strife in the community. At one point the struggle was a seven-way dispute involving the following participants:

- two landowning families in a long-term conflict (family #1 and family #2)
- a lower-caste group (the Blue caste or Blues), who had been the tenant farmers of family #2, but who over the past twenty years had been working their way out of servitude, which was resisted by family #2
- a renegade member of family #1—a son who had a reputation for being temperamental, litigious, prone to violence, and radically individualist, often rejecting the normal local behavior of respecting the decisions of elders
- two government departments opposing each other's decisions
- an unscrupulous contractor attempting to have his own work stopped.

The families and the Blues owned the property touching on the school's east and north sides.

Soccer Field Incident

One son in family #1 had been part of most of the community participation process to prepare for construction. He had been present in meetings to learn the construction plan and give design input, and he knew all about the project's conflict resolution agreement procedures and the significance of the Committee-Contractor Agreement. Soon after construction of the school started, however, he suddenly decided to ignore these agreements and raised a subject unheard of up to that point.

This school had an unusually large plot of land that included a soccer field. The son did not believe that the soccer field's size would be maintained after reconstruction, despite reassurances from the PERRP construction managers, who showed him detailed site plans. All the region's soccer teams depended on this playing field. It was the only regulation-size soccer field in the district, and he was certain that the new school was so large it would take up some of the field, making it no longer suitable for the regular tournaments that had been held here for years.

The school committee held meetings with family #1 and this son to try to convince him to believe the construction managers. Still, he became increasingly agitated and started making threats against the project and construction. Despite attempts by the committee and his own elders to get him to stop protesting, he ignored them and applied to the court to stop construction. If a court stay order were issued, it would stop construction and lead to many other problems in the community, including conflict over the stoppage. In the meantime, the threat of violence persisted.

As elders, construction managers, committee members, social mobilizers, and this man met on the school ground to try to discuss the matter, the man's equally agitated brother showed up and began swinging an axe at the people. Fortunately, a local policeman who happened to be nearby and in uniform diverted the brother with the axe, allowing discussion to continue on the site.

The social mobilizers realized that the problem was that the man had not understood the technical drawing of the school and site plans. They got the project engineers and surveyors to lay out on the ground the actual location, size, and orientation of the planned soccer field. When they installed pegs joined by rope all around the perimeters of the field and the planned school, at last the man and his friends were convinced. The court application was withdrawn, with no negative effect on construction.

Block the Windows

A couple of months later the same man raised another issue, making it into a crisis and again—without the committee or his elders knowing about it—he applied to court to stop construction. The matter he was concerned about was that the upstairs windows of this boys' school would look directly into the neighboring compound where he lived. He said this was an interference in his privacy and he would not tolerate it.

His repeated aggressive behavior was an embarrassment to his elders and the surrounding community, as they by then were familiar with the project's process and dialogue-based conflict resolution procedures. They knew that PERRP took measures at other schools to install glass block visual barriers in upstairs windows so that there was no view into private property. Yet even after being taken to a nearby PERRP school so he could see the visual barrier for himself, the man would not relent. The case made it to the first court hearing, but the judge dismissed his request for a stay order as unfounded when committee members attended the hearing, showing photos and evidence of the visual barriers, which were already planned for their school, at the other PERRP-built school.

Access Path Dispute and Rapid Cultural Change
The most complicated issue to solve was over a walking path that neighbors would use to go around or through the school ground. On the surface, this dispute was about the path, but underlying that was the long historical struggle between family #2 and the Blues, neither of which was willing to yield to the other. The situation was further complicated by an unscrupulous contractor. Once again, this dispute could have grown and resulted in stopping the by then almost completed construction, but it was resolved by the social team working in partnership with the engineers, committee members, elders, the Department of Education, and the district coordination officer.

As stated elsewhere, in construction and any development work where there is community participation, it is necessary to understand the community. This is challenging enough where the community is static, but even more difficult and crucial when change is occurring, as was the case in this location.

Rapid cultural change was occurring in this rural conservative community. The formerly highly oppressed people of the Blue caste were working their way out of subjugation to the current generation of wealthy landowning families, including family #2. The Blues now openly and defiantly opposed family #2. While the rise of the Blues began roughly two decades earlier, it was rapidly accelerated by the earthquake: locals said that the status quo changed in only three seconds. See two anecdotes "Low Caste . . . ," page 71.

This change began with a few Blues breaking free of their bonds, becoming entrepreneurs and helping other Blues do the same. They were increasing their level of education and moving away from traditional ways of life. Due to their own initiatives, in many but not all locations in the region, the Blues were out from under the thumb of their former landlords. A few had even become well-off. Not surprisingly, this in itself created mutual hostility.

Such cultural change, where a low caste moves up relatively quickly to rival the higher caste, is rare. The Blues were said to have recently and rapidly escalated their own status by pooling the relief money they had received from the government to rebuild earthquake-destroyed homes, using their collective resources to buy property and start businesses. Their ability to turn relief money into development money deserves more in-depth study. The earthquake only lasted three seconds, but for this one oppressed group, it might have brought their freedom. A sure sign of moving up in status is that people in the region had elected a Blue person in the last five elections.

If the argument over the access path had happened a few decades ago, the story would be very different. Now, however, the Blues would boldly stand up for what they wanted.

In the 1980s, the school ground had been enlarged to include the regulation-size soccer pitch, as discussed above. Until that time, the Blues had walked through the unfenced school ground to get to the main road. But when the sports field was put in, a solid boundary wall was added, blocking their route to the road. At that time, there was a dispute over the wall, because over half a century earlier, when the school was first built by the British, there had been a formal agreement with the government allowing free passage across school land. As the Blues had no power when the new field and wall were built, they gave in. Their access route was moved to a rough track on the outside of the wall, between it and a nearby stream.

In the intervening years, when a member of family #2 found that the school wall deflected some of the stream water onto his property, he belligerently installed a stone masonry wall on his side to deflect the water back toward the school wall. Then, in heavy flooding the year before school construction started, his deflection wall resulted in the foot track being washed away and the boundary wall being damaged. Now there was no path at all, and the only road access required walking through the water—a dangerous and inconvenient route.

The dispute arose again when the construction contractor was about to start installing a chain-link fence on the perimeter of the school ground, on the side of the field facing land owned by the Blues and by family #2. The Blues appealed to the construction contractor to not install the fence and instead leave the ground open so that they could have a safe walking route again.

Here, the unscrupulous contractor saw the chance to buy time. He had work elsewhere and wanted an excuse to slow down or stop work here, so he suggested to the Blues that they get a court stay order about the fence.

That way, he could get out of this construction for a while and they maybe could get the fence stopped. With his encouragement, the Blues proceeded through official channels to build their case, going to the Revenue Department to get the historical records and, through their political connections, they sought to influence the district coordination officer to stop the plan to put in a chain-link fence.

Once these old legal documents were found, the district coordination officer ordered his Revenue Department to demarcate the path that had, and still would, pass through the middle of the school's sports ground. To reinforce this idea, the Blues went ahead and also filed an application with the court for a stay order to stop construction and give them back an access route. They named as defendants the Department of Education, the head master, and the secretly colluding contractor.

The social mobilizers had already held several urgent meetings to resolve this issue. Construction of the school building was almost finished and a stay order would stop it from being completed. On getting news of the court application, the mobilizers immediately asked for a meeting that would include the contractor, PERRP engineers, and representatives from the Department of Education, the Blues, and both landholding families.

In this meeting, the Department of Education representatives rejected the district coordination officer's order. They argued that, since another flood might further damage the boundary wall, the boundary line and damaged section should be moved inward twenty feet in one corner, again allowing a path to go around the outside of the wall. They suggested that a retaining wall should be put between the path and stream. Into the fray again stepped the same adult son of family #1, so protective of the soccer field, who hotly contested both ideas: he refused to allow anyone to use "his" field as a pathway, and he opposed moving the wall inward.

After much discussion it was a relief that agreement was finally reached. All parties agreed that, along one end of the school ground, facing land owned by both the Blues and family #2, the chain-link fence would be installed with a small gap so people could walk through across the field. The parties involved wrote a resolution, and everyone signing it, attesting that they had reached agreement. Family #1 assured all stakeholders that their son would not continue his legal actions. The signed agreement was to be taken to the court to withdraw the case—or at least that was the idea.

Outside the courtroom the day the case was to be heard, social mobilizers watched as the calculating contractor still urged the Blues to persist in the case. If the Blues persisted and won, it could have bought the contractor a great deal of time. At first the Blues' representative resisted the contractor's pressure, but then he saw the opportunity and made a counterdemand: he would go into the courtroom and continue to press for a stay order—

despite the signed agreement—if the contractor agreed to build the Blues a new road, one that was unrelated to the school construction. When the contractor balked at committing to this new construction, the representative stalled. The social mobilizers wondered: Would he proceed into court to withdraw the case? Was the case to stop construction going to be dropped or not?

In the last few moments before being called to appear before the judge, another influential community member stepped in and informed the Blues' representative that, if he did not drop the case as had been agreed, then he would seek punishment from the Blues' own politician, who was the man's personal friend. Finally, the representative had the case withdrawn.

With all this facilitation, in the end everybody—except the contractor—got what they wanted: construction continued and was completed without a single day lost; the soccer playing field was still regulation size; the Blues got free access across the field; and family #2 was happy to have the wall moved away from their land.

Each of the construction sites in PERRP had difficulties to overcome and achievements to celebrate. If I had written up all seventy-seven sites in this much detail, they would not be dissimilar—they would simply involve different blocs of power and different issues. While reconstruction projects by other implementing agencies were halted over issues as complex as the one described above—being dragged through the courts and sometimes never resolved—with the anthropological approaches and community participation in PERRP, each incident was solved peacefully with no loss to local people or to construction time.

Conclusion

This final chapter first draws some conclusions about the state of disasters in general, their predicted growth, and the needs for the future. It raises some of the challenges faced and discusses who has roles to play in confronting them, but the emphasis is on the importance and benefits of bringing affected communities into infrastructure reconstruction as part of the planning and implementation process. I then present conclusions from the PERRP project. I focus on how a structured community participation process benefitted both this infrastructure reconstruction project and the local communities, listing several significant and practical benefits. This chapter closes with three batches of recommendations—first, for donor agencies, policy makers, implementing agencies, and aid and reconstruction planners; second, more specific recommendations for implementing agencies on integrating the social and technical elements of the work; and finally, specific recommendations for social teams.

General Conclusions

Around the world, disasters are growing (and are predicted to keep growing) in number and intensity, suggesting that there will also be an increase in the need for reconstruction and related agencies, skills, and services.

Construction is about more than steel and cement, and this is especially true in disaster reconstruction scenarios. Not only have buildings and other infrastructure been destroyed—possibly taking many lives, creating loss and trauma—but the community and sociocultural foundations may also have been shaken. The reconstruction planning process should therefore be part of broader recovery efforts—in addition to replacing lost infrastructure, NGOs and aid agencies should also help local institutions recover and support local capacity development.

In many locations, even without a disaster, challenges in infrastructure construction result in projects being slow, stalled, or even abandoned.

The burgeoning literature on infrastructure construction worldwide features wide-ranging discussions on the problems and challenges to construction, and there is general agreement that in developing countries the construction industry is plagued with certain common issues (Mir, Tanvir, and Durrani 2007: 1). The issues could be categorized as managerial, technical, financial, policy related, procedural, environmental, or legal. They may become manifest at the construction site in innumerable ways: a lack of skilled contractors, defective contract documents, corrupt contracting procedures, poor foreign exchange procedures, and so on. Still, in the literature, there is little mention of the local people and the issues they may be facing, or the ways in which construction and the people may have an impact on each other. Few studies focus on how some of the most serious problems in construction emerge from interactions between construction sites and the local people. Moreover, even in the disaster studies literature, the sociocultural side of infrastructure reconstruction is barely mentioned. There is a need for much further research on the kinds of realities, problems, and needs that arise from interactions between construction sites and their sociocultural contexts.

At the same time, the subject of local people and their communities—wherever they may be in the world—is highly complex. As chapter 3 discusses, communities are composed of subgroups that are often divided by such factors as ethnicity, clans, beliefs, race, or political alliances, resulting in some people holding power, leaving others with little or none. For community participation to occur on a representative basis, it is necessary to know who are the dominant and who are the dominated. Sociocultural specialists must ask: What is the local social structure? How can power be shifted and shared so that participation is representative of the community?

Communities are far from being quaint, harmonious, and unified places—a common misconception. Rather, conflict is common in communities around the world. It may be subtle, overt, or predominant. Conflicts in communities often stem from multiple causes arising out of the above community divisions; for construction, some of the problems may come from these underlying social causes. Moreover, projects such as construction can easily spark conflict due to the money, jobs, and other opportunities they bring. Something as seemingly simple as the arrival of a construction contractor can ignite reaction, as such events frequently occur without local consultation, and so local people can react against them. Contractors often impose or act in other ways that are not accepted, resulting in violence, court stay orders, or other actions that lead to long, costly delays. In the reconstruction process in Pakistan such tension was one of the main causes of slow or halted construction.

Who is part of this scene, and who may have roles to play? Families, NGOs, and governments will likely continue to work on rebuilding housing and other small-scale facilities. However, reconstruction of large public infrastructure is the realm of large commercial design and construction companies, and of NGOs with similar advanced capabilities, due to their expertise. As disasters increase, demand for their services and those of related for-profit or nonprofit consulting and facilitation services will also likely grow. Governments, donor agencies, policy makers, and aid planners need to lead the way in involving sociocultural specialists in infrastructure projects. Such specialists include practitioners, researchers, academics, and consultants, as well as students across the full gamut of sociocultural and technical fields: disaster, development, and conflict resolution studies, and architects, engineers, and construction managers.

Structured, representative, guided community participation can make a significant difference in disaster reconstruction projects, as it can help improve project efficiency and effectiveness while significantly enhancing local capacities for recovery and development. For this to occur, such disaster reconstruction projects need to include a social program and adapt it for each situation, drawing on examples such as PERRP.

Conclusions from PERRP

A year after the earthquake, when the PERRP team arrived in Pakistan to start work, reconstruction in the country was already in trouble. Hundreds of implementing agencies were working in different sectors of disaster relief, and over fifty agencies were present to carry out hundreds of projects to reconstruct thousands of buildings. Yet, among these many agencies, there were common complaints that many of their sites were already stalled, unable to proceed. This pace of reconstruction and completion never significantly improved. Even by the twelfth anniversary of the quake, the media reported that only a fraction of the planned reconstruction had been completed: thousands of schools had not been rebuilt, and "concrete skeletons of unfinished schools litter[ed]" the earthquake zone (Naviwala 2017).

Early on, the implementing agencies identified two main categories of problems: inept local contractors and conflict. Some of the hurdles included cost overruns, high worker turnover, and contractors' attempts to manipulate projects, to change designs, or to use different materials than had been agreed upon. Yet most problems were of a social nature: often people in the local communities were already fighting over other problems, but then got into conflict with the contractors, resulting in violence, sabotage, blocked access to the construction sites, and court stay orders. These social problems caused long costly delays in construction and, sometimes, even abandonment. When the people's ideas and issues are unknown or ignored, construction projects are at risk; when these factors are carefully considered, however, the opposite result can occur. As shown in PERRP, it is possible for a construction project to prevent or mitigate many social problems by involving the local people. Community participation in reconstruction can thus benefit both the construction project and the people and their recovery.

Of all the agencies working in reconstruction in postquake Pakistan, PERRP was the only project that had a dedicated social team with a structured community participation program that focused exclusively on reconstruction. Other projects left this work—including problems between contractors and community members—either to technical personnel who lacked time and relevant skills or to government departments, which often did not respond effectively. Some of the agencies had teams of social mobilizers, but these teams were busy with work in other sectors—in water and sanitation, health, livelihoods, and so on. When problems inevitably arose, solutions were attempted on an ad hoc basis, which often did not work.

Benefits of Community Participation to the Project and to Local People

As demonstrated in PERRP, strong construction management and structured community participation can save a great deal of time and prevent many problems while also significantly adding to local capacities.

- As a result of PERRP approaches, no court stay orders were issued, only eight out of the project's fifty thousand construction days were lost to conflict, and all but two of the seventy-seven schools and health units constructed were completed on or ahead of schedule.
- PERRP led communities to form representative committees with three main purposes: to prevent or solve community problems related to construction, to help the schools improve education, and to maintain the new buildings—this last purpose being held in shared responsibility with the government.
- While much reconstruction stalled over land issues, PERRP's first assignment to each committee was to have the land issues settled before construction could proceed. This was achieved in only one day at each site, well before design or construction even started. This first step saved enormous amounts of time throughout the project,

and it also resolved land disputes that had festered for years, giving relief to those affected.
- Various tools developed within the social team, which are listed in the recommendations below, increased cooperation and reduced the flare-ups of conflict that were common in the other reconstruction efforts.
- On a day-to-day basis, with close coordination and agreements between the technical and social components, the committees were able to anticipate the needs of the contractors and have help ready—for example, to lend extra land or provide a water supply.
- Although being from poor communities, committees contributed thousands of volunteer hours and mobilized resources with significant cash value.
- Community input to design helped improve the functioning and cultural suitability of the buildings, and saved costly design mistakes.
- The cost to include a social team was a small fraction of the project budget—the PERRP social team constituted only 6 percent of the project personnel—while the costs saved by the social team, although not calculated, would have been enormous.
- Through creating a friendly, respectful partnership, there was goodwill among the local people, contractors, project staff, clients, and local government officials. It was a win-win situation.
- For local people, such participation was a new experience. One of the most common comments by community members to social mobilizers was: "Before this project, nobody had ever asked us to participate to do anything. When you first started talking to us about having our community participate, we did not know what you meant, but now we understand and like it a lot. We wish others would ask us too!"

As detailed in chapter 3, communities in this region and project were notable for their stratified layers of power. Each community and subcommunity was hierarchical and heterogenous, with divisions into social groups based on caste, kinship, ethnicity, tribal group, sect, political affiliations, and a host of other factors. Tensions and conflict were common, fanned by the region's history of war and continuing frictions. Even before the disaster, the earthquake zone was among the poorest areas in Pakistan.

Even so, members of those communities also had strong capacities on which PERRP capitalized: a strong desire for recovery and development, a willingness to organize and work with the project, influential people and customs for conflict resolution, and skills from other experiences that they could bring to reconstruction. The PERRP social team deliberately looked for these strengths and capacities; even in the most divided or conflictual situations, there may be people or customs that can support reconstruction work—a fact too often overlooked. The idea is to identify the local strengths and then ensure that they are recognized and put to work in the project process.

PERRP was a rare if not unprecedented opportunity for local communities to choose representatives from different social groups to form committees to work with the project. The committees were then led through a structured, step-by-step process supporting the technical work before, during, and after construction. Capacities were built in areas such as planning, communications, participatory decision-making, resource mobilization, group formation and management, conflict prevention and resolution, data collection and monitoring, and earthquake-resistant construction.

As committees developed their skills and succeeded in their project duties, their profiles and respect in their communities rose, drawing in more willingness to participate and contribute. Each step in the process increased committee members' confidence and prominence, and committees took initiative to contribute—clear signs of renewed vision and empowerment. This community participation demonstrated how people and communities—even those with deep divisions—can work together to achieve a common goal.

In addition to ending with a beautiful new building in the shortest possible time, which would benefit generations to come, each community's exposure to this new experience had the potential for long-lasting impact. For roughly three to four years in each community—the duration of the construction—local people had an experience that would raise their expectations about how other projects should be managed and how they could participate in them. Although the committees ceased to function once the project was completed, members could carry all these new skills and experiences to other endeavors.

Lessons Learned and Recommendations from PERRP

For Donors, Reconstruction Planners, and Implementing Agencies

- A social component should be included in every disaster reconstruction project, but for participation to happen at the "bottom" in a such a project, its initiation may need to come from the "top." In PERRP, community participation was a prerequisite required by the donor, USAID; and the implementing agency, CDM Smith, put it into practice from top management downward.

- Given that disaster reconstruction takes place within wide sociocultural contexts that have strong implications for the project, a social component with sociocultural experts should routinely be included alongside the technical team—the architects, designers, and engineering, environmental, and other technical specialists—and the project's other professionals in human resources, finance, information management, and so on.
- Get past the rhetoric. For decades already, no matter the sector, donor agencies have expected or required levels of local participation, but it is often vaguely stated and applied in name only, with little accountability. As part of a project bidding process or proposal preparation, potential implementing agencies should present specific plans that detail how they intend to include a community participation program: its purposes, activities, and key progress indicators, as well as information on how it will be carried out and monitored. As part of the regular reporting on the project as a whole, donors should require reporting on the sociocultural team's progress. Along with compliance expected for such matters as building standards, accessibility for the disabled, environmental concerns, anti-corruption practices, financial accounting, and health and safety regulations, there needs to be at least a basic framework—including guidelines, standards, and compliance requirements—for participation by the stakeholders.
- To emphasize that local participation is an integral part of the project, make the head of the social program a member of the senior management team. Like other members of this team, the head of the social program should be responsible for both high-level decision-making and their team's work in the field. Have the senior management team speak with a unified, consistent voice in all matters, including community participation.
- Plan for follow-through and sustainability, physically and institutionally. If the donor expects long-term operation and maintenance of the newly built facilities, they should make agreements and plans for this at the earliest stages with owners or authorities. It may be unrealistic for the end users—for instance, the teachers, parents, and students of a government-owned school—to take much or any responsibility for their facility if the owner is not engaged to play a part. Create incentives for ongoing institutional support.
- Design and construction companies that can demonstrate practical know-how—not only to "build back better," but also to "empower local authorities and communities" (UNDRR, n.d.a)—will be reflecting the some of the most valued skills among international disas-

ter authorities, donors, planners, and policy makers, which will give them a competitive edge.

For Social-Technical Integration

As part of the windup of the PERRP project, some debriefing and evaluation exercises were held internally. One of those exercises, described in chapter 6, was a focus group consisting of selected project engineers and construction managers, who provided their observations and comparisons of construction management inside and outside of PERRP. A second focus group met to analyze PERRP; this focus group, comprising the same eleven engineers and twelve members of the social team, had a combined total of over five hundred years of experience in construction and community mobilization in Pakistan and the region. The key topic discussed in those sessions was, if another disaster occurred somewhere, and you were asked for advice on construction/community matters, what would you recommend?

For the project engineers and construction managers in PERRP, it was a new experience to have a social component and structured community participation, but having the component was unanimously recommended as it made their work easier and got better results. These two focus groups also provided recommendations specific to the integration of technical and sociocultural teams.

- Accept that some of the challenges on a construction or reconstruction site come from negative interactions between the construction team and the people who live in the vicinity. Local complaints should be heard and considered valid, and they should receive a fair, quick response. When such occurrences are ignored, they can cause untold loss to the local people and can delay construction.
- Do not expect a reconstruction project's technical or management staff to be able to solve problems with local people. Having a social team frees up the engineers and other technical personnel to concentrate on their own specialized work.
- Communicate. Social and technical specialists may have no experience of working together and may even resist it. Be open about this with each other and decide how the work will be divided but coordinated.
- Plan for the technical and social staff to be trained together so they can better learn from each other and increase their understanding of and support for each other's roles. They should work as counterparts, advancing together on a joint plan.

- Specify steps. As each construction job is different, the engineer and construction managers need to specify their step-by-step critical path for design and construction. From that list, the social specialists can plan the step-by-step community participation process to facilitate design and construction.
- Take a holistic look together. With the social and technical teams, look ahead for all the things that could go wrong in design or construction that involve local people. Take both a problem-based and a capacity-driven approach. Do not wait to react to problems; instead, foresee what they will be, and then plan ahead, using capacities to the maximum to prevent problems or resolve them if they occur.
- Develop tools. The participation, management, and conflict prevention tools that the focus groups identified as the most helpful in PERRP were the Committee-Contractor Agreements, codes of conduct, and communication protocols that separated but coordinated the work. For all parties, cooperation was facilitated by having grievance procedures that both got fair responses and were simple and quick.
- Encourage both the social and technical teams to do no harm and to be culturally sensitive and conflict sensitive.
- Solicit design input by community members in order to generate local interest, develop designs that suit the end users, and avoid cultural mistakes that will have a negative impact on usage of the new buildings.

For Sociocultural Specialists and Community Participation Teams

In addition to providing recommendations for technical and sociocultural team integration, the focus groups also developed specific recommendations for the sociocultural aspects of disaster reconstruction work.

- Whether the social team is working in-house or is subcontracted, the requirements are the same. Social team members have two main functions: to work closely with their counterpart construction managers, and to work with the community as a capacity builder, facilitator, and advocate.
- For social team members, hire local people from the same regions, cultures, and language groups as those where projects will be carried out. This creates jobs for disaster survivors and ensures that local knowledge will be high from the start.
- To build understanding of the community, social team members need to figure out many aspects of the local community, and must do so in a specified amount of time to prepare for design and con-

struction. Topics needing research include the project contexts, the culture, the power structure, the status of conflict and collaboration, the dividers and connectors, the stakeholder groups, and the local capacities, strengths, and resources, as wells as local weaknesses, risks, problems, and vulnerabilities.
- Once the local power structure is known, figure out what is feasible in order to get the most representative participation from the community members and the widest sharing of power.
- Plan specific details of participation. Based on knowledge of the community and the step-by-step critical path for design and the construction technical process, ask: What needs to happen, in what order, by when? Who will participate, how, and what will they do? Who has what responsibilities? How will these steps be synchronized with the schedule for design and construction?
- From the beginning, choose ways to work that will increase the likelihood that community participation and power sharing will be sustained once the project is finished. This could mean continuing with the same form of community committee or organization; or it could mean a change to other forms where power will still be shared, where those normally excluded will be included, and where assistance will be concentrated in the places that need it most. For this to occur, ensure project exit planning to encourage follow-through by government institutions, NGOs, the committees themselves, or other entities. Include and prepare them for this role from the start.
- To get participation at the community level in each location, either partner with a suitable existing community-based group that is representative of the community, or activate a new representative group that fits in the existing legal framework. That group's main roles should be to help prevent losses for local people and to prevent and solve community-related problems that might affect construction.
- Be clear and realistic about expectations. A project's social team needs to be clear and specific when speaking with local people about expectations for their participation. The project can be demanding but within reasonable limits. An observant, analytical social team will be able to assess what are reasonable limits, keeping in mind that poor communities often underestimate their own abilities and resources. An important part of the participatory process is to have confidence in the people and instill self-confidence in them.
- Have participatory performance monitoring. Having the local people participate in their own performance monitoring gives community people a voice and raises their expectations of what should be achieved.

APPENDIX

Schools and Health Facilities Constructed in the Pakistan Earthquake Reconstruction and Recovery Project (2006–2013)

Schools Constructed in Mansehra District, Khyber Pakhtunkhwa Province			
1	Government Boys' Primary School Paras	18	Government Boys' High School Khawari
2	Government Girls' Middle School Paras	19	Government Girls' High School Khawari
3	Government Girls' Primary School Paras	20	Government Boys' Primary School Khawari
4	Government Boys' High School Paras	21	Government Girls' High School Behali
5	Government Boys' Primary School Mohandri	22	Government Girls' Primary School Behali
6	Government Boys' High School Mohandri	23	Government Boys' Higher Secondary School Parhina
7	Government Boys' High School Bherkund	24	Government Boys' Higher Secondary School Mansehra #1
8	Government Boys' Primary School Ahl	25	Government Boys' Higher Secondary School Jabori
9	Government Boys' High School Ahl	26	Government Boys' Higher Secondary School Jared
10	Government Boys' Primary School Trappi	27	Government Boys' Primary School Kaghan
11	Government Boys' High School Trappi	28	Government Boys' High School Kaghan
12	Government Boys' High School Nokot	29	Government Girls' High School Kaghan
13	Government Boys' High School Afzalabad	30	Government Boys' Primary School Naran
14	Government Girls' High School Afzalabad	31	Government Boys' High School Naran
15	Government Boys' High School Mansehra #2	32	Government Girls High School Trangri Bala
16	Government Boys' High School Gurwal	33	Government Boys' Higher Secondary School Kewai
17	Government Boys' High School Bandi Parao	34	Government Boys' Middle School Nika Pani

Schools Constructed in Bagh District, Azad Jammu and Kashmir			
1	Government Girls' Middle School Kahna Mohri	15	Government Boys' High School Kafal Garh
2	Government Girls' Middle School Noman Pura	16	Government Boys' High School Burka Mehra
3	Government Boys' Primary School Pehl	17	Government Girls' High School Thub
4	Government Boys' Middle School Chaknari	18	Government Girls' High School Dhal Qazian
5	Government Boys' Middle School Koteri Najam Khan	19	Government Boys' High School Dhal Qazian
6	Government Girls' Middle School Basouti	20	Government Girls' High School Mahldara
7	Government Girls' High School Chatter #2	21	Government Boys' High School Kahouta
8	Government Boys High School Dharray	22	Government Girls' Higher Sec. School Kharal Abbasian
9	Government Girls' High School Chowki	23	Government Boys' Higher Secondary School Birpani
10	Government Girls' Inter College Rerra	24	Government Boys' High School Pinyali
11	Government Boys' Higher Secondary School Rerra	25	Government Girls' High School Juglari
12	Government Boys' High School Harighel	26	Government Girls' Gehl Rawli
13	Government Boys' High School Arja	27	Government Girls' High School Savor Mutwali
14	Government Girls' Inter College Arja		

Health Facilities Constructed in Bagh District, Azad Jammu and Kashmir			
1	Thana Headquarters Hospital, Dhirkot	9	Basic Health Unit Kotli
2	Basic Health Unit Harighel	10	Basic Health Unit Chanjal
3	Basic Health Unit Khawaja Ratnoi	11	Basic Health Unit Sohawa
4	Basic Health Unit Bani Minhassan	12	Basic Health Unit Sahlian
5	Basic Health Unit Kala Mola	13	Basic Health Unit Neela Butt
6	Basic Health Unit Hallan Shamali	14	Basic Health Unit Seri Peeran
7	Basic Health Unit Raikot	15	Basic Health Unit Thub
8	Basic Health Unit Chowki	16	Basic Health Unit Rerra

References

ADB (Asian Development Bank) and WB (World Bank). 2005. "Pakistan 2005 Earthquake: Preliminary Damage and Needs Assessment." Islamabad, Pakistan. Retrieved 5 October 2017 from https://www.gfdrr.org/sites/default/files/publication/pda-2005-pakistan.pdf.

Agrawal, Arun R. 1999. "Enchantment and Disenchantment: The Role of Community in Natural Resource Conservation." *World Development* 17(4): 629–49.

AHKRC. 2010. *Islands of Hope, Recollections of Dr. Akhter Hameed Khan*. Compiled by Akhter Hameed Khan Resource Centre. Lahore, Karachi, Islamabad: Vanguard Books.

Ahmed, Mughees. 2009. "Local Bodies or Local Biradari System: An Analysis of the Role of the Biradari in the Local Bodies System of the Punjab." *Pakistan Journal of History and Culture* 30(1): 81–92. Retrieved 13 March 2022 from http://www.nihcr.edu.pk/Latest_English_Journal/Local-Bodies.pdf.

Aijazi, Omer. 2020. "What about *Insāniyat*? Morality and Ethics in the *Pahars* of Kashmir." *Himalaya* 40(1): 30–48. Retrieved 25 May 2021 from https://digitalcommons.macalester.edu/himalaya/vol40/iss1/8.

AIT (Asian Institute for Technology). 2010. "Risk Management in the Pakistan Construction Industry: A Contractor's Perspective." *Professional Project Management Education*. Retrieved 30 January 2018 from http://professionalprojectmanagement.blogspot.ca/2010/05/risk-management-in-pakistan.html.

Alavi, Hamza. 1971. "The Politics of Dependence: A Village in West Punjab." *South Asian Review* 4(2): 111–28.

———. 2001. "The Two Biradiris: Kinship in Rural West Punjab: Subsistence Economy and the Effect of Internal Migration." In *Muslim Communities of South Asia: Culture, Society and Power*, 3rd edition, ed. T. N. Madan. New Delhi: Manohar.

Aliani, Shahbano. 2009. "Caste in Pakistan: The Elephant in the Room." *The Red Diary*. Retrieved 10 November 2018 from https://reddiarypk.wordpress.com/2009/08/25/caste-in-pakistan/.

Alif Ailaan and SDPI. 2016. *Alif Ailaan Pakistan District Education Rankings 2016*. Islamabad: Alif Ailaan. Retrieved 25 July 2018 from https://d3n8a8pro7vhmx.cloudfront.net/alifailaan/pages/537/attachments/original/1474368820/Pakistan_District_Education_Rankings_2016_Full_Report.pdf?1474368820.

Amnesty International. 2001. "Pakistan, Azad Jammu and Kashmir, Torture or Ill Treatment/Arbitrary Detention/Possible Prisoners of Conscience," 14 June, Index number: ASA 33/014/2001. Retrieved 13 March 2022 from https://www.amnesty.org/en/documents/asa33/014/2001/en/.

Anderson, Mary B. 1999. *Do No Harm: How Aid Can Support Peace—or War*. Boulder and London: Lynne Rienner Publishers.

Anderson, Mary B., and Peter J. Woodrow. 1989. *Rising from the Ashes: Development Strategies in Times of Disaster*. Boulder and San Francisco: Westview Press.

ANGOC (Asian Nongovernment Organization Coalition). 2019. *State of Land Rights and Land Governance in Eight Asian Countries*. Asian NGO Coalition for Agrarian Reform and Rural Development. Retrieved 11 February 2020 from https://angoc.org/wp-content/uploads/2019/07/State_of_Land_Rights__Land_Governance.pdf.

Annan, Kofi. 2005. "Secretary-General's Press Conference" United Nations, 10 October, Geneva, Switzerland. Retrieved 13 March 2022 from https://www.thenewhumanitarian.org/fr/node/198070.

Anwar, Shahzad. 2018. "Faulty Land Records Primary Cause of Homicide in AJK." *Express Tribune*, 22 February. Retrieved 10 December 2018 from https://tribune.com.pk/story/1641597/1-faulty-land-records-primary-cause-homicide-ajk/.

Archer, David, and Sara Cottingham. 1996. *REFLECT: Regenerated Freirean Literacy Through Empowering Community Techniques*. London: ActionAid.

Azhar, Nida, Rizwan U. Farooqui, and Syed M. Ahmed. 2008. "Cost Overrun Factors in Construction Industry of Pakistan." *First International Conference on Construction in Developing Countries (ICCIDC-I)*, Karachi, Pakistan, 4–5 August. Retrieved 30 January 2018 from https://www.researchgate.net/publication/277987526_Cost_Overrun_Factors_In_Construction_Industry_of_Pakistan.

Barenstein, Jennifer E. Duyne, and Esther Leemann, eds. 2012. *Post-Disaster Reconstruction and Change: Communities' Perspectives*. Boca Raton, FL: CRC Press.

Bengali, Kaiser. 2010. *Land Tenure: Issues in Housing Reconstruction and Income Poverty, Case Study of Earthquake Affected Areas in Hazara*. Sustainable Development Policy Institute. Retrieved 17 July 2020 from https://landportal.org/fr/library/resources/eldisa69952/land-tenure-issues-housing-reconstruction-and-income-poverty-case.

Bentley, Leslie. 1999. "A Brief Biography of Paulo Freire." *Pedagogy and the Theatre of the Oppressed*. Retrieved 12 September 2018 from https://ptoweb.org/aboutpto/a-brief-biography-of-paulo-freire/.

Bernardi, Fabrizio, Juan J. Gonzalez, and Miguel Requena. 2006. "The Sociology of Social Structure." In *21st Century Sociology: A Reference Handbook*, ed. B. Bryant and D. Peck, 162–70. Newbury: Sage. Retrieved 13 March 2022 from https://www.researchgate.net/publication/310912518_THE_SOCIOLOGY_OF_SOCIAL_STRUCTURE.

Birukou, Aliaksandr, Enrico Banzieri, Paolo Giogini, and Fausto Giunchiglia. 2013. "A Formal Definition of Culture." In *Models for Intercultural Collaboration and Negotiation*, ed. Katia Sycara, Michele Gelfand, and Allison Abbe, 1–26. Dordrecht: Springer.

Block, Peter. 2008. *Community: The Structure of Belonging*. San Francisco: Berrett-Koehler Publishers.

Bokhari, Ashfak. 2016. "Resistance to Digitization of Land Records." *The Dawn*, 25 April. Retrieved 9 December 2018 from https://www.dawn.com/news/1254162.

Bosher, L. S., and A. R. J. Dainty. 2011. "Disaster Risk Reduction and 'Built-In' Resilience: Towards Overarching Principles of Construction Practice." *Disasters: Journal of Disaster Studies, Policy and Management* 35(1): 1–18. Retrieved 13 March 2022 from http://citeseerx.ist.psu.edu/viewdoc/download?doi=10.1.1.955.9672&rep=rep1&type=pdf.

Braine, Theresa. 2006. "Was 2005 the Year of Natural Disasters?" *Bulletin of the World Health Organization* 84 (1): 4–6. Retrieved 24 February 2020 from https://apps.who.int/iris/handle/10665/269551.

Brenner, Sabrina. 2017. "Teaching Cultural Sensitivity at Architecture Schools for More Sustainable Buildings." In *Design for Sustainable Culture, Perspectives and Education: Perspectives, Practices and Education*, ed. Astrid Skjerven and Janne Beate Reitan, 197–213. New York: Routledge.

Brett, Edwin Allan. 1996. "The Participatory Principle in Development Projects: The Costs and Benefits of Cooperation." *Public Administration and Development* 20(3): 5–19.

Bruce, John. 2013. "Land and Conflict: Land Disputes and Land Conflicts." *USAID*. Retrieved 19 December 2018. https://www.land-links.org/issue-brief/land-disputes-and-land-conflict/.

Buggy, Lisa, and Karen Elizabeth McNamara. 2015. "The Need to Reinterpret 'Community' for Climate Change Adaptation: A Case Study of Pele Island, Vanuatu." *Climate and Development* 8(3): 270–80. Retrieved 13 March 2022 from https://doi.org/10.1080/17565529.2015.1041445.

Bulmer, Mark, Tony Farquhar, Masud Roshan, Sadar Saeed Akhtar, and Sajjad Karamat Wahla. 2007. "Landslide Hazards After the 2005 Kashmir Earthquake." *Eos, Transactions American Geophysical Union* 88(5): 53–55.

Button, Gregory V., and Mark Schuller, eds. 2016. *Contextualizing Disaster*. Catastrophes in Context, Volume 1. New York: Berghahn Books.

Callan, Hilary. n.d. "Social and Cultural Anthropology." *Discover Anthropology*. Retrieved 3 July 2018 from https://discoveranthropology.org.uk/about-anthropology/what-is-anthropology/social-and-cultural-anthropology.html.

Cambridge Dictionary. n.d. "Community." *Cambridge Academic Content Dictionary*. Retrieved 19 March 2022 from https://dictionary.cambridge.org/dictionary/english/community.

Canada: Immigration and Refugee Board of Canada. 1997. "Azad Kashmir and Northern Areas." Retrieved 4 December 2017 from http://www.refworld.org/docid/3ae6a83ac.html.

Cannon, Terry. 2014. "Why Do We Pretend There Is 'Community'? Problems of Community Based-Adaptation (CBA) and Community Based Disaster Reduction (CBDRR)." *IDS Povertics*, 23 April 2014. Retrieved 25 February 2020 from http://vulnerabilityandpoverty.blogspot.com/2014/04/why-do-we-pretend-there-is-community.html.

Cannon, Terry, Alexandra Titz, and Fred Kruger. 2014. "The Myth of Community?" In *World Disasters Report: Focus on Culture and Risk*. Geneva: International Federation of Red Cross and Red Crescent Societies.

Cannon, Terry, Fred Kruger, and Greg Bankoff. 2014. "The Links between Culture and Risk." In *World Disasters Report: Focus on Culture and Risk*. Geneva: International Federation of Red Cross and Red Crescent Societies.

Cannon, Terry, Fred Kruger, Greg Bankoff, and Lisa Schipper. 2014. "Putting Culture at the Center of Risk Reduction." In *World Disasters Report: Focus on Culture and Risk*. Geneva: International Federation of Red Cross and Red Crescent Societies.

Cernea, Michael M. 1985. *Putting People First: Sociological Variables in Rural Development*. Oxford: Oxford University Press.

Chambers, Robert. 1974. *Managing Rural Development: Ideas and Experience from East Africa*. Uppsala: Scandinavian Institute of African Studies. Retrieved 18 July 2020 from http://nai.diva-portal.org/smash/get/diva2:278970/FULLTEXT01.

———. 1983. *Rural Development: Putting the Last First*. Essex: Longman Group Limited.

———. 1994a. "The Origins and Practice of Participatory Rural Appraisal." *World Development* 22(7): 953–69. Retrieved 12 March 2019 from https://www.sciencedirect.com/science/article/abs/pii/0305750X94901414.

———. 1994b. "Participatory Rural Appraisal: Analysis of Experience." *World Development* 22(9): 1253–68.

———. 1997. *Whose Reality Counts? Putting the First Last.* London: Intermediate Technology Development Group.

———. 2005. *Ideas for Development.* London: Earthscan.

———. 2017. *Can We Know Better? Reflections for Development.* Warwickshire: Practical Action Publishing.

Chan, Adrian D. C., and Jonathan Fishbein. 2009. "A Global Engineer for the Global Community." *Journal of Policy Engagement* 1(2), 4–9. Retrieved 25 April 2019 from http://my2.ewb.ca/site_media/static/attachments/group_topics_group topic/61681/Global percent20Engineering.pdf.

Chevalier, Jacques M. and Daniel J. Buckles. 2008. "A Guide to Collaborative Inquiry and Social Engagement." New Delhi: Sage. Retrieved 16 February 2018 from https://idl-bnc-idrc.dspacedirect.org/bitstream/handle/10625/35977/IDL-35977.pdf.

Chmutina, Ksenia, Jason Von Meding, J. C. Gaillard, and Lee Bosher. 2017. "Why Natural Disasters Aren't All Natural." Open Democracy Net. Retrieved 13 March 2022 from https://www.opendemocracy.net/en/why-natural-disasters-arent-all-that-natural/.

Choi, Jin Ouk, Ghada M. Gad, Jennifer S. Shane, and Kelly C. Strong. 2015. "Culture and Organizational Culture in the Construction Industry: A Literature Review." Canadian Society for Civil Engineering, 5th International/11th Construction Specialty Conference, University of British Columbia, Vancouver, Canada, 7–10 June 2015. Retrieved 24 April 2019 from https://open.library.ubc.ca/cIRcle/collections/52660/items/1.0076488.

Cohen, John M., and Norman T. Uphoff. 1977. *Rural Development Participation: Concepts and Measures for Project Design, Implementation and Evaluation.* Ithaca: Cornell University Center for International Studies.

———. 1980. "Participation's Place in Rural Development: Seeking Clarity Through Specificity." *World Development* 8(3): 213–35. Retrieved 11 January 2020 at https://ideas.repec.org/a/eee/wdevel/v8y1980i3p213-235.html.

Conflict Sensitivity Consortium. 2012. *How to Guide to Conflict Sensitivity.* Retrieved 21 March 2018 from https://conflictsensitivity.org/wp-content/uploads/2015/04/6602_HowToGuide_CSF_WEB_3.pdf.

Cooke, Bill, and Uma Kothari, eds. 2001. *Participation: The New Tyranny?* London: Zed Books.

Cornwall, Andrea, and Ian Scoones, eds. 2011. *Revolutionizing Development: Reflections on the Work of Robert Chambers.* London: Earthscan.

"Cuba Doubles Pakistan Quake Medical Team to 200." 2005. Reuters, 21 October. Retrieved 12 October 2017 from https://reliefweb.int/report/pakistan/cuba-doubles-pakistan-quake-medical-team-200.

Dainty, Andrew, Stuart Green, and Barbara Bagilhole, eds. 2007. *People and Culture in Construction: A Reader.* London: Routledge.

Davidson, Colin H., Cassidy Johnson, Gonzalo Lizarralde, Nese Dikmen, and Alicia Sliwinski. 2007. "Truths and Myths about Community Participation in Post-Disaster Housing Projects." *Habitat International* 31(1): 100–15. Retrieved 24 July 2018 from https://www.sciencedirect.com/science/article/pii/S0197397506000348.

"Decades of Military Rule." 2018. *Development and Cooperation*, 1 February. Retrieved 13 March 2022 from https://www.dandc.eu/en/article/brief-history-military-rule-pakistan.

Dreyer, Lynette. n.d. *Disappointments of Participation: Find the Correct Role for Community Participation*. Retrieved 12 March 2019 from http://citeseerx.ist.psu.edu/viewdoc/download?doi=10.1.1.526.966&rep=rep1&type=pdf.

Durrani, Ahmad Jan, Amr Salah Elnashi, Youssef M. A. Hashash, Sung Jig Kim, and Arif Masud. 2005. "The Kashmir Earthquake of October 8, 2005: A Quick Look Report." Mid-America Earthquake Center, University of Illinois at Urbana-Champaign. Report No. 05-04. Retrieved 14 July 2018 from https://www.ideals.illinois.edu/bitstream/handle/2142/8937/Report05-04.pdf.

EERI (Earthquake Engineering Research Institute). 2006. "Special Earthquake Report: Learning from Earthquakes: The Kashmir Earthquake of October 8, 2005. Impacts in Pakistan." Retrieved 14 July 2018 from https://www.eeri.org/products-page/other-special-reports/.

Eriksen, Thomas H. 2001. *Small Places, Large Issues: An Introduction to Social and Cultural Anthropology*, 2nd edition. London: Pluto Press.

"Extensive Drive Launched Against Land Mafia in AJK: Farooq." 2017. *Associated Press of Pakistan*, 29 January. Retrieved 13 March 2022 from https://www.app.com.pk/national/extensive-drive-launched-against-land-mafia-in-ajk-farooq/.

Faas, A. J., and Elizabeth K. Marino. 2020. "Mythopolitics of 'Community': An Unstable but Necessary Category." *Disaster Prevention and Management: An International Journal* 29(4): 481–84. Retrieved 25 February 2021 from https://doi.org/10.1108/DPM-04-2020-0101.

Fals-Borda, Orlando. 1995. "Research for Social Justice: Some North-South Convergences." Plenary Address at the Southern Sociological Society Meeting, 8 April. Retrieved 27 January 2017 from http://comm-org.wisc.edu/si/falsborda.htm.

"Four Killed Over Land Dispute in Mianwali." 2018. *Geo News*, 21 January. Retrieved 9 December 2018 from https://www.geo.tv/latest/177922-four-killed-over-land-dispute-in-mianwali.

Freedom House. 2011. "Freedom in the World 2011—Kashmir [Pakistan]." Retrieved 8 July 2020 from https://www.refworld.org/docid/4e4cd6552954.html.

———. 2017. "Freedom in the World 2004—Kashmir [Pakistan]." Retrieved 28 June 2020 from https://www.refworld.org/docid/473c549cc.html.

Friedman, Steven. 1993. *The Elusive "Community": The Dynamics of Negotiated Urban Development*. Research Report No. 28. Johannesburg: Center for Policy Studies. Retrieved 31 January 2019 from https://books.google.ca/books/about/The_elusive_community.html?id=Igg0AQAAIAAJ&redir_esc=y.

Friere, Paulo. 1970. *Pedagogy of the Oppressed*, 30th Anniversary Edition, 2005, trans. Myra Bergman Ramos. New York: Continuum. Retrieved 24 March 2020 from https://envs.ucsc.edu/internships/internship-readings/freire-pedagogy-of-the-oppressed.pdf.

"The Future of Kashmir." 2011. *BBC News*. Retrieved 16 January 2018 from http://news.bbc.co.uk/2/shared/spl/hi/south_asia/03/kashmir_future/html/.

Gardezi, S. Shujaa Safdar, Irfan Anjum Manarvi, and S. Jamal Safdar Gardezi. 2013. "Time Extension Factors in Construction Industry of Pakistan." Fourth International Symposium on Infrastructure Engineering in Developing Countries. Retrieved 10 July 2018 from https://ac.els-cdn.com/S1877705814009990/1-s2.0-S1877705814009990-main.pdf.

Gazdar, Haris. 2007. "Class, Caste or Race: Veils Over Social Oppression in Pakistan." *Economic and Political Weekly*, 13 January: 86–88.

Gilani, Ijaz, Aized H. Mir, and Ermeena Malik. 2007. *Local Stakeholder's Perception Survey*. Pakistan Infrastructure Implementation Capacity Assessment (PIICA). Discussion Paper Series Technical Note 2. Report No.43186. South Asia Sustainable Development Unit, World Bank. Retrieved 13 March 2022 from https://openknowledge.worldbank.org/handle/10986/19610?locale-attribute=es.

Glass, Juniper. 2015. *Decades of Change: A Short History of International Development Organizations in Canada*. Retrieved 20 April 2020 from http://thephilanthropist.ca/2015/05/decades-of-change-a-short-history-of-international-development-organizations-in-canada/.

Government of AJ&K. 2018. "AJK at a Glance." Planning and Development Department. Retrieved 13 March 2022 from https://opendata.com.pk/dataset/bureau-of-statistics_ajk/resource/55dac734-129e-458d-9afc-ffe0ccbf2bd1.

Greenwood, Davydd J., William F. Whyte, and Ira Harkavy. 1991. "Participatory Action Research, as a Process and as a Goal." *Human Relations* 46(2): 175–92. Retrieved 13 March 2022 from https://doi.org/10.1177/001872679304600203.

Hafeez, Abdul, and Khurshid Ahmed. 2014. "Azad Jammu and Kashmir Agriculture Policy: A Ten Year Perspective." Retrieved 13 March 2022 from https://www.academia.edu/35438817/AZAD_JAMMU_AND_KASHMIR_AGRICULTURE_POLICY_A_Ten_Years_Perspective.

Hagan, Ross, and Haroon Shuaib. 2014. "Pakistan Reconstructed." *USAID Frontlines: Online Edition*, January/February. Retrieved 17 September 2017 from https://2012-2017.usaid.gov/news-information/frontlines/energy-infrastructure/pakistan-reconstructed.

Haiplik, Brenda. 2007. "The Education Cluster in Pakistan." *Forced Migration Review* 29: 40–42. Retrieved 17 July 2020 from https://www.fmreview.org/humanitarianreform/haiplik.

Hampton, Jerry. n.d. "Group Dynamics and Community Building," Definition 3. Retrieved 5 September 2018 from www.community4me.com/comm_definitions.html.

Harrell-Bond, Barbara E. 1986. *Imposing Aid Emergency Assistance to Refugees*. New York: Oxford University Press.

Hart R. A. 1992. "Children's Participation: From Tokenism to Citizenship," UNICEF Innocenti Essays, No. 4, Florence.

Harty, Chris. 2008. "Sociology and Construction Management Research: Issues, Approaches and Implications." Innovative Construction Research Center, School of Construction Management, University of Reading. *Proceedings 24th Annual ARCOM Conference*: 1–3. Retrieved 26 April 2019 from https://www.researchgate.net/publication/264887390_Sociology_and_construction_management_research_Issues_approaches_and_implications.

Harvey, Peter, Sohrab Baghri, and Bob Reed. 2005. *Emergency Sanitation: Assessment and Program Design*. Water, Engineering and Development Centre (WEDC) Publications, Loughborough University, Leicestershire, UK. Retrieved 15 July 2020 from https://ec.europa.eu/echo/files/evaluation/watsan2005/annex_files/WEDC/es/ES01CD.pdf.

Hasan, Arif. 2009. *The Unplanned Revolution: Observations on the Processes of Socio-Economic Change in Pakistan*. Oxford: Oxford University Press.

Hasseeb, M., Xinhai-Lu, Aneesa Bibi, Maloof-ud-Dyian, and Wahab Rabbani. 2011. "Causes and Effects of Delays in Large Construction Projects in Pakistan." *Kuwait Chapter of Arabian Journal of Business and Management Review* 1(4): 18–42. Retrieved 30 January 2018 from https://www.arabianjbmr.com/pdfs/KD_VOL_1_4/3.pdf.

Hayat, Fatima Akram. 2017. "The Relationship Between Access to Toilets and School Enrolment in Pakistan." Master's thesis, Georgetown University. Retrieved 24 July 2018 from https://repository.library.georgetown.edu/bitstream/handle/10822/1044655/Hayat_georgetown_0076M_13782.pdf?sequence=1.

"Hayat Khan Says He Is Premier of Graveyard." 2005. Reuters, 11 October. Retrieved 22 May 2020 from https://gulfnews.com/world/asia/pakistan/hayat-khan-says-he-is-premier-of-graveyard-1.303920.

Hedberg, T. 2001. "The Role of the Global Engineer." In *Educating the Engineer for the 21st Century*, ed. D. Weichert, B. Rauhut, and R. Schmidt, 7–13. Dordrecht, Netherlands: Springer. Retrieved 31 July 2018 from https://link.springer.com/chapter/10.1007/0-306-48394-7_2.

Hendry, Joy. 2008. *An Introduction to Social Anthropology: Sharing Our Worlds*, 2nd edition. London and New York: Palgrave MacMillan.

———. 2016. *An Introduction to Social Anthropology*. London: Palgrave MacMillan.

Herbert, Jacques, and Maurice Strong. 1980. *The Great Building Bee: Canada, A Hope for the Third World*. Toronto: General Publishing Company.

Heron, J. 1995. *Cooperative Inquiry: Research into the Human Condition*. London: Sage.

Hickey, Samuel, and Giles Mohan. 2004. "Towards Participation as Transformation: Critical Themes and Challenges." In *Participation: Tyranny to Transformation? Exploring New Approaches to Participation in Development*, ed. Samuel Hickey and Giles Mohan. London: Zed Books.

Hidayat, B., and C. Egbu. 2010. "A Literature Review of the Role of Project Management in Post-Disaster Reconstruction." 26th Annual ARCOM Conference, 6–8 September 2010, Leeds, UK, Association of Researchers in Construction Management, 1269–78. Retrieved 14 January 2020 from http://usir.salford.ac.uk/id/eprint/10144/.

Hoffman, Susanna M. 2020. "The Scope and Importance of Anthropology and Its Core Concept of Culture in Closing the Disaster Knowledge to Policy and Practice Gap." In *Disaster Upon Disaster: Exploring the Gap between Knowledge, Policy and Practice*, ed. Susanna M. Hoffman and Roberto Barrios, Catastrophes in Context, Volume 2. New York: Berghahn.

Hoffman, Susanna M., and Roberto E. Barrios, eds. 2020. *Disaster Upon Disaster: Exploring the Gap Between Knowledge, Policy and Practice*, Catastrophes in Context, Volume 2. New York: Berghahn.

Hoffman, Susanna M., and Anthony Oliver-Smith, eds. 2002. *Catastrophe & Culture. The Anthropology of Disaster*. Santa Fe: School of American Research Press.

Hofstede, Geert. 2011. "Dimensionalizing Cultures: The Hofstede Model in Context." *Online Readings in Psychology and Culture*, Unit 2. Retrieved 13 March 2022 from http://mchmielecki.pbworks.com/w/file/fetch/64591689/hofstede_dobre.pdf.

Home Office, Government of United Kingdom. 2017. "Country Policy and Information Note Pakistan: Land Disputes." Retrieved 14 March 2022 from https://www.landportal.org/library/resources/country-policy-and-information-note-pakistan-land-disputes.

HRCP (Human Rights Commission of Pakistan). 2010. "The Upheaval in AJK Judiciary: Report of an HRCP Fact Finding Mission." HRCP Report, April/May. Retrieved 4 January 2018 from http://hrcp-web.org/hrcpweb/wp-content/pdf/ff/9.pdf.

Human Rights Watch. 2006. "With Friends like These . . .": Human Rights Violations in Azad Kashmir. Retrieved 17 November 2017 from https://www.hrw.org/report/2006/09/20/friends-these/human-rights-violations-azad-kashmir.

———. 2016. "'This Crooked System': Police Abuse and Reform in Pakistan (Summary)." Retrieved 13 December 2018 from https://www.refworld.org/docid/57e8d0f64.html.

IDS (Institute for Development Studies). n.d. "Website Participatory Methods. Learn and Empower." University of Sussex. Retrieved 4 May 2018 from https://www.participatorymethods.org.

IFRC (International Federation of Red Cross and Red Crescent Societies). 2014. World Disasters Report: Focus on Culture and Risk. Geneva: IFRC. Retrieved 13 March 2022 from https://reliefweb.int/report/world/world-disasters-report-2014-focus-culture-and-risk.

"India Threatens £10 Million Fine for Mapmakers Who Don't Toe the Line on Disputed Territories." 2016. The Telegraph, 6 May. Retrieved 11 November 2017 from http://www.telegraph.co.uk/news/2016/05/06/india-threatens-10m-fine-for-mapmakers-who-dont-toe-line-on-displ/.

"Interview with Amos Rapoport." 1992. Architecture & Behavior 8(1): 93–102. Retrieved 31 March 2019 from https://www.epfl.ch/labs/lasur/wp-content/uploads/2018/05/RAPOPORT_en-v8n1.pdf.

Jalal, Ayesha. 1995. Democracy and Authoritarianism in South Asia: A Comparative and Historical Perspective. Cambridge: Cambridge University Press.

———. 2005. "Pakistan: A State with a Split Personality." Interview on Qantara website. Retrieved 22 July 2020 from https://en.qantara.de/content/interview-ayesha-jalal-pakistan-a-state-with-a-split-personality.

Jha, Abhas K., Jennifer Duyne Barenstein, Priscilla M. Phelps, Daniel Pittet, and Stephen Sena. 2010. Safer Homes, Stronger Communities: A Handbook for Reconstructing after Natural Disasters. World Bank Open Knowledge Repository. Retrieved 20 April 2020 from https://openknowledge.worldbank.org/handle/10986/2409.

Jigyasu, Rohit. 2013. "Forword." In Post-Disaster Reconstruction and Change: Communities' Perspectives, ed. Jennifer E. Duyne Barenstein and Esther Leemann. Boca Raton, FL: CRC Press.

"Kashmir and the Politics of Water." 2011. Al Jazeera, 1 August. Retrieved 13 January 2008 from http://www.aljazeera.com/indepth/spotlight/kashmirtheforgottenconflict/2011/07/20117812154478992.html.

"The Kashmir Earthquake." 2005. The Washington Post, 12 October. Retrieved 9 October 2017 from http://www.washingtonpost.com/wp-dyn/content/article/2005/10/11/AR2005101101727.html.

"Kashmir's Earthquake: A Humanitarian Failure." 2005. The Economist, 29 October. https://www w.economist.com/leaders/2005/10/27/a-humanitarian-failure.

Keesing, Roger M. 1981. Cultural Anthropology: A Contemporary Perspective. New York: Holt, Rinehart and Winston.

Khan, Akhter Hameed. 1998. Orangi Pilot Project: Personal Reminiscences of Change. Oxford: Oxford University Press.

———. 2010. Islands of Hope: Recollections of Dr. Akhter Hameed Khan. Akhter Hameed Khan Resource Center. Karachi: Vanguard Books.

Khan, Azam. 2013. "Constituency Profile: For Mansehra Seats, It's the Mosque that Matters." *Express Tribune Pakistan*, 20 April. Retrieved 13 March 2022 from https://tribune.com.pk/story/538043/constituency-profile-for-mansehra-seats-its-the-mosque-that-matters/.

Khan, Ilyas. 2018. "The Kashmiri Property Rows that Date Back to British India." *BBC News*, 20 March. Retrieved 7 December 2018 from https://www.bbc.com/news/world-asia-india-4282091.

Khan, Sardar Abdul Hameed. 2016. *The Azad Jammu and Kashmir Land Laws*. Federal Law House. Retrieved 5 December 2018 from http://www.federallawhouse.com/wp-content/uploads/2017/04/Title-Printline-and-Table-of-Contents.pdf.

Khan, Shoaib Sultan. 1990. "The Aga Khan Rural Support Programme." In *MIMAR 34: Architecture in Development*. London: Concept Media Ltd.

Khan, Shoaib Sultan, and Mahmood Hasan Khan. 2009. *The Aga Khan Rural Support Programme: A Journey Through Grassroots Development*. New York: Oxford University Press.

Kivrak, Serkan, Andrew Ross, and Gokhan Arslan. 2008. "Effects of Cultural Differences in Construction Projects: An Investigation Among UK Construction Professionals." International Conference on Multi-National Construction Projects, "Securing High Performance through Cultural Awareness and Dispute Avoidance," 21–23 November 2008, Shanghai, China. Retrieved 20 April 2019 from https://www.irb.fraunhofer.de/CIBlibrary/search-quick-result-list.jsp?A&idSuche=CIB+DC12193.

Klint, Louise Munk, Emma Wong, Ming Jiang, Terry De Lacy, David Harrison, and Dale Dominey-Howes. 2011. "Climate Change Adaptation in the Pacific Island Tourism Sector: Analysing the Policy Environment in Vanuatu." *Current Issues in Tourism* 15(3): 247–74. Retrieved 13 March 2022 from https://doi.org/10.1080/13683500.2011.608841.

Kokab, Tabinda. 2015. "The Disaster That Liberated Me." *BBC News Magazine*. Retrieved 19 October 2017 from http://www.bbc.com/news/magazine-34459110.

Kumar, Somesh. 2002. *Methods for Community Participation: A Complete Guide for Practitioners*. London: ITDG Publishing.

"Land Management: AJK to Launch Electronic Land Records." 2016. *The Express Tribune*, 3 January. Retrieved 8 December 2018 from https://tribune.com.pk/story/1020988/land-management-ajk-to-launch-electronic-land-records/.

Leach, Melissa, Robin Mearns, and Ian Scoones. 1997. "Challenges to Community-Based Sustainable Development: Dynamics, Entitlements, Institutions." *IDS Bulletin* 28(4): 4–14. Retrieved 20 May 2020 from https://onlinelibrary.wiley.com/doi/epdf/10.1111/j.1759-5436.1997.mp28004002.x.

Leal, Pablo Alejandro. 2011. "Participation: The Ascendancy of a Buzzword in the Neo-Liberal Era." In *The Participation Reader*, ed. Andrea Cornwall, 70–85. London: Zed Books.

Loach, Kristen, Jennifer Rowley, and Jillian Griffiths. 2017. "Cultural Sustainability as a Strategy for the Survival of Museums and Libraries." *International Journal of Cultural Policy* 23(2): 186–98. Retrieved 20 March 2019 from https://www.tandfonline.com/doi/full/10.1080/10286632.2016.1184657.

Mahadevia, Darshini. 2009. "Social Protection in Asian Cities." In *Regional Trends, Issues and Practices in Rural Poverty Reduction*. United Nations Environmental and Social Commission for Asia and the Pacific (ESCAP).

Malik, Hasnaat. 2016. "Illegal Dispossession Act: Illegal Occupants Will Serve a Decade in Jail, Says Supreme Court." *Express Tribune*, 20 July. Retrieved 5 December 2018 from https://tribune.com.pk/story/1145383/illegal-dispossession-act-illegal-occupants-will-serve-decade-jail-says-sc/.

Manzoor, Usman. 2015. "Mistakes in Rehabilitation of 2005 Quake Should Not Be Repeated." *The International News*, 27 October. Retrieved 14 October 2017 from https://www.thenews.com.pk/print/69774-mistakes-in-rehabilitation-of-2005-quake-should-not-be-repeated.

Maru, Vivek. 2014. "Law and Disorder: Rough Justice Rules in the Developing World." *The Guardian*, 7 February. Retrieved 13 December 2018 from https://www.theguardian.com/global-development/poverty-matters/2014/feb/07/rough-justice-rules-in-developing-world.

Masnuri, Ghazala, and Rao Vijayendra. 2004. "Community-Based and Driven Development: A Critical Review." *World Bank Research Observer* 19(1): 1–40. Retrieved 10 December 2019 from https://elibrary.worldbank.org/doi/abs/10.1093/wbro/lkh012.

Memmott, Paul, and Cathy Keys. 2015. "Redefining Architecture to Accommodate Cultural Difference: Designing for Cultural Sustainability." *Architectural Science Review* 58(4): 278–89.

Merriam-Webster. n.d. "Community." *Merriam-Webster.com* dictionary. Retrieved 19 March 2022 from https://www.merriam-webster.com/dictionary/community.

Middleton, Neil, and Phil O'Keefe. 1998. *Disaster and Development: The Politics of Humanitarian Aid*. London and Chicago: Pluto Press.

Mir, Aized H., Mehreen Tanvir, Amer Z. Durrani. 2007. "Development of Construction Industry—A Literature Review." Pakistan Infrastructure Implementation Capacity Assessment, World Bank Discussion Paper Series: Technical Note 1. Report No. 43185. Retrieved 12 July 2018 from https://openknowledge.worldbank.org/bitstream/handle/10986/7743/431850PNT0REPL10A0Literature0Review.pdf;sequence=1.

Mohmand, S. K., and Haris Gazdar. 2007. "Social Structures in Rural Pakistan." Asian Development Bank, TA 4319-PAK, Determinants and Drivers of Poverty Reduction and ADB's Contribution in Rural Pakistan. Retrieved 17 March 2020 from http://www.researchcollective.org/Documents/Social_Structure_in_Rural_Pakistan.pdf.

Monaghan, J., and P. Just. 2000. *Social and Cultural Anthropology: A Very Short Introduction*. Oxford: Oxford University Press.

Mulligan, Martin. 2015. "On Ambivalence and Hope in the Restless Search for Community: How to Work with the Idea of Community in the Global Age." *Sociology* 49(2): 340–55.

Murphy Thomas, Jane. 1994. *Project Brief, Aga Khan Rural Support Programme*. Geneva: Aga Khan Foundation.

———. 1995. *Management for Development, Managing and Running an NGO*. Peshawar: Mawafaq Foundation.

———. 2004. *Social Organizer's Manual for Afghanistan*. Kabul: Aga Khan Development Network.

———. 2007. *Guidebook for Social Mobilizers*. Pakistan Earthquake Reconstruction and Recovery Program.

———. 2012a. "Community Participation and Construction." Pakistan Earthquake Reconstruction and Recovery Program. Unpublished monograph.

———. 2012b. *Participation Index Study: Community Participation and Construction*. Report to USAID, Pakistan Earthquake Reconstruction and Recovery Program.

———. 2013a. *Assessment of School Committees in the Punjab and Khyber Pakhtunkhwa Province, Pakistan*. Bonn: GIZ Basic Education Program (German Corporation for International Cooperation).

———. 2013b. *Get Off My Land, Please! A Primer for Community Participation and Construction*. Training document for engineers.

———. 2020. "Disaster Theory versus Practice? It Is a Long Rocky Road: A Practitioner's View from the Ground." In *Disaster Upon Disaster: Exploring the Gap Between Knowledge, Policy and Practice*, ed. Susanna M. Hoffman and Roberto E. Barrios, Catastrophes in Context, Volume 2. New York: Berghahn.

NAPA (National Association for the Practice of Anthropology). n.d. "About." Retrieved 14 May 2019 from https://www.practicinganthropology.org/discover/about/.

Naqash, Tariq. 2015. "Remembering Oct 8, 2005: The Day the Earth Shook." *Dawn*, 8 October. Retrieved 4 October 2017 from https://www.dawn.com/news/1211695.

Naqvi, Syed Mohsin. 2005. "Pakistan Aid Pledges to Top $5.8 Billion." *CNN World*, 19 November. Retrieved 30 October 2017 from http://www.cnn.com/2005/WORLD/asiapcf/11/19/quake.pakistan.aid/.

Narayan, Deepa. 1995. "The Contribution of People's Participation: Evidence from 121 Rural Water Supply Projects." Environmentally Sustainable Development Occasional Paper Series, The World Bank.

NATO (North Atlantic Treaty Organization). 2010. "Pakistan Earthquake Relief Operation." Retrieved 18 February 2020 from https://www.nato.int/cps/en/natohq/topics_50070.htm.

Naviwala, Nadia. 2016. *Pakistan's Education Crisis: The Real Story*. Washington, DC: Woodrow Wilson International Center for Scholars. Retrieved 13 March 2022 from https://eric.ed.gov/?q=source%3A%22Woodrow+Wilson+International+Center+for+Scholars%22&id=ED570671.

———. 2017. "Kashmir Earthquake: 'What Happened to the 12 years and $6 billion?'" *The New Humanitarian*, 12 May. Retrieved 14 June 2018 from https://www.thenewhumanitarian.org/feature/2017/05/12/kashmir-earthquake-what-happened-12-years-and-6-billion.

New Pak Historian. 2018. "Languages, Religion, Tribes and Castes of the Hazara Region." Retrieved 5 October 2018 from https://newpakhistorian.wordpress.com/2018/04/17/languages-religion-tribes-and-castes-of-the-hazara-region/.

Nuclear Threat Initiative. 2019. "Pakistan: Nuclear." Retrieved 25 March 2020 from https://www.nti.org/learn/countries/pakistan/nuclear/.

Oakley, Peter. 1991. "The Concept of Participation in Development." *Landscape and Urban Planning* 20(1–3): 115–122. Retrieved 13 March 2022 from https://doi.org/10.1016/0169-2046(91)90100-Z.

Oakley, Peter, and WHO (World Health Organization). 1989. *Community Involvement in Health Development: An Examination of the Critical Issues*. Geneva: WHO.

ODA (Overseas Development Administration). 1995. *A Guide to Social Analysis for Projects in Developing Countries*. London: Overseas Development Administration.

OER Services. n.d. "Five Stages of Team Development." *Principles of Management*. Retrieved 13 March 2022 from https://courses.lumenlearning.com/suny-principlesmanagement/chapter/reading-the-five-stages-of-team-development/.

Okui, Olico. 2004. "Community Participation: An Abused Concept?" *Health Policy and Development* 2: 7–10. Retrieved 16 November 2019 from http://www.bioline.org.br/pdf?hp04003.

Oliver-Smith, Anthony. 1999. "Peru's Five Hundred-Year Earthquake: Vulnerability in Historical Context." In *Angry Earth, Disaster in Anthropological Perspective*, ed. Anthony Oliver-Smith and Susanna M. Hoffman. New York: Routledge.

———. 2005. "Communities after Catastrophe: Reconstructing the Material, Reconstructing the Social." In *Community Building in the Twenty-First Century*, ed. Stanley E. Hyland. Sante Fe: School of American Research.

———. 2014. "Climate Change, Displacement and Resettlement." In *Land Solutions for Climate Displacement*, ed. Scott Leckie, 53–109. New York: Routledge.

Oliver-Smith, Anthony, and Susanna M. Hoffman. 1999. *Angry Earth: Disaster in Anthropological Perspective*. New York: Routledge.

———. 2002. "Why Anthropologists Should Study Disasters." In *Catastrophe and Culture: The Anthropology of Disaster*, ed. Anthony Oliver-Smith and Susanna M. Hoffman. Sante Fe: School of American Research Press.

Opoku, Alex. 2015. "The Role of Culture in a Sustainable Built Environment." In *Sustainable Operations Management: Measuring Operations Performance*, ed. Andrea Chiarini, 37–52. Switzerland: Springer. Retrieved 13 March 2022 from: https://doi.org/10.1007/978-3-319-14002-5_3.

"Pakistan: UN Quake Relief Moves into Higher Gear with Emergency Food Deliveries." 2005. *UN News Center*, 10 October. Retrieved 13 October 2017 from http://www.un.org/apps/news/story.asp?NewsID=16152&Cr=Pakistan&Cr1=#.WeEFdkyZOt8.

Palliyaguru, Roshani, Dilanthi Amaratunga, and Richard Haigh. 2010. "Integration of Disaster Risk Reduction into the Infrastructure Reconstruction Sector: Policy vs. Practice Gaps." *International Journal of Disaster Resilience in the Built Environment* 1(3): 277–96. Retrieved 13 March 2022 from https://doi.org/10.1108/17595901011080878.

PERRP (Pakistan Earthquake Reconstruction and Recovery Program). 2011/2012. "Pakistan Reconstruction Program." 24-page annual project brochure.

———. 2013. "Pakistan Reconstruction Program (Earthquake Component)." 28-page annual project brochure.

Pink, Sarah, Dylan Tutt, and Andrew Dainty. 2013. "Ethnographic Research in the Construction Industry." In *Introducing Ethnographic Research in the Construction Industry*, ed. Sarah Pink, Dylan Tutt, and Andrew Dainty. New York: Routledge.

Pretty, Jules N., Irene Guijt, Ian Scoones, and John Thompson. 1995. *Participatory Learning and Action: A Trainer's Guide*. London: International Institute for Environment and Development.

Price, Gareth. 2017. "Is India Getting Serious about Dialogue in Kashmir?" Chatham House website, 30 October. Retrieved 17 January 2018 from https://www.chathamhouse.org/expert/comment/india-getting-serious-about-dialogue-kashmir.

Price, Gareth, and Farzana Shaik. 2016. "Pakistan Faces International Isolation after Kashmir Incident." Chatham House website, 27 September. Retrieved 17 January 2018 from https://www.chathamhouse.org/expert/comment/pakistan-faces-international-isolation-after-kashmir-incident.

Qadir, Ihsan. 2017. "Patwaris to Protest against Land Record Digitization." *Pakistan Today*, 18 August. Retrieved 9 December 2018 from https://www.pakistantoday.com.pk/2017/08/18/patwaris-to-protest-against-land-record-digitisation/.

"Quake 'is UN's worst nightmare.'" 2005. *BBC News Front Page*, 20 October. Retrieved 6 October 2017 from http://news.bbc.co.uk/2/hi/south_asia/4358902.stm.

Quinion, Michael. 2008. *-Ologies and -Isms: A Dictionary of Word Beginnings and Endings*. Oxford: Oxford University Press. Retrieved 27 June 2018 from https://www.thefreedictionary.com/social+anthropology.

Rahnema, M. 1997. "Participation." In *The Development Dictionary: A Guide to Knowledge as Power*, ed. W. Sachs. Hyderabad: Orient Longman.

Rapoport, Amos. 1980. "Cross Cultural Aspects of Environmental Design." In *Human Behavior and Environment: Advances in Theory and Research*, ed. I. Altman, A. Rapoport, and J. F. Wohlwill, 7–46. New York: Plenum.

———. 2005. *Culture, Architecture and Design*. Chicago: Locke Science Publishing Co. Inc.

Reason, Peter, and Hilary Bradbury. 2012. *The Sage Handbook of Action Research, Participative Inquiry and Practice*. London: Sage. Retrieved 13 March 2022 from https://uk.sagepub.com/en-gb/eur/the-sage-handbook-of-action-research/book228865.

Rehmat, Adnan. 2006. "Building Media Capacities to Improve Disaster Response: Lessons from Pakistan." Humanitarian Practice Network. Retrieved 12 May 2020 from https://internews.org/wp-content/uploads/2021/04/hpn_rehmat_20060427.pdf.

Rietbergen-McCracken, Jennifer, and Deepa Narayan. 1998. "Participation and Social Assessment: Tools and Techniques." Washington, DC: International Bank for Reconstruction and Development, World Bank.

Roy, Arundhati. 2008. "Land and Freedom." *The Guardian*, 22 August. Retrieved 9 December 2018 from https://www.theguardian.com/world/2008/aug/22/kashmir.india.

Satterthwaite, D., D. Bajracharya, R. Hart, C. Levy, D. Ross, J. Smit, and C. Stephen, 1995. "Children, Environment and Sustainable Development." New York: UNICEF, Environment Division.

Satti, Jahangir Ahmad. 1990. "Pakistan Certainly has a Caste System." *New York Times*, 8 December, Section 1, p. 24. Retrieved 10 November 2018 from https://www.nytimes.com/1990/12/08/opinion/l-pakistan-certainly-has-a-caste-system-224690.html.

Saxena, N. C. 2011. "What Is Meant by People's Participation?" In *The Participation Reader*, ed. Andrea Cornwall. London: Zed Books.

Sayid, Aizad. 2012. "Pakistan Azad Kashmir 2005 Earthquake Devastation and Relief Camp." Video, 1:47:00, https://youtu.be/9TwP1ta5_aw.

Schuller, Mark. 2012. *Killing with Kindness: Haiti, International Aid, and NGOs*. New Brunswick: Rutgers University Press.

Schuller, Mark, Lacey Benedeck, Halle Boddy, Katelyn Kramer, Evan Blankenberger, Ardyn Cieslak, and Christine Jenkins. 2020. "'Imagining a More Just World.' Interview with Julie Maldonado." *Annals of Anthropological Practice* 44(1): 6–13.

Sengupta, Somini. 2005. "U.N. Appeals for $550 million to Help Pakistan Quake Survivors." *New York Times*, 26 October. Retrieved 20 October 2017 from http://www.nytimes.com/2005/10/26/international/asia/un-appeals-for-550-million-to-help-pakistan-quake.html.

Shafiq, Sumaira. 2015. "Pakistan's Policy Toward Kashmir Dispute (2001–2014)." *Margalla Papers* 19(2). Retrieved 13 March 2022 from https://www.studocu.com/row/document/university-of-engineering-and-technology-taxila/pakistan-studies/07-pakistans-policy/17249493.

Shah, Murtaza Ali. 2017. "UN Human Rights Commissioner 'Remotely Monitoring' Kashmir LOC Situation." *Geo News*, 15 September. Retrieved 8 January 2018 from https://www.geo.tv/latest/158245-un-commissioner-says-remote-monitoring-kashmir-loc-situation.

Shahid, Kunwar Khuldune. 2015. "Religion's View on Earthquakes." *The Nation*, 29 October. Retrieved 13 March 2022 from https://nation.com.pk/29-Oct-2015/religion-s-view-on-earthquakes.

Shapan, Adnan. 1992. *People's Participation, NGOs and Flood Action Plan*. Dhaka, Bangladesh: Research and Advisory Services. Retrieved 15 February 2019 from https://www.worldcat.org/title/peoples-participation-ngos-and-the-flood-action-plan-an-independent-review/oclc/30474940.

Skjerven, Astrid. 2017. "Design Research." In *Design for a Sustainable Culture: Perspectives, Practices and Education*, ed. Astrid Skjerven and Janne Beate Reitan, 1–10. London: Routledge.

Sliwinski, Alicia. 2010. "The Politics of Participation, Involving Communities and Post-Disaster Reconstruction." In *Rebuilding after Disasters: From Emergency to Sustainability*, ed. G Lizarralde, C. Johnson, and C. Davidson. London: Spon Press. Retrieved 28 April 2020 from https://wlu-ca.academia.edu/AliciaSliwinski.

Snedden, Christopher. 2012. *The Untold Story of the People of Azad Kashmir*. London: Hurst & Company.

———. 2015. *Understanding Kashmir and Kashmiris*. London: Hurst & Company.

"Social Structure." n.d. *Sociology Guide: A Student's Guide to Sociology*. Retrieved 15 February 2020 from https://www.sociologyguide.com/social-structure/index.php.

Sökefeld, Martin. 2015. "At the Margins of Pakistan: Political Relationships between Gilgit-Baltistan and Azad Jammu and Kashmir." In *Pakistan's Political Labyrinths: Military, Society and Terror*, ed. Ravi Kalia, 174–88. London: Routledge India.

Stebbins, Robert. 1987. *Sociology: The Study of Society*. New York: Harper and Row.

Stein, Judith. n.d. "Using the Stages of Team Development." Cambridge, MA: Massachusetts Institute of Technology Human Resources. Retrieved 23 April 2020 from https://hr.mit.edu/learning-topics/teams/articles/stages-development.

Stiefel, Matthias, and Marshall Wolfe. 2011. "The Many Faces of Participation." In *The Participation Reader*, ed. Andrea Cornwall. London: Zed Books.

Titz, Alexandra, Terry Cannon, and Fred Kruger. 2018. "Uncovering 'Community': Challenging an Elusive Concept in Development and Disaster Related Work." *Societies* 8(3): 71. Retrieved 31 January 2020 from https://www.mdpi.com/2075-4698/8/3/71.

Tylor, Edward B. 1871. *Primitive Culture: Research into the Development of Mythology, Philosophy, Religion, Art and Customs*, Volume 1. London: John Murray.

Ul Haque, Nadeem, 2009. "Eminent Domain." *The Nation*, 30 June. Retrieved 6 April 2020 from https://nation.com.pk/30-Jun-2009/eminent-domain.

UN (United Nations). 1987. *Our Common Future: United Nations General Assembly Report of the World Commission on Environment and Development*. Retrieved 15 February 2017 from https://www.are.admin.ch/are/en/home/sustainable-development/international-cooperation/2030agenda/un-_-milestones-in-sustainable-development/1987—brundtland-report.html.

UNDRR (United Nations Office for Disaster Risk Reduction). n.d.a. "What is the Sendai Framework for Disaster Risk Reduction?" Retrieved 4 March 2022 from https://www.undrr.org/implementing-sendai-framework/what-sf.

———. n.d.b. "Key Concept: Capacity." *Prevention Web*. Retrieved 4 March 2022 from https://www.preventionweb.net/risk/capacity.

———. 2015. *Chart of the Sendai Framework of Disaster Risk Reduction*. Retrieved 26 February 2022 from https://www.undrr.org/publication/chart-sendai-framework-disaster-risk-reduction-2015-2030.

UNFAO (United Nations Food and Agriculture Organization). n.d. *Participatory Development: Guidelines on Beneficiary Participation in Agriculture and Rural Development*. Retrieved 16 July 2021 from http://www.fao.org/3/ad817e/ad817e01.htm#TopOfPage.

UN HABITAT (United Nations Human Settlements Programme). 2012. *A Guide on Land and Property Rights in Pakistan*, 2nd edition. United Nations Human Settlement Program. Retrieved 10 December 2018 from http://www.ndma.gov.pk/Publications/A percent20Guide percent20on percent20Land percent20and percent20 Property percent20Rights percent20in percent20Pakistan percent202012.pdf.

UNHCR (United Nations High Commissioner for Refugees). 2008. "The Context, Concepts and Guiding Principles." In *A Community-Based Approach in UNHCR Operations*. Retrieved 23 August 2021 from https://www.unhcr.org/47f0a6712.html.

UNICEF (United Nations Children's Fund). 2014. "Lack of Toilets Dangerous for Everyone, UNICEF Says." News release, 19 November. Retrieved 16 July 2018 from http://www.unicef.org/media/media_77952.html.

———. 2016. *Conflict Sensitivity and Peacebuilding Programming Guide*. Retrieved 8 November 2018 from https://www.unicef.org/media/59156/file.

UNISDR (United Nations International Strategy for Disaster Reduction). 2009. Terminology on Disaster Risk Reduction. Retrieved 13 March 2022 from https://www.unisdr.org/files/7817_UNISDRTerminologyEnglish.pdf.

Uphoff, Norman, Milton J. Esman, and Anirudh Krishna. 1998. *Reasons for Success: Learning from Instructive Experiences in Rural Development*. Connecticut: Kumarian Press.

USAID (United States Agency for International Development). 2016. *Country Profile: Property Rights & Resource Governance—Pakistan*. Retrieved 5 December 2018 from https://www.land-links.org/wp-content/uploads/2016/09/USAID_Land_Tenure_Pakistan_Profile_0.pdf.

USAID (United States Agency for International Development) Office of Inspector General. 2012. *Audit of USAID/Pakistan's Reconstruction Program in Earthquake-Affected Areas*. Retrieved 17 Aug 2021 from https://oig.usaid.gov/sites/default/files/2018-06/g-391-12-007-p.pdf.

US Department of State. 2005. "US Response to the Pakistan Earthquake Disaster." US Department of State Archive. Retrieved 15 August 2018 from https://2001-2009.state.gov/r/pa/prs/ps/2005/57890.htm.

Usman, Ahmed. 2011. "Social Stratification in a Punjabi Village of Pakistan: The Dynamics between Caste, Gender and Violence." PhD dissertation, University of Leeds, School of Sociology and Social Policy. Retrieved 20 November 2018 from http://etheses.whiterose.ac.uk/21130/1/582096.pdf.

Waldheim, Kurt. 1974. "Popular Participation and Its Practical Implications for Development." UN Document No. E/CN. 5/496.

"What is Anthropology?" n.d. American Anthropological Association. Retrieved 18 June 2018 from https://www.americananthro.org/AdvanceYourCareer/Content.aspx?ItemNumber=2150.

"What Is Social Anthropology?" n.d. University of Cambridge Department of Social Anthropology. Retrieved 28 June 2018 from https://www.socanth.cam.ac.uk/prospective-students/prospective-undergraduates/what-is-socanth.

"What Is Social Anthropology?" n.d. University of Manchester Department of Social Anthropology. Retrieved 27 June 2018 from https://www.socialsciences.manchester.ac.uk/social-anthropology/study/what-is-social-anthropology/.

White, Sarah C. 1996. "Depoliticising Development: The Uses and Abuses of Participation." *Development in Practice* 6(1): 6–15. Retrieved 1 May 2014 from https://doi.org/10.1080/0961452961000157564.

Wilder, Andrew. 2008. "Humanitarian Agenda 2015: Perceptions of the Pakistan Earthquake Response." Feinstein International Center. Retrieved 14 September 2019 from https://fic.tufts.edu/wp-content/uploads/HA2015-Pakistan-Earthquake-Response.pdf.

———. 2010. "Aid and Stability in Pakistan: Lessons from the 2005 Earthquake Response." *Disasters* 34(s3): S406–S426.

World Bank. n.d. "Technical Note 1: Development of Construction Industry: A Literature Review." Washington, DC.

———. 1994. *The World Bank and Participation*. Washington, DC. Retrieved 22 April 2019 from http://documents.worldbank.org/curated/en/627501467990056231/The-World-Bank-and-Participation.

———. 1996a. *Improving Basic Education in Pakistan: Community Participation, System Accountability and Efficiency*. Report-14960-PAK. Washington, DC.

———. 1996b. *World Bank Participation Sourcebook*. International Bank for Reconstruction and Development. Washington, DC. Retrieved 18 July 2020 at http://documents1.worldbank.org/curated/en/289471468741587739/pdf/multi-page.pdf.

———. 2004. *World Development Report: Making Services Work for the Poor People*. Washington DC.

———. 2017. "In Pakistan and Beyond, Land Records Get a Digital Upgrade." *World Bank News*, 20 September. Retrieved 17 January 2018 from https://www.worldbank.org/en/news/feature/2017/09/20/in-pakistan-and-beyond-land-records-get-a-digital-upgrade.

———. 2018. "School Enrollment, Primary, Male (% Gross)—Pakistan." Retrieved 17 January 2018 from https://data.worldbank.org/indicator/SE.PRM.ENRR.MA?locations=PK.

World Bank Group. 2014. "Pakistan Earthquake 2005: The Case of the Centralized Recovery Planning and Decentralized Implementation." Retrieved 12 October 2017 from https://reliefweb.int/sites/reliefweb.int/files/resources/Pakistan percent20Earthquake percent202005_0.pdf.

World Summit for Social Development Program of Action. 1995. "Chapter 2: Eradication of Poverty, Basis for Action and Objectives." Copenhagen. Retrieved 7 February 2017 from http://www.un.org/esa/socdev/wssd/text-version/agreements/poach2.htm.

Yousaf, Nasim. 2014. "Aktar Hameed Khan: A Legendary Social Scientist." *Education about Asia* 19(3). Retrieved 18 September 2018 from http://aas2.asian-studies.org/EAA/EAA-Archives/19/3/1327.pdf.

Zaidi, S. Akbar. 2008. "Social and Structural Transformations in Pakistan." *Economic and Political Weekly*, May 17. Retrieved 26 November 2018 from https://www.epw.in/journal/2008/20/letter-south-asia-columns/social-and-structural-transformations-pakistan.html.

Zaman, Mohammad Q. 1999. "Vulnerability, Disaster and Survival in Bangladesh: Three Case Studies." In *Angry Earth, Disaster in Anthropological Perspective*, ed. Anthony Oliver-Smith and Susanna M. Hoffman. New York: Routledge.

Index

Afghanistan, 12, 13, 15–16, 113
Afghan refugee camps, in Pakistan, 12, 112–14
Aga Khan Rural Support Program (AKRSP), 35, 87–88, 136
analysis. *See also* capacities/vulnerabilities analysis
   communities, 103, 140–41
   construction management comparative, 235–39
   engineer focus group, 235–39
   of power structures, 124–25
   of social structure, 81, 99–100, 122, 124–25, 141, 145
   stakeholder, 142–44
   "What Could Go Wrong?," 149–55
Anderson, Mary B., 47, 88–89, 136
Annan, Kofi, 21
anthropologists, on culturally sensitive design, 239
anthropology. *See also* social anthropology
   foundations of, 268–69
   as problem solving, 270, 272–74
   realities for the sociocultural expert in reconstruction, 271
   social anthropological approaches applied in PERRP, 272
   social anthropology of reconstruction, 265
Asian Institute of Technology, 223
author's reflections, 11
Azad Jammu and Kashmir (AJ&K), 2, 8, 16, 44
   first book fairs in, 255–57, 259, 263
   KP compared to, 53–54, 62
   media regarding, 20, 21, 45, 256
   political power structure impacting, 25
   social mobilizer work in, 139–40

Bangladesh, 82, 104–7, 267–68
Barrios, Roberto, 1
beneficiaries, 31, 62, 84, 122, 145
Bherkund, snake infestation in, 171–72
Bin Laden, Osama, 45, 46
biradari (unity group), 54, 55–56, 97, 123
book fairs, 255–57, 259, 263
book sourcing, for Library Challenge, 253–57, 259–60
boundary, lines and walls, 36, 64, 182, 240–41

cadastral survey, 36, 181–83
capacities
   approach, 28, 100, 258, 284–85
   committees building, 187–88, 285
   power and, 100–102
capacities/vulnerabilities analysis
   conflict/collaboration/security findings in, 148–49
   and conflict sensitivity analysis, 144–49
   physical/material findings in, 146, 148
case studies, influential, 87–88
castes, 37, 50, 54, 56, 60, 66, 154. *See also biradari*; social structure
   politicization of, 55
CDM Constructors Inc. (CCI), 10, 23
CDM Smith, xv, 10, 23, 143, 144, 177, 232, 236
   educational facility design-build honor award to, 212
   Library Challenge regarding, 253, 255, 257
Chambers, Robert, 87, 89, 109, 110, 136
CIDA (Canadian International Development Agency), 104–6
code of conduct, for construction workers, 153, 155, 157, 177, 180, 186

Committee-Contractor Agreements, 69,
78, 170, 193–94, 244
  conflict prevention with, 155
  exercise, 155
  as step in community participation,
185
committees, 10, 29. See also Parent
Teacher Councils; School
Management Committees
  benefits for committee members,
164
  capacity building of, 187–88, 285
  community participation social steps
regarding, 180, 184–85, 187–88,
190
  community participation three-step
process for, 131–33
  conflict prevention of, 154
  conflict resolution facilitated by,
161–62, 207–8
  contractor pre-bid visit hosted by, 184
  coordinated social and technical step
duties of, 177–78, 190
  decision-making of, 161
  design input, 184
  dissolution of, 165–66
  duties in step-by-step process, 177,
178–90
  exit plan developed with, 188, 190
  final inspection participation of, 189
  formation and collaboration of, 154
  gifts in kind and cash initiatives of,
162–63
  Library Challenge involvement of, 253,
254–55, 257–58, 259
  members, 123, 133, 164, 166
  membership purposes and criteria,
133
  participation and contribution of,
160–64
  PERRP construction schedule
regarding, 33
  power arrangements impacted by, 52
  PTC/SMC guideline changes to shift
and share power, 131–32
  representativeness of, 132, 133, 161
  school event organization by, 163–64
  temporary land arrangement
organized by, 183

communication protocol, viii, 78, 102,
125, 139, 152–56
  conflict prevention of, 154
  with grievance procedures, 29, 154,
180, 191–93, 197, 247–48
  integration tools, 191–93
communities in PERRP, 3, 27, 82, 115,
247, 269, 281. See also power;
social structure
  analysis, 103, 140–55
  beneficiaries, 31, 62, 84, 122, 145
  capacities approach with, 28, 100
  conflict prevention by, 249–51
  critical perspectives on, 95–96, 97–100
  design input of, 216–19, 240–44
  exercises to develop understanding
of, 116
  by geography, 122–23
  heterogeneity of, 58
  how they participated and
contributed, 155–63
  informal leaders, elders, notables,
62-3, 120–21, 128, 131–33
  land issue prevention with, 35–37
  leader perspectives in, 151–52
  Library Challenge comments of, 261
  local moderators in, 101
  member benefits, 164
  "myth" argument on, 9, 97–99, 100,
102
  participation/contribution monitoring
of, 155–64
  power, 100–102, 106, see also power
arrangements, see also power
blocs, see also power structures
  rival factions in, 75
  semantics regarding, 102–3
  shunning threatened by, 71–72
  by social composition, 123
  as stakeholders, 224–25, 226
"community." See also power; social
structure
  analysis, 103
  arguments about semantics, 102
  communities real but highly complex,
99–102
  community as myth, 9, 97–99
  critical perspectives on, 95–102
  definitions, meanings, language, 96

community participation, 9, 11, 123, 166, 238–39, 252, 280, 286, 289. *See also* participation index
  approaches by NGOs, 135
  benefits of participation, 283–85
  committee three-step process for, 131–33
  in conflict prevention, 78–81
  critical perspectives on, 95–96
  decision makers understanding lack of, 92, 93
  in decision-making, 84, 85
  emergence of, 82–86
  grievance procedures, 29
  health officials' opposition to, 110–11
  influencers, thinkers, books, case studies, 86–89
  issues regarding, what went wrong?, 92–94
  in land issue management, 36, 37
  opposition to, 92–93, 108, 110–12
  phrase misuse of, 90–91
  planning and implementation of, 6
  and power, 93, 124–31
  starting it in PERRP, 33–37
  use and misuse of phrase "community participation," 90
  what went wrong and why?, 92–93
community participation social steps
  before, during, at end of construction, 177–91
  committees regarding, 180, 184–85, 187–88, 190
  communication protocol and grievance procedures, 29, 154, 180, 191–93, 197, 247–48
  construction workers "code of conduct," 153, 155, 157, 177, 180, 186
  contractors, 184–85, 190
  at end of construction, 189–90
  exit plan, 188, 190
  in land issue settlement process, 181–83, 205–6
  operation, management and maintenance, 186–87, 188, 189
  participation/contribution monitoring of, 156–58
  public handover and inauguration, 189–90
  rapid social assessment, 34–35, 178
  temporary land arrangement, 183
  willingness resolution for, 179–80, 204–5
complaints, 29, 78–81
conclusions, 283
  benefits of community participation to project and local people, 283
  lessons learned in PERRP, 285
conflict and collaboration, 28, 281
  contractors regarding, 155, 185, 248, 249–51
  "do no harm" approach to, 48, 88–89, 136, 155, 185
  "do no harm" guidelines for contractors, 155
  historical causes of, 43–48
  informal leaders, elders, notables, 48, 60, 62–3, 120–1, 128–9, 138
  local customs for conflict prevention, resolution, 12, 63, 147, 148–49
  peace compared to, 47
  sensitivity, 48, 144–49, 153–54
  underlying social causes of, 3, 5, 50, 206–7, 274–79
  "War on Terror," 45–46
conflict prevention and resolution, 12, 63, 147, 148–49
  committees facilitating, 161–62, 207–8
  community participation in, 78–81
  social team on, 81
conflict prevention in PERRP, 12, 63, 147, 148, 161–62
  analysis of "What Could Go Wrong?," 149–55
  Committee-Contractor Agreements, 155
  committee formation and collaboration, 154
  communication protocol and grievance procedures, 154
  by communities and social mobilizers, 249–51
  construction workers' code of conduct, 155
conscientização (conscientization), 86–87

construction, 27, 220–51, 269, 282–83.
See also contexts, reconstruction
site; contractors
  destruction causes of, 221–22
  industry, 3–4, 223
  inward focus of, 38, 265–66
  local stakeholders ignored in, 224–25, 226
  Pakistan and international challenges in, 222–26
  perceptions of, 150–51, 267–68
  sites, 167, 228, 229–30, 234
  sociocultural approach to, 225–26
  studies on, 223–24
  workers "code of conduct," 153, 155, 157, 177, 180, 186
construction, PERRP, 9–10, 31, 220. See also community participation; community participation social steps; contractors
  communities viewing, 234, 235
  "construction" versus "reconstruction" in PERRP, 9
  corruption prevention, 232–33
  cost control, 238
  engineer focus group analysis for, 235–39
  feasibility assessments of, 34, 228–29
  final site selection for, 229–30
  health and safety, 237
  individual opposing, 275–76
  leadership and communications, 238
  management comparative analysis of, 235–39
  monitoring, quality control, quality assurance and supervision, 231–32, 237
  operation and maintenance, 233–34
  organization and management of, 228–39
  Pakistan and international challenges for, 222–26
  payments, 238
  scheduling, 32–33, 221, 230–31, 237
  subcontracts for, 230
  technical challenges in, 226–28
contexts, reconstruction site, 38–81
  disaster risk reduction, 42
  gender roles, 61–62
  history, international relations, conflict and collaboration, 43–48
  human rights situation, 46
  independence and partitioning, 43
  language, 60
  local power structures and informal leaders, 62–63
  power and culture, 48–50, 53–56
  power arrangements in, 51–53
  religion and beliefs, 57, 58–59
  security environment, 45–48
  social anthropology regarding, 265–68
  social structure, 48–50
  vulnerability, 28, 42, 144–49
  "War on Terror," 45–46
contractors, 10, 27, 32–33, 135, 151, 195, 196, 206, 281
  cleanup and restorations by, 190
  Committee-Contractor Agreements influence, 69, 78, 155, 170, 185, 193–94, 244
  committee hosted pre-bid visit, 184
  conflict regarding, 155, 185, 248, 249–51
  contracts and scope of work for, 236
  corruption prevention, 232–33
  cultural breach by, 68–69, 273
  "do no harm" guidelines for, 155, 185
  eminent domain attitude, 224–25
  liability defects period, 190
  payments to, 238
  perspectives of, 152, 223
  power bloc of, 131
  scheduling incentivizing, 231
  social component briefing for, 184–85
  subcontracts to, 230
  unscrupulous contractor, 277–79
corruption prevention, 232–33
court
  cases, 5, 26, 28–29, 63, 66, 69, 78, 153, 181, 206
  stay order, 28, 277–79
  system, 65–66
critical perspectives, on "community" and "participation," 95–103
cultural change, 57, 74, 154, 274, 276–79
cultural norms, 56–58, 72, 73, 137
  of gender roles and purdah, 61–62
  of language, 60

of local power structures and informal
leaders, 62–63
serious breach of cultural norms, 68–69
social structure and power regarding,
53–56
culture, 4, 9, 42, 48, 49, 56, 57–58, 72, 268
power and, 48–50, 53–56
social structure regarding, 48–51,
53–56
"why didn't you just tell them to
change their culture?," 73

decision makers
community participation
understanding lack of, 92, 93
decision-making
of committees, 161
community participation in, 84, 85
of informal leaders *jirgas*, 128
Department of Education officers, 205–6,
278
Department of Health officials, 110–11
Design-Build Institute of America, 212
design of buildings
anthropologists on, 239
architects' perspectives on, 213–14,
239
committees input on, 184
culturally sensitive design, 213–20,
242–43
end user and community input to,
216–19, 240–44
in Pakistan, 215
post-disaster opportunities for, 212
rationale and process of, 216–18
stakeholder consultation for, 212
subcontracts for, 230
sustainability, 219–20
disaster reconstruction. *See specific
topics*
Disaster Risk Reduction (DRR), 40, 42,
52, 53, 57, 59, 175
disasters, 1
changes after, 266–67
disaster risk reduction (DRR), 40, 52,
57, 59
"disasters" and "hazards," 40–41
disaster studies, 1, 3, 281
guiding principles of DRR, 42

opportunities after, 212
and reconstruction, 5, 7, 9, 21, 23, 28
Sendai framework, 42
vulnerability regarding, 42
Do No Harm (Anderson), 88–89. *See also*
conflict and collaboration
"do no harm" approach, to conflict, 48,
88–89, 136, 155, 185

earthquake, in Pakistan in 2005, 15–22
Earthquake Engineering Research
Institute (EERI) study, 222
Earthquake Reconstruction and
Rehabilitation Authority (ERRA),
24, 26, 117, 172, 173, 229
Egeland, Jan, 16
elite capture, 91, 98, 102, 153, 164, 195
from construction site access
blockage, 167
of decision-making, 127
prevention of, 129, 167
by some head teachers, 127
eminent domain, 67, 131, 224
empowerment, 43, 53, 85, 94, 145, 169,
252, 258
encroachment, 67, 71, 118, 153
engineers, 36
AJ&K government road maintenance
department executive, 170–71,
248
coordinated social and technical steps,
176
PERRP focus group of, 235–39
perspectives of, 150–51
relationship building with social team,
198–204, 208–10
training together with social
mobilizers, 195–97
ethnicities, 37, 50, 54, 55, 56, 60, 66, 76
exercises
capacities/vulnerabilities and conflict
sensitivity analysis, 144–49
case studies integration tools, 195–96
Committee-Contractor Agreement,
155
committee formation and
collaboration, 154
communication protocol and
grievance procedures, 154

for communities, 116
conflict sensitivity, 153–54
construction workers "code of conduct," 155
social mobilizers and engineers training, 195–96
stakeholder analysis, 142–44
"What Could Go Wrong?" analysis, 149–55

Federal Relief Commission, 23
flash floods, 244
focus groups, 235–39, 287–89
Freire, Paulo, 86–87, 136

geological impact of the earthquake, 16
gender roles, 61–62
gender separation. See purdah
girls' education, 169–70
girls' schools, culturally sensitive design for, 240–41
glass blocks, in windows, 242, 275–76
government, Pakistan, 23–25, 43–48
    Kerry-Lugar bill, 30–31
    military and civilian rule of, 44
Government Boys' Schools
    Higher Secondary School Jared, xii, 246, 256
    Higher Secondary School Rerra, 190
    High School in Flat Land, 274–79
    Primary and High School Mohandri, 19, 228, 245, 261
    Primary School Phel, 52
Government Girls' Schools
    High School Chatter #2, xiii, 139
    High School Juglari, xiii, 164
    High School Kheral Abbasian, xii, 17, 171
    Middle School Kahna Mohri, 32
    Primary and Middle Schools Paras, 169
Grameen Bank, 84
graves, respect for, 243
grievance procedures, 29, 154, 180, 191–93, 197, 205, 208, 247–48

Hagan, Ross, 23, 29, 203
Harrell-Bond, Barbara, 84
"hazards" and "disasters," 40–41
head teacher
    parents protest against, 168–69
    power bloc of, 126–28
    SMCs and PTCs adversarial relationship with, 127
health facilities, 74–75, 110–11, 247
Hoffman, Susanna M., 1, 2, 41, 57
hostel, for students, 246
hotel association, 250
human impact of the earthquake, 20
human rights situation, 46, 51, 55, 66

independence and partitioning, 43
Indian Administered Kashmir (IAK), 43
informal leaders, 121, 127
    cultural norms of, 62–63
    power bloc of, 128–29
integration tools of social and technical components
    case studies exercise, 195–96
    of Committee-Contractor Agreements, 69, 78, 155, 170, 185, 193–94, 244
    communication protocol and grievance procedures, 191–93
    social mobilizers and engineers training together, 195–97
    and training, 191–97
international development field, 83–84
International Security Assistance Force (ISAF), 16, 22

jirga (community-based decision-making body), 128

Kashmir issue, 43–45
kateeb (religious leader), 79, 250
Kerry-Lugar bill, 30–31
key terms, 9
Khan, Ahktar Hameed, 88
Khan, Mohammad Zaffar, 26
Khan, Sultan Shoaib, 87, 88
Khyber Pakhtunkhwa province (KP), 8, 16, 25, 128
kinship groups, 37, 50, 54, 55, 56, 60, 66, 76

Lahore International Bookfair, 256
land
    administration, laws, police, court system, 65–66, 181–83
    patwari culture, 65–66, 181–83

patwaris (land record officers), 37, 66, 72, 118, 181–82
  shortages of land, 227
  temporary arrangement of, 183
land issues, 26, 33, 35–37, 63, 118, 195–96
  in Bangladesh embankment alignment, 105, 106
  from boundary lines, 36, 64
  cadastral survey regarding, 36, 181–83
  construction sites eliminated due to, 229
  eminent domain, 67, 224–25
  encroachment, 67, 71, 118, 153
  land grab, 67
  PERRP land issue settlement process, 181–83, 205–6
  Perspective matters, 75–76
  prevention, 35–37, 170
  understanding social nature of, 67–68
landowners, local
  power blocs of, 129
  as stakeholders, 133
languages
  as cultural norm, 60
  multilingual project area, 60
  social mobilizer language skills, 137–38
leadership, 71
  of community leaders, 151–52
  of informal leaders, 62–63, 121, 127, 128–29
  in PERRP construction, 238
Library Challenge, 6–7, 252
  book fairs for, 255–57, 259, 263
  book sourcing for, 253–57, 259–60
  CDM Smith regarding, 253, 255, 257
  committee involvement in, 253, 254–55, 257–58, 259
  community on, 261
  libraries established for, 257–59
  library management training for, 260
  presentation of, 254–55
  related activities introduced by, 261
  students engaging with, 261, 262–64
Line of Control, 44
local government, 37, 181
local, national and international assistance, 20–22
"local" trouble over use of, 246–47

MacLeod, Robert, xv, 203
media coverage, 20, 21, 45, 256
Memmott, Paul, 214
men. *See also* purdah; women
  in committees, 77–78
  participation rate by gender, 161
Mid-America Earthquake Center (MAE), 24, 222
monitoring
  of committee member benefits, 164
  of communities, 155–64
  for community participation social steps, 156–58
  of participation and contribution forms, 160–64
  participation index periodic performance assessment for, 158
  PERRP construction, 231–32, 237
  social component, 156–58
mountainous areas, 32, 245
Murphys' Corners, 11
Muzaffarabad, damage to, 18–19
"myth" argument, community, 9, 97–99, 100, 102

National Association for the Practice of Anthropology (NAPA), 270
NATO (North Atlantic Treaty Organization), 22
NGOs (non-governmental organizations), 21–22, 24, 83, 85, 120–21, 137
  ineffective community participation of, 135
  lack of coordination, 116–17

Oakley, Peter, 86, 88
Oliver-Smith, Anthony, xv, 2, 41, 57, 95–96
Orangi Pilot Project (OPP), 88

parents
  power blocs of, 130
  school involvement of, 168–69
Parent Teacher Councils (PTCs), School Management Committees (SMCs), 121
  guideline changes shifting and sharing power, 131–32

head teacher adversarial relationship
    with, 127
  women in, 77–78
participant observer approach, 124, 225,
    269, 272
participation index, 160
  methodology, 158–59
  periodic participatory performance
    assessment, 158
participatory rural appraisal (PRA), 87
patwaris (land record officers), 65–66,
    181–83. *See also* land issues
peace. *See also* conflict and collaboration
  conflict compared to, 47
Pedagogy of the Oppressed (Freire), 87
Personal Reminiscences of Change (Khan,
    Ahktar Hameed), 88
police, 65–66, 90
politicization, 46, 55–56, 140
power, 12, 70, 115
  and capacity, 100–102
  communities, 100–102, 106
  and community participation, 93,
    124–31
  cultural norms regarding, 53–56
  culture and, 48–50, 53–56
  of individuals, 69
  power and culture, 48
  PTC and SMC guidelines shifting and
    sharing, 131–32
  shifting and sharing, 131–34
power arrangements, 51
  committees impacting, 52
  in communities, 12, 98, 125–26
  identification of, 69–70
  in reconstruction site contexts, 51–53
power blocs
  in communities, 125–26
  of contractors, 131
  of head teacher, 126–28
  of informal leaders, notables, elders,
    and elites, 128–29
  of landowners outside school land, 129
  of parents and students, 130
  of project, 130
power structures, 25, 111
  analyzing the power structure, why
    and how, 124–25
  in communities, 102–3, 126

cultural norms of, 62–63
  semantics regarding, 102–3
purdah (gender separation), 48, 60–62,
    73, 120, 138, 180
  culturally sensitive design regarding,
    215, 219
  cultural norms of, 61–62
  gender roles and purdah, 61
  offense against, 68

Al-Qaeda, 45

Rapoport, Amos, 95, 96, 211, 214
reading, Library Challenge inspiring, 261,
    262–64
reconstruction rates, status "concrete
    skeletons of unfinished school,"
    25
"reconstruction" *versus* "construction"
    in PERRP, 9
relationship building. *See also* social-
    technical integration
  among engineers and social
    mobilizers, 198–203
  stages of, 199–200, 202–3
  "stay in your lanes" approach for,
    201–2
  team building and development,
    199–203
religion, and beliefs, 57–59
response to the earthquake by
    governments of US and Pakistan,
    23
Richter scale, 16, 17
*Rising From the Ashes: Development
    Strategies in Times of Disaster*
    (Anderson and Woodrow), 88

School Management Committees
    (SMCs), Parent Teacher Councils
    (PTCs), 121
  guideline changes to shift and share
    power, 131–32
  head teacher adversarial relationship
    with, 127
  power leveraged by, 70
schools, 171. *See also* Library Challenge
  access path dispute, 276–79
  attendance factors for, 61, 215

above clouds, 52, 70
committees event organization for, 163–64
culturally sensitive design for, 240–41
culture regarding, 68–69, 239, 273
data on, 26
destruction of, 17, 18, 19
final site selection of, 229–30
incompletion of, 25–26
landowners bordering, 129
outside, 25–26, 32, 34
parents involvement in, 168–69
student on, 243
security environment, 30, 45–48, 148–49Selim, Tarek, xv
semantics, power structures regarding, 102–3
Sendai Framework, 42
senior management team, 13, 35, 116, 119, 120, 136, 143, 228
social-technical integration of, 134–35, 203, 204, 286
sociocultural expertise in, 134–35, 203, 286
stakeholder analysis responsibilities of, 144
shunning, 71–72
SMCs. See School Management Committees
soccer field, 242–43, 275
social anthropology of reconstruction, 265
examples of real-world problems solved, 272
people and change in post-disaster scenario, 266
perceptions of construction and reconstruction, 267, 269
realities for the sociocultural expert in reconstruction, 271
reconstruction sites cannot be divorced from surroundings, 265
social anthropological approaches applied in PERRP, 272
social assessment, rapid, 34–35, 178
social component of PERRP, 11, 115–74, 286. See also social team
committee dissolution end of project, 165–66

community participation/contributions monitoring as, 155–64
contractors briefed for, 184–85
of land issues, 67–68
monitoring, 156–58
Part 1: "At the Community Level," 116
Part 2: "Social Team and Process," 134
Part 3: "Monitoring Participation and Contributions," 155
participation index participatory performance assessment, 158
social component, community level, 116–18, 122–24. See also power
relationships and trust building, 119–20
social team decision for, 120–21
social mobilizers, 33, 62, 278. See also social team
conflict prevention by, 249–51
determining number needed, 136–37
engineers partnership with, 138, 139, 195–203, 204, 208–10, 217–18, 232
relationship building with engineers, 198–204, 208–10
roles of, 138
selection of, 136–37
skills and qualifications, experience, multilingual abilities, 137–38
training of, 139
training together with engineers, 195–97
social structure, 71. See also castes
analysis of, 81, 99–100, 122, 124–25, 141, 145
biradari, 54, 55–56, 97, 123
committee dissolution impacted by, 165–66
cultural norms regarding, 53–56
culture and, 48–51, 53–56
ethnicities and kinship groups, 37, 50, 54, 55, 56, 60, 66, 76
power regarding, 53–56
reconstruction site contexts, 48–50
social team, 5, 11, 25, 27, 134, 174, 235, 288–89. See also social mobilizers
capacities approach proposed by, 28
community level social component decision of, 120–21

on conflict resolution, 81
coordinated social and technical steps for, 176–78, 190
duties and responsibilities, 138
formation of, 134–35, 136–37
on land issue prevention, 36–37
on preventative measures, 6
process of, 134–39
social process and community analysis, 140–41
trust built by, 24
social-technical integration, 175–210. *See also* community participation social steps; integration tools; relationship building
Committee-Contractor Agreements, 69, 78, 155, 170, 185, 193–94, 244
construction schedule shared emphasis, 32–33
construction workers "code of conduct," 153, 155, 157, 177, 180, 186
coordinated social and technical steps, 176–91
counterpart system, 125, 143, 287–88
joint communications and reporting, 204
Part 1: "Coordinated Social and Technical Steps," 176
Part 2: "Community Participation in PERRP—The Step-by-Step Process," 178
Part 3: "Integration Tools and Training," 191
Part 4: "Relationship Building, Engineers and Social Mobilizers," 198
partnership of social mobilizers and engineers, 138, 139, 195–203, 204, 208–10, 217–18, 232
relationship building, engineers and social mobilizers, 198–203
of senior management, 134–35, 203, 204, 286
"stay in your lanes" approach for, 201–2
top down management to get bottom-up participation, 203, 285

sociocultural considerations in construction, 225–26
sociocultural expertise, in senior management team, 134–35, 203, 286
sociocultural specialists, 8, 49–50, 106, 266, 271, 288–89
staff, in PERRP, 31, 228, 260
stakeholders, 122
analysis exercise, 142–44
communities invisible to some as stakeholders, 224–26
design input by, 212
importance of recognizing, 142–44
local landowners as, 133
"stay in your lanes" approach, 201–2
students, 130, 134, 143, 219, 243
death rate of, 15, 19
hostel for, 246
Library Challenge engagement of, 261, 262–64
reading, 261, 262–64
subcontracts, 230

Taliban, 13, 25, 45, 46, 62, 114
technical component, 8, 11, 211–12. *See also* construction, PERRP; design
challenges of, 172–73, 226–28
shortages impacting, 227–28
step-by-step process, 177
topography, altitude and climate, 227, 244–45
toilets, 215, 239, 240, 243
trust, 24, 31, 119–20

UBC (Uniform Building Code) 1997, 222
UNESCO World Heritage sites, 222
United Nations (UN), 21, 83
United Nations Office of Disaster Risk Reduction (UNDRR), 42
United States government
Kerry-Lugar bill policy change of, 30–31
response to earthquake, 23–25
Urdu, 60, 96–97, 255–56
USAID (United States Agency for International Development), 8, 9, 23, 30, 31, 34, 64, 119, 130, 134, 172, 173
Kerry-Lugar bill impacts of, 30–31

social component initiated by, 134–35
sociocultural expertise included in senior management, 203

Vanuatu, 49
vulnerabilities, 28, 42, 144–49. *See also* capacities/vulnerabilities analysis

"War on Terror," 45–46
Washington Association of Professional Anthropologists (WAPA), xvi
"What Could Go Wrong?" analysis exercise, 149–55
willingness resolution, 179–80, 204–5
windows, glass blocks in, 242, 275–76
"*With Friends Like These . . .*" (Human Rights Watch), 46
women, 196. *See also* men; *purdah*
   in committees, 62
   participation rate by gender, 161
World Bank Group, 24, 223, 224

www.ingramcontent.com/pod-product-compliance
Lightning Source LLC
Chambersburg PA
CBHW070802040426
42333CB00061B/1796